2023 Nelson's Pediatric Antimicrobial Therapy

29th Edition

John S. Bradley, MD
Editor in Chief

John D. Nelson, MD
Emeritus

Elizabeth D. Barnett, MD
Joseph B. Cantey, MD, MPH
David W. Kimberlin, MD
Paul E. Palumbo, MD
Jason Sauberan, PharmD
J. Howard Smart, MD
William J. Steinbach, MD
Contributing Editors

American Academy of Pediatrics

DEDICATED TO THE HEALTH OF ALL CHILDREN®

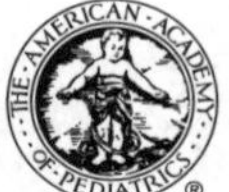

American Academy of Pediatrics Publishing Staff

Mary Lou White, *Chief Product and Services Officer/SVP, Membership, Marketing, and Publishing*
Mark Grimes, *Vice President, Publishing*
Cheryl Firestone, *Senior Manager, Digital Publishing*
Mary Kelly, *Senior Editor, Professional and Clinical Publishing*
Caroline Heller, PhD, *Editorial Assistant*
Shannan Martin, *Production Manager, Consumer Publications*
Amanda Helmholz, *Medical Copy Editor*
Mary Louise Carr, MBA, *Marketing Manager, Clinical Publications*

Published by the American Academy of Pediatrics
345 Park Blvd
Itasca, IL 60143
Telephone: 630/626-6000
Facsimile: 847/434-8000
www.aap.org

The American Academy of Pediatrics is an organization of 67,000 primary care pediatricians, pediatric medical subspecialists, and pediatric surgical specialists dedicated to the health, safety, and well-being of all infants, children, adolescents, and young adults.

While every effort has been made to ensure the accuracy of this publication, the American Academy of Pediatrics does not guarantee that it is accurate, complete, or without error.

The recommendations in this publication do not indicate an exclusive course of treatment or serve as a standard of medical care. Variations, taking into account individual circumstances, may be appropriate.

Statements and opinions expressed are those of the authors and not necessarily those of the American Academy of Pediatrics.

Any websites, brand names, products, or manufacturers are mentioned for informational and identification purposes only and do not imply an endorsement by the American Academy of Pediatrics (AAP). The AAP is not responsible for the content of external resources. Information was current at the time of publication.

The publishers have made every effort to trace the copyright holders for borrowed materials. If they have inadvertently overlooked any, they will be pleased to make the necessary arrangements at the first opportunity.

This publication has been developed by the American Academy of Pediatrics. The contributors are expert authorities in the field of pediatrics. No commercial involvement of any kind has been solicited or accepted in the development of the content of this publication. Disclosures: Dr Kimberlin disclosed a principal investigator relationship with Gilead. Dr Palumbo disclosed financial relationships with Gilead Sciences and Janssen Pharmaceutical Companies.

Every effort has been made to ensure that the drug selection and dosages set forth in this publication are in accordance with current recommendations and practice at the time of publication. It is the responsibility of the health care professional to check the package insert of each drug for any change in indications or dosage and for added warnings and precautions and to review newly published, peer-reviewed data in the medical literature for current data on safety and efficacy.

Please visit www.aap.org/errata for an up-to-date list of any applicable errata for this publication.

Special discounts are available for bulk purchases of this publication. Email Special Sales at nationalaccounts@aap.org for more information.

Printed in the United States of America

9-488/0223 1 2 3 4 5 6 7 8 9 10
MA1076
ISSN: 2164-9278 (print)
ISSN: 2164-9286 (electronic)
ISBN: 978-1-61002-650-5
eBook: 978-1-61002-651-2

Editor in Chief

John S. Bradley, MD, FAAP
Distinguished Professor of Pediatrics
Division of Infectious Diseases, Department of Pediatrics
University of California, San Diego, School of Medicine
Medical Director, Division of Infectious Diseases, Rady Children's Hospital San Diego
San Diego, CA
Lead editor: Chapters 1, 3, 4, 11, 12, 14, and 15

Emeritus

John D. Nelson, MD
Professor Emeritus of Pediatrics
The University of Texas
Southwestern Medical Center at Dallas
Southwestern Medical School
Dallas, TX

Contributing Editors

Elizabeth D. Barnett, MD, FAAP
Professor of Pediatrics
Boston University Aram V. Chobanian & Edward Avedisian School of Medicine
Division of Pediatric Infectious Diseases
Director, International Clinic
Boston Medical Center
Boston, MA
Lead editor: Chapters 9 and 10

Joseph B. Cantey, MD, MPH, FAAP
Assistant Professor of Pediatrics
Divisions of Pediatric Infectious Diseases and Neonatology/Perinatal Medicine
University of Texas Health Science Center at San Antonio
San Antonio, TX
Lead editor: Chapters 2 and 17

David W. Kimberlin, MD, FAAP
Professor of Pediatrics
Co-director, Division of Pediatric Infectious Diseases
University of Alabama at Birmingham
Birmingham, AL
Lead editor: Chapters 7 and 8

Paul E. Palumbo, MD
Professor of Pediatrics and Medicine
Geisel School of Medicine at Dartmouth
Director, International Pediatric HIV Program
Dartmouth-Hitchcock Medical Center
Lebanon, NH
Lead editor: HIV treatment

Contributing Editors *(continued)*

Jason Sauberan, PharmD
Neonatal Research Institute
Sharp Mary Birch Hospital for Women & Newborns
Rady Children's Hospital San Diego
San Diego, CA
Lead editor: Chapters 2, 3, 13, and 18

J. Howard Smart, MD, FAAP
Chairman, Department of Pediatrics
Sharp Rees-Stealy Medical Group
Assistant Clinical Professor of Pediatrics
University of California, San Diego, School of Medicine
San Diego, CA
Lead editor: App development

William J. Steinbach, MD, FAAP
Robert H. Fiser, Jr, MD, Endowed Chair in Pediatrics
Chair, Department of Pediatrics
Associate Dean for Child Health
University of Arkansas for Medical Sciences
Pediatrician-in-Chief, Arkansas Children's
Little Rock, AR
Lead editor: Chapters 5 and 6

Additional Contributor

Christopher R. Cannavino, MD
Divisions of Infectious Diseases and Hospital Medicine
University of California, San Diego (UCSD)
Rady Children's Hospital San Diego
Associate Professor of Clinical Pediatrics
Director, UCSD Pediatric Infectious Disease Fellowship Program
Associate Director, UCSD Pediatric Residency Program
Director, Pediatric Medical Student Education, UCSD School of Medicine
San Diego, CA
Lead editor: Chapter 16

Equity, Diversity, and Inclusion Statement

The American Academy of Pediatrics is committed to principles of equity, diversity, and inclusion in its publishing program. Editorial boards, author selections, and author transitions (publication succession plans) are designed to include diverse voices that reflect society as a whole. Editor and author teams are encouraged to actively seek out diverse authors and reviewers at all stages of the editorial process. Publishing staff are committed to promoting equity, diversity, and inclusion in all aspects of publication writing, review, and production.

Contents

Introduction

Welcome to the 29th edition of *Nelson's Pediatric Antimicrobial Therapy*, the third edition written during the COVID-19 pandemic, which continues to significantly affect our lives and our practice of pediatrics. Thank goodness that COVID-19 vaccines are available for all children older than 6 months! All the other pediatric infections (particularly viral infections) are now coming back with a vengeance, as all of you are experiencing. We maintain close contact between our American Academy of Pediatrics (AAP) Publishing colleagues and our group of editors, who continue to provide clinical care and conduct research while creating policy for pediatric COVID-19 on both local and national levels.

The chapters have all been updated, supported by the medical literature and by our opinions and justifications when the literature does not provide answers. More than 100 new citations and updates to web pages are again provided to support recommendations. The *Nelson's* app has continued to evolve, particularly the search functions, under Dr Howard Smart's direction (he uses the app in his pediatric practice), and it is easier for me to find information on the app than in the print book. Howard wishes to keep improving the app, so if anyone has some thoughts on how we can make it even easier for you to find information, please just let us know at nelsonabx@aap.org. Peter Lynch, senior manager, publishing acquisitions and digital strategy, has been very supportive of the digital presence of *Nelson's*, including the app; we are still trying to get the app into some of the most often used electronic medical records (EMRs) so you can look up infections, antimicrobials, and doses while updating a child's EMR. As new important information becomes available (eg, as new drugs are approved), we share that information with Howard to add to the app and it is periodically "pushed out" to the registered users. We continue to appreciate the ongoing advice of our digitally savvy colleagues, Dr Juan Chaparro (a pediatric infectious disease specialist at Nationwide Children's Hospital in Columbus, OH) and Dr Daniel Sklansky (a pediatric hospitalist at the University of Wisconsin–Madison), who share their medical informatics expertise with us to improve our digital user experience and who continue to work with Peter to explore options for the app in EMRs.

We are quite fortunate to have nationally/internationally recognized editors who are experts in each field contribute to the *Nelson's* chapters, both the clinical chapters and the mini-educational chapters on why they picked specific agents within a class to use for therapy. Dr Chris Cannavino (double board certified in hospital medicine and infectious diseases) continues to update his chapter on antibiotic allergies.

We continue to work closely with the AAP, and many of us have close connections with the AAP Committee on Infectious Diseases, particularly Dr David Kimberlin, the editor of the *Red Book*. Although *Nelson's* is published by the AAP, it is not actually AAP policy (in contrast to the *Red Book*), so we are able to share personal observations that may not be possible in an AAP publication that requires approval by the AAP Board of Directors.

We continue to provide grading of our recommendations—our assessment of how strongly we feel about a recommendation and the strength of the evidence to support our recommendation (noted in the Table). This is not the GRADE (*G*rading of *R*ecommendations *A*ssessment, *D*evelopment, and *E*valuation) method but certainly uses the concepts on which GRADE is based: the strength of recommendation and level of evidence. As with GRADE, we review the literature (and the most important manuscripts are referenced), but importantly, we work within the context of professional society recommendations (eg, the AAP) and our experience.

Strength of Recommendation	Description
A	Strongly recommended
B	Recommended as a good choice
C	One option for therapy that is adequate, perhaps among many other adequate therapies
Level of Evidence	**Description**
I	Based on well-designed, prospective, randomized, and controlled studies in an appropriate population of children
II	Based on data derived from prospectively collected, small comparative trials, or noncomparative prospective trials, or reasonable retrospective data from clinical trials in children, or data from other populations (eg, adults)
III	Based on case reports, case series, consensus statements, or expert opinion for situations in which sound data do not exist

As we state each year, many of the recommendations by the editors for specific situations have not been systematically evaluated in controlled, prospective, comparative clinical trials.

Mary Kelly, senior editor, professional and clinical publishing, continues to do an impressive job organizing the editors and being an outstanding advocate for us and the clinician-users of the book, making sure that all the COVID-19 delays (including paper shortages for the print publication) do not stop the *Nelson's* editors from meeting our deadlines!

It has been a privilege to work with all our friends at AAP Publishing, particularly during the COVID-19 pandemic. Our ability to share our book at professional society meetings and publisher meetings was greatly affected by COVID-19 as we all tried to work from home (unless we were in the hospital or clinics). We have started to plan for the future of *Nelson's* with AAP colleagues, trying to make the book more relevant for clinicians in both outpatient and inpatient settings. A particular thanks to Mary Kelly and Peter Lynch, highlighted above; to Mark Grimes, vice president, publishing; to Jeff Mahony, senior director, professional and consumer publishing; and to the ever-enthusiastic Linda Smessaert, director, marketing. We will be reengaging with Barrett Winston, senior manager, publishing acquisitions and business development, as we look to create our long-term vision of John Nelson's book. We are all truly honored to keep his goals of providing better care to children as our focus in the evolving book and app.

We continue to be very interested in learning from readers and users ways to improve *Nelson's*! Please feel free to share your suggestions with us at nelsonabx@aap.org. Fosfomycin, a very early cell wall synthesis inhibitor, is our molecule of the year.

Hopefully, all of you are safe. We are looking forward to collaborating with everyone at meetings again, even if some of us may still be wearing masks.

John S. Bradley, MD
July 2022

Notable Changes to *2023 Nelson's Pediatric Antimicrobial Therapy*, 29th Edition

We are quite grateful to Dr Howard Smart for the continual upgrading of the *Nelson's* app search function. We will be linking "similar" terms for each disease entity, based on National Library of Medicine search libraries, so the different terminology used by clinicians better matches the terminology used by an editor (eg, "suppurative lymphadenitis" vs "cervical lymph node abscess").

Bacterial/Mycobacterial Infections and Antibiotics

Last year, we shifted our recommendation for serious, invasive methicillin-resistant *Staphylococcus aureus* (MRSA) infections from vancomycin to ceftaroline, US Food and Drug Administration (FDA) approved for all pediatric age-groups, including neonates. We are still holding off on recommendations for MRSA endocarditis and central nervous system infections, as the US companies that have owned the antibiotic (Cerexa/Forest/Actavis/Allergan/AbbVie) have not supported prospective pediatric clinical trials for these indications. We do select antibiotics based on safety, and it is nice to forgo our monitoring of renal function and vancomycin serum concentrations in the treatment of coagulase-negative and coagulase-positive staphylococci that are methicillin resistant.

Many new antibiotics are coming out for treatment of multidrug-resistant (MDR) gram-negative bacilli, particularly serine-based carbapenemase-producing organisms. So far, only one is approved for children (ceftazidime/avibactam), but others are not far behind. Some of the new beta-lactam/beta-lactamase inhibitors for metallo-beta-lactamases are now in clinical trials.

Bacteriophages are now becoming options for treatment of MDR bacteria. Resistance can develop quickly, and combination therapy (>1 bacteriophage, given in combination with antibiotics) seems to be the best option. No bacteriophages are FDA approved for human use at this time.

Dalbavancin, a once-weekly lipoglycopeptide antibiotic for MRSA infections, was approved for children this past year and has found a place in long-term parenteral MRSA infection treatment as an option for children in whom long-term central catheters are not a good option. Other anti-MRSA antibiotics are still under study in children.

New guidelines for treatment of latent tuberculosis infection (now just called "infection") with once-weekly prophylaxis for 12 weeks, and for shorter courses of treatment of pediatric tuberculosis disease, are now being recommended.

New guidelines for treatment of pediatric osteomyelitis are now recommending only 3 to 4 weeks of treatment of uncomplicated methicillin-susceptible *S aureus* bone infection.

Fungal Infections and Antifungal Agents

New global guidelines for treatment of endemic mycoses (including blastomycosis, coccidioidomycosis, histoplasmosis, paracoccidioidomycosis, and sporotrichosis) were recently published in an attempt to harmonize diagnosis and management ("One World, One Guideline").

New additional studies with ibrexafungerp (Brexafemme), a new oral triterpenoid antifungal with activity against *Candida* have been published. Current FDA approved indication is for vulvovaginal *Candida* in post-menarchal females.

Viral Infections and Antiviral Agents

HIV and hepatitis C virus (HCV) are 2 areas in which change continues to be very rapid. Current recommendations about HIV and antiretrovirals, including those for the treatment of newborns exposed to HIV, are posted on ClinicalInfo.HIV.gov (https://clinicalinfo.hiv.gov), which is continually updated. Current recommendations on treatment of HCV are posted on www.hcvguidelines.org/unique-populations/children. There are now 3 HCV antiviral treatments approved for use down to 3 years of age: (1) sofosbuvir (Sovaldi) and sofosbuvir in a fixed-dose combination tablet with ledipasvir (Harvoni); (2) sofosbuvir/velpatasvir (Epclusa); and (3) glecaprevir/pibrentasvir (Mavyret). In addition, elbasvir with grazoprevir (Zepatier) is now approved down to 12 years of age.

Remdesivir, a nucleoside antiviral that inhibits viral RNA polymerases, was authorized for emergency use on May 1, 2020, for the treatment of hospitalized children who have documented or suspected COVID-19 and require supplemental oxygen. It now is approved for use in patients 28 days or older and at least 3 kg in weight with positive results of direct SARS-CoV-2 viral testing, who are hospitalized or who are not hospitalized and have mild to moderate COVID-19 and risk factors for progression to severe COVID-19. Nirmatrelvir/ritonavir (Paxlovid) has Emergency Use Authorization (EUA) from the FDA for the treatment of mild to moderate COVID-19 in people 12 years or older and 40 kg or more in weight; it has numerous drug-drug interactions, so the listing on the FDA or Pfizer website should be reviewed before prescribing. In addition, molnupiravir has EUA from the FDA for the treatment of mild to moderate COVID-19 in adults 18 years or older.

Next, a new cytomegalovirus (CMV) antiviral drug, maribavir, has been approved for the treatment of adults and pediatric patients (aged ≥12 years and weighing at least 35 kg) with posttransplant CMV infection/disease that is refractory to treatment (with or without genotypic resistance) with ganciclovir, valganciclovir, cidofovir, or foscarnet. Following letermovir, this is the second new CMV antiviral with a novel mechanism of action to be approved in the past few years.

Finally, Cabenuva (an injectable, long-acting combination of cabotegravir and rilpivirine) has recently been approved for HIV treatment in 12- to 18-year-olds. It requires an oral lead-in dosing period followed by dual injections every 2 months for treatment of HIV infection. The complexity of this strategy supports the initiation and management by a pediatric/adult HIV specialty team.

Parasitic Infections and Antiparasitic Agents

We continue to encourage readers faced with diagnosing and treating children with malaria and uncommon parasitic infections to contact the Centers for Disease Control and Prevention (CDC) for consultation about management and antiparasitic drug availability (770/488-7100). We have updated the sections on leishmaniasis and human African trypanosomiasis, but readers are encouraged to check current guidelines and seek expert advice if treating patients with these conditions, due to the evolving nature of the management of these conditions. Availability and sources of drugs to treat parasitic infections change frequently (sodium stibogluconate is no longer available, intravenous artesunate is no longer provided by the CDC, and fexinidazole has been approved by the FDA), so clinicians are encouraged to check recent sources of information for the most up-to-date recommendations.

1. Antimicrobial Therapy According to Clinical Syndromes

NOTES

- This chapter should be considered guidance for a typical patient. Dosage recommendations are for patients with normal hydration, renal, and hepatic function. Because the dose required is based on the exposure of the antibiotic to the pathogen at the site of infection, higher dosages may be necessary if the antibiotic does not penetrate well into the infected tissue (eg, meningitis) or if the child eliminates the antibiotic from the body more quickly than average. Higher dosages/longer courses may also be needed if the child is immunocompromised and the immune system cannot help resolve the infection. It is becoming more apparent that the host contributes significantly to microbiological and clinical cure above and beyond the antimicrobial-attributable effect. Most of the doses reviewed and approved by the US Food and Drug Administration (FDA) are from the original clinical trials for drug registration, unless a safety issue becomes apparent when the label is modified or in cases in which the original industry sponsor of an antibiotic wishes to pursue approval for additional infection sites ("indications") and conducts new prospective clinical trials to share with the FDA. The original sponsor of the drug may not have studied all pathogens at all sites of infection in neonates, infants, and children. The FDA carefully reviews data presented to it but is not required to review the entire literature on each antibiotic and update the package labels. If the FDA has not reviewed data for a specific indication (eg, ampicillin for group A streptococcal cellulitis), there is usually no opinion about whether the drug may or may not work. Ampicillin is not "approved" for skin and soft tissue infections caused by any bacteria. That does not mean that the drug does not work or is unsafe; rather, data on safety and efficacy have not been presented to the FDA to expand the package label. The editors will provide suggestions for clinical situations that may not have been reviewed and approved by the FDA. These recommendations are considered *off-label,* signifying that safety and efficacy data have not been reviewed by the FDA at its high level of rigor.

- Duration of treatment should be individualized. Durations recommended are based on the literature, common practice, and general experience. Critical evaluations of the duration of therapy have been carried out in very few infectious diseases. In general, a more extended period of treatment should be used (1) for tissues in which antibiotic concentrations may be relatively low (eg, undrained abscess, central nervous system [CNS] infection); (2) for tissues in which repair following infection-mediated damage is slow (eg, bone); (3) when the organisms are less susceptible; (4) when a relapse of infection is unacceptable (eg, CNS infections); or (5) when the host is immunocompromised in some way. An assessment after therapy will ensure that your selection of antibiotic, dose, and duration of treatment was appropriate. Until prospective, comparative studies are performed for different durations, we cannot assign a specific increased risk of failure for shorter courses. We support the need for these studies in an outpatient or inpatient controlled clinical research setting.

- Our approach to therapy is continuing to move away from the concept that "one dose fits all." In addition to the dose that provides antibiotic exposure and host immunocompetence, the concept of *target attainment* is being better defined. The severity of illness and the willingness of the practitioner to accept a certain rate of failure need to be considered; hence, broad-spectrum, high-dose treatment is used for a child in florid septic shock (where you need to be right virtually 100% of the time), compared with the child with impetigo (where a treatment that is approximately 70% effective is acceptable, as you can see the child back in the office in a few days and alter the therapy as necessary).
- Diseases in this chapter are arranged by body systems. Please consult Chapter 3 for an alphabetized listing of bacterial and mycobacterial pathogens and uncommon organisms not included in this chapter.
- A more detailed description of treatment options for methicillin-resistant *Staphylococcus aureus* (MRSA) infections and multidrug-resistant gram-negative bacilli infections, including a stepwise approach to increasingly broad-spectrum agents, is provided in Chapter 12. Although, in the past, vancomycin has been the mainstay of therapy for invasive MRSA, it is nephrotoxic and ototoxic, and it requires monitoring renal function and serum drug concentrations. Its use against organisms with a minimal inhibitory concentration of 2 or greater may not provide adequate exposure for a cure with safe, realistic pediatric doses. Ceftaroline, the first MRSA-active beta-lactam antibiotic approved by the FDA for adults in 2010, children in 2016, and neonates in 2019, is as effective for most staphylococcal tissue site infections (no controlled data on CNS infections) as vancomycin, but safer, and should be considered preferred therapy over vancomycin.
- **Abbreviations:** AAP, American Academy of Pediatrics; ACOG, American College of Obstetricians and Gynecologists; ADH, antidiuretic hormone; AFB, acid-fast bacilli; AHA, American Heart Association; ALT, alanine transaminase; AmB, amphotericin B; amox/clav, amoxicillin/clavulanate; AOM, acute otitis media; ARF, acute rheumatic fever; AST, aspartate transaminase; AUC:MIC, area under the curve (the mathematically calculated area below the serum concentration-versus-time curve) to minimum inhibitory concentration; BAL, bronchoalveolar lavage; bid, twice daily; BL, beta-lactamase; CA-MRSA, community-associated methicillin-resistant *Staphylococcus aureus;* cap, capsule; CDC, Centers for Disease Control and Prevention; cephalosporin-R, cephalosporin-resistant; CF, cystic fibrosis; CMV, cytomegalovirus; CNS, central nervous system; CRP, C-reactive protein; CSD, cat-scratch disease; CSF, cerebrospinal fluid; CT, computed tomography; DAT, diphtheria antitoxin; div, divided; DOT, directly observed therapy; EBV, Epstein-Barr virus; ESBL, extended-spectrum beta-lactamase; ESR, erythrocyte sedimentation rate; ETEC, enterotoxin-producing *Escherichia coli;* FDA, US Food and Drug Administration; GC, *Neisseria gonorrhoeae;* gentamicin-S, gentamicin-susceptible; GI, gastrointestinal; HACEK, *Haemophilus aphrophilus, Aggregatibacter* (formerly *Actinobacillus*) *actinomycetemcomitans, Cardiobacterium hominis, Eikenella corrodens, Kingella* species; HSV, herpes simplex

virus; HUS, hemolytic uremic syndrome; I&D, incision and drainage; ID, infectious disease; IDSA, Infectious Diseases Society of America; IM, intramuscular; INH, isoniazid; IV, intravenous; IVIG, intravenous immune globulin; KPC, *Klebsiella pneumoniae* carbapenemase; L-AmB, liposomal amphotericin B; LFT, liver function test; LP, lumbar puncture; max, maximum; MDR, multidrug resistant; MIS-C, multisystem inflammatory syndrome in children; MRI, magnetic resonance imaging; MRSA, methicillin-resistant *S aureus;* MRSE, methicillin-resistant *Staphylococcus epidermidis;* MSM, men who have sex with men; MSSA, methicillin-susceptible *S aureus;* MSSE, methicillin-sensitive *S epidermidis;* ophth, ophthalmic; PCR, polymerase chain reaction; PCV13, Prevnar 13-valent pneumococcal conjugate vaccine; pen-R, penicillin-resistant; pen-S, penicillin-susceptible; PIDS, Pediatric Infectious Diseases Society; PIMS-TS, pediatric inflammatory multisystem syndrome temporally associated with SARS-CoV-2; pip/tazo, piperacillin/tazobactam; PMA, postmenstrual age; PO, orally; PPD, purified protein derivative; PZA, pyrazinamide; q, every; qd, once daily; qid, 4 times daily; qod, every other day; RIVUR, Randomized Intervention for Children with Vesicoureteral Reflux; RSV, respiratory syncytial virus; RT-PCR, real-time polymerase chain reaction; soln, solution; SPAG-2, small particle aerosol generator-2; spp, species; staph, staphylococcal; STEC, Shiga toxin–producing *E coli;* STI, sexually transmitted infection; strep, streptococcal; tab, tablet; TB, tuberculosis; Td, tetanus, diphtheria; Tdap, tetanus, diphtheria, acellular pertussis; tid, 3 times daily; TIG, tetanus immune globulin; tol/taz, ceftolozane/tazobactam; TMP/SMX, trimethoprim/sulfamethoxazole; ULN, upper limit of normal; UTI, urinary tract infection; VDRL, Venereal Disease Research Laboratories; WBC, white blood cell.

A. SKIN AND SOFT TISSUE INFECTIONS

Clinical Diagnosis	Therapy (evidence grade)	Comments
NOTE: CA-MRSA (see Chapter 12) is prevalent in most areas of the world but is now decreasing, rather than increasing.[1,2] Recommendations for staph infections are given for these scenarios: standard MSSA and CA-MRSA. Antibiotic recommendations "for CA-MRSA" should be used for (1) empiric therapy in regions with >5%–10% of invasive staph caused by MRSA; (2) clinical suspicion of CA-MRSA; and (3) documented CA-MRSA infections. "Standard recommendations" refer to treatment of MSSA. Oxacillin/nafcillin are considered equivalent agents. For MSSA causing most skin and soft tissue infections and bone/joint infections, first-generation cephalosporins (ie, cephalothin, cefazolin, cephalexin) are considered equivalent to oxacillin/methicillin, but for MSSA infections in other tissues (eg, endocarditis), cephalosporins other than first generation may not be equivalent (need more high-quality data to know with better certainty). Before using clindamycin for empiric therapy, please check your local susceptibility data for *Staphylococcus aureus* (MSSA and MRSA), as resistance can be as high as 40% in some locations. For MRSA skin infections caused by susceptible organisms, clindamycin and TMP/SMX provide similar clinical cure rates.		
Adenitis, acute bacterial[3–7] (*S aureus,* including CA-MRSA, and group A streptococcus; consider *Bartonella* [CSD] for subacute adenitis.)[8] Also called "suppurative adenitis" or "lymph node abscess"	Empiric therapy Standard: oxacillin/nafcillin 150 mg/kg/day IV div q6h OR cefazolin 100 mg/kg/day IV div q8h (AI), OR cephalexin 50–75 mg/kg/day PO div tid CA-MRSA: clindamycin 30 mg/kg/day IV or PO (AI) div q8h OR ceftaroline: 2 mo–<2 y, 24 mg/kg/day IV div q8h; ≥2 y, 36 mg/kg/day IV div q8h (max single dose 400 mg); >33 kg, either 400 mg/dose IV q8h or 600 mg/dose IV q12h (BI), OR vancomycin 40 mg/kg/day IV q8h (BII), OR daptomycin: 1–<2 y, 10 mg/kg IV qd; 2–6 y, 9 mg/kg IV qd; 7–11 y, 7 mg/kg qd; 12–17 y, 5 mg/kg qd (BI) CSD: azithromycin 12 mg/kg qd (max 500 mg) for 5 days (BIII)	May need surgical drainage for staph/strep infection; not usually needed for CSD. Additional antibiotics may not be required after drainage of mild to moderate suppurative adenitis caused by staph/strep. For oral therapy for MSSA: cephalexin or amox/clav. For CA-MRSA: clindamycin, TMP/SMX, or linezolid. For oral therapy for group A strep: amoxicillin or penicillin V. Daptomycin should be avoided in infants until age 1 y due to potential neurotoxicity. Total IV + PO therapy for 7–10 days. For CSD: this is the same high dose of azithromycin that is recommended routinely and FDA approved for strep pharyngitis.

Adenitis, nontuberculous (atypical) mycobacterial[9–14] Also called "subacute lymphadenitis"	Excision is usually curative (BII); azithromycin PO OR clarithromycin PO for 6–12 wk (with or without rifampin or ethambutol) if susceptible (BII).	Antibiotic susceptibility patterns are quite variable; cultures should guide therapy: excision >97% effective; medical treatment 60%–70% effective. No well-controlled trials are available. With surgical and medical therapy, children usually achieve symptomatic cure within 6 mo.[12] For more resistant organisms, other antibiotics may be active, including TMP/SMX, fluoroquinolones, doxycycline, or, for parenteral therapy, amikacin, meropenem, or cefoxitin. See Chapter 3 for specific mycobacterial pathogens.
Adenitis, tuberculous[15,16] (*Mycobacterium tuberculosis* and *Mycobacterium bovis*)	INH 10–15 mg/kg/day (max 300 mg) PO, IV qd, for 6 mo AND rifampin 15–20 mg/kg/day (max 600 mg) PO, IV qd, for 6 mo AND PZA 30–40 mg/kg/day PO qd for first 2 mo of therapy (BI); if suspected multidrug resistance, add ethambutol 15–25 mg/kg/day PO qd. Twice-weekly dosing after initial response (2–4 wk): INH 20–30 mg/kg/day (max 900 mg) PO AND rifampin 15–20 mg/kg/day (max 600 mg) PO AND PZA 50 mg/kg/day PO qd (max 2 g)	Surgical excision is not usually indicated because organisms are treatable. Adenitis caused by *M bovis* (unpasteurized dairy product ingestion) is uniformly resistant to PZA. Treat 9–12 mo with INH and rifampin if susceptible (BII). No contraindication to fine-needle aspirate of the node for diagnosis.
Anthrax, cutaneous[17]	Empiric therapy: ciprofloxacin 20–30 mg/kg/day PO div bid OR doxycycline 4.4 mg/kg/day (max 200 mg) PO div bid (regardless of age) (AIII)	If susceptible, amoxicillin or clindamycin (BIII). Ciprofloxacin and levofloxacin are FDA approved for inhalational anthrax for children >6 mo and should be effective for skin infection (BIII).

A. SKIN AND SOFT TISSUE INFECTIONS *(continued)*

Clinical Diagnosis	Therapy (evidence grade)	Comments
Bites, dog and cat[3,18–24] (*Pasteurella multocida; S aureus,* including CA-MRSA; *Streptococcus* spp, anaerobes; *Capnocytophaga canimorsus,* particularly in asplenic hosts)	Amox/clav 45 mg/kg/day PO div tid (amox/clav 7:1; see Aminopenicillins in Chapter 4) for 5–10 days (AII). For hospitalized children, use ampicillin AND clindamycin (BII) OR ceftriaxone AND clindamycin (BII).	Amox/clav has good *Pasteurella,* MSSA, and anaerobic coverage but lacks MRSA coverage. Ampicillin/amoxicillin plus clindamycin has good *Pasteurella,* MSSA, MRSA, and anaerobic coverage. For IV therapy options: ceftaroline has good *Pasteurella,* MSSA, and MRSA coverage but lacks *Bacteroides fragilis* anaerobic coverage.[23] Ampicillin/sulbactam, meropenem, and pip/tazo lack MRSA coverage. Consider rabies prophylaxis[24] for bites from at-risk animals that were not provoked (observe animal for 10 days, if possible) (AI); state and local public health departments and the CDC can provide advice on risk and management (www.cdc.gov/rabies/resources/contacts.html; reviewed July 29, 2022; accessed September 21, 2022); consider tetanus prophylaxis. For penicillin allergy, ciprofloxacin (for *Pasteurella*) plus clindamycin (BIII). Tigecycline or doxycycline may be considered for *Pasteurella* coverage.
Bites, human[3,20,21,25] (*Eikenella corrodens; S aureus,* including CA-MRSA; *Streptococcus* spp, anaerobes)	Amox/clav 45 mg/kg/day PO div tid (amox/clav 7:1; see Aminopenicillins in Chapter 4) for 5–10 days (AII). For hospitalized children, use ampicillin and clindamycin (BII) OR ceftriaxone and clindamycin (BII).	Human bites have a very high infection rate (do not routinely close open wounds). Amox/clav has good *Eikenella,* MSSA, and anaerobic coverage but lacks MRSA coverage. Ampicillin/sulbactam and meropenem lack MRSA coverage. For penicillin allergy, moxifloxacin can be used.[25]

Bullous impetigo[3,4,6,26] (usually *S aureus*, including CA-MRSA)	Standard: cephalexin 50–75 mg/kg/day PO div tid OR amox/clav 45 mg/kg/day PO div tid (CII) CA-MRSA: clindamycin 30 mg/kg/day PO div tid OR TMP/SMX 8 mg/kg/day of TMP PO div bid; for 5–7 days (CI)	For topical therapy if mild infection: mupirocin or retapamulin ointment
Cellulitis of unknown etiology (usually *S aureus*, including CA-MRSA, or group A streptococcus)[3,4,26–29]	IV empiric therapy for non-facial cellulitis Standard: oxacillin/nafcillin 150 mg/kg/day IV div q6h OR cefazolin 100 mg/kg/day IV div q8h (BII) CA-MRSA: clindamycin 30 mg/kg/day IV div q8h OR ceftaroline: 2 mo–<2 y, 24 mg/kg/day IV div q8h; ≥2 y, 36 mg/kg/day IV div q8h (max single dose 400 mg); >33 kg, either 400 mg/dose IV q8h or 600 mg/dose IV q12h (BI) OR vancomycin 40 mg/kg/day IV q8h (BII) OR daptomycin: 1–<2 y, 10 mg/kg IV qd; 2–6 y, 9 mg/kg IV qd; 7–11 y, 7 mg/kg qd; 12–17 y, 5 mg/kg qd (BI) For oral therapy for MSSA: cephalexin (AII) OR amox/clav 45 mg/kg/day PO div tid (BII); for CA-MRSA: clindamycin (BII), TMP/SMX (AII), or linezolid (BII)	For periorbital or buccal cellulitis, also consider *Streptococcus pneumoniae* or *Haemophilus influenzae* type b in unimmunized infants. Periorbital swelling that looks like cellulitis may occur with severe sinusitis in older children. Total IV + PO therapy for 7–10 days. Because nonsuppurative cellulitis is most often caused by group A streptococcus, cephalexin alone is usually effective. In adults, a prospective, randomized study of non-purulent cellulitis did not show that the addition of TMP/SMX improved outcomes over cephalexin alone.[28]
Cellulitis, buccal (for unimmunized infants and preschool children, *H influenzae* type b)[30]	Ceftriaxone 50 mg/kg/day (AI) IV, IM q24h, for 2–7 days parenteral therapy before switch to oral (BII)	Rule out meningitis (larger dosages may then be needed). For penicillin allergy, levofloxacin IV/PO covers pathogens, but no clinical data available. Oral therapy: amoxicillin if BL negative; amox/clav or oral second- or third-generation cephalosporin if BL positive.
Cellulitis, erysipelas (streptococcus)[3,4,7,31]	Penicillin G 100,000–200,000 U/kg/day IV div q4–6h (BII) initially, then penicillin V 100 mg/kg/day PO div qid (BIII) OR amoxicillin 50 mg/kg/day PO div tid (BIII) for 10 days	Clindamycin is also effective for most strains of group A streptococcus. Few well-designed prospective studies exist to provide evidence for recommendations.[31]

A. SKIN AND SOFT TISSUE INFECTIONS *(continued)*

Clinical Diagnosis	Therapy (evidence grade)	Comments
Gas gangrene (See Necrotizing fasciitis later in this table.)		
Impetigo (*S aureus*, including CA-MRSA; occasionally group A streptococcus)[3–7,32]	Mupirocin OR retapamulin topically (BII) to lesions tid; OR for more extensive lesions, oral therapy Standard: cephalexin 50–75 mg/kg/day PO div tid OR amox/clav 45 mg/kg/day PO div tid (AII) CA-MRSA: clindamycin 30 mg/kg/day (CII) PO div tid OR TMP/SMX 8 mg/kg/day of TMP PO div bid (AI); for 5–7 days	A meta-analysis suggests that topical therapy is as effective as oral therapy, but many studies did not specify outcomes based on pathogen susceptibilities.[32]
Ludwig angina[33] (mixed oral aerobes/anaerobes)	Penicillin G 200,000–250,000 U/kg/day IV div q6h AND clindamycin 40 mg/kg/day IV div q8h (CIII)	Alternatives: ceftriaxone/clindamycin; meropenem, imipenem or pip/tazo if gram-negative aerobic bacilli also suspected (CIII); high risk of respiratory tract obstruction from inflammatory edema
Lymphadenitis (See Adenitis, acute bacterial, earlier in this table.)		
Lymphangitis (usually group A streptococcus, rarely *S aureus*)[3,4,7]	Penicillin G 200,000 U/kg/day IV div q6h (BII) initially, then penicillin V 100 mg/kg/day PO div qid OR amoxicillin 50 mg/kg/day PO div tid for 10 days	Cefazolin IV (for group A strep or MSSA infection) or clindamycin IV (for group A strep, most MSSA and MRSA) For mild disease, penicillin V 50 mg/kg/day PO div qid for 10 days
Myositis, suppurative[34] (*S aureus*, including CA-MRSA; synonyms: tropical myositis, pyomyositis, muscle abscess)	Standard: oxacillin/nafcillin 150 mg/kg/day IV div q6h OR cefazolin 100 mg/kg/day IV div q8h (CII) CA-MRSA: clindamycin 40 mg/kg/day IV div q8h OR ceftaroline: 2 mo–<2 y, 24 mg/kg/day IV div q8h; ≥2 y, 36 mg/kg/day IV div q8h (max single dose 400 mg); >33 kg, either 400 mg/dose IV q8h or 600 mg/dose IV q12h (BI) OR vancomycin 40 mg/kg/day IV q8h (CIII) OR daptomycin: 1–<2 y, 10 mg/kg IV qd; 2–6 y, 9 mg/kg IV qd; 7–11 y, 7 mg/kg qd; 12–17 y, 5 mg/kg qd (BIII)	Surgical debridement is usually necessary. For disseminated MRSA infection, may require aggressive, emergent debridement; use clindamycin to help decrease toxin production (BIII); consider IVIG to bind bacterial toxins for life-threatening disease (CIII); abscesses may develop with CA-MRSA while on therapy. With infection caused by MRSA, highly associated with Panton-Valentine leukocidin.[35]

Necrotizing fasciitis (Pathogens vary depending on the age of the child and location of infection. Single pathogen: group A streptococcus; *Clostridia* spp, *S aureus* [including CA-MRSA], *Pseudomonas aeruginosa, Vibrio* spp, *Aeromonas* spp. Multiple pathogen, mixed aerobic/anaerobic synergistic fasciitis: any organism[s]: above, plus gram-negative bacilli, plus *Bacteroides* spp, and other anaerobes.)[3,36–38]	Empiric therapy: ceftazidime 150 mg/kg/day IV div q8h, or cefepime 150 mg/kg/day IV div q8h AND clindamycin 40 mg/kg/day IV div q8h (BIII); OR meropenem 60 mg/kg/day IV div q8h; OR pip/tazo 400 mg/kg/day pip component IV div q6h (AIII). ADD vancomycin OR ceftaroline for suspected CA-MRSA, pending culture results (AIII). Mixed aerobic/anaerobic/gram-negative: meropenem or pip/tazo AND clindamycin (AIII).	Aggressive emergent wound debridement (AII). ADD clindamycin to inhibit synthesis of toxins during the first few days of therapy (AIII). If CA-MRSA identified and susceptible to clindamycin, additional vancomycin is not required. Consider IVIG to bind bacterial toxins for life-threatening disease (BIII). Value of hyperbaric oxygen is not established (CIII).[39,40] Focus definitive antimicrobial therapy based on culture results. For documented group A strep infection: penicillin G 200,000–250,000 U/kg/day div q6h AND clindamycin 40 mg/kg/day div q8h (AIII).
Pyoderma, cutaneous abscesses (*S aureus*, including CA-MRSA; group A streptococcus)[4,6,7,26,27,41]	Standard: cephalexin 50–75 mg/kg/day PO div tid OR amox/clav 45 mg/kg/day PO div tid (BII) CA-MRSA: clindamycin 30 mg/kg/day PO div tid (BII) OR TMP/SMX 8 mg/kg/day of TMP PO div bid (AI)	I&D when indicated; IV for serious infections. With decreasing MRSA infection, approaches to prevention of recurrent MRSA infection include the use of baths with chlorhexidine soap daily or qod (BIII) OR the use of bleach baths twice weekly (½ cup of bleach per full bathtub) (BII). Decolonization with nasal mupirocin in a specific child may also be helpful; decolonization of the entire family may be important in certain situations.[42]
Rat-bite fever (*Streptobacillus moniliformis, Spirillum minus*)[43,44]	Penicillin G 100,000–200,000 U/kg/day IV div q6h (BII) for 7–10 days; for endocarditis, ADD gentamicin for 4–6 wk (CIII). For mild disease, oral therapy with amox/clav (CIII).	Organisms are normal oral flora for rodents. One does not require a bite to get infected. High rate of associated endocarditis. With this uncommon infection, no prospective comparative outcomes data exist. Alternatives: doxycycline; second- and third-generation cephalosporins (CIII).

A. SKIN AND SOFT TISSUE INFECTIONS *(continued)*

Clinical Diagnosis	Therapy (evidence grade)	Comments
Staphylococcal scalded skin syndrome (*S aureus* [MSSA, occasionally CA-MRSA])[45,46]	Standard: oxacillin 150 mg/kg/day IV div q6h OR cefazolin 100 mg/kg/day IV div q8h (CII) CA-MRSA: clindamycin 30 mg/kg/day IV div q8h (CIII) OR ceftaroline OR daptomycin	Burow or Zephiran compresses for oozing skin and intertriginous areas. Corticosteroids are contraindicated. Surgical debridement should be discouraged.

B. SKELETAL INFECTIONS

Clinical Diagnosis	Therapy (evidence grade)	Comments
NOTE: CA-MRSA infections (see Chapter 12) are decreasing in most areas of the world. However, even during the era of widespread MRSA infection, skeletal infections caused by MRSA were less common than skin infections. Recommendations are given for CA-MRSA and MSSA. Antibiotic recommendations for empiric therapy should include CA-MRSA when suspected or documented, while treatment of MSSA with beta-lactam antibiotics is preferred over clindamycin. During the past few years, clindamycin resistance in both MSSA and MRSA has remained stable at 10%–20%, with higher resistance reported by laboratories that report clindamycin-susceptible but D-test–positive strains (methylase-inducible) as resistant. Please check your local susceptibility data for *Staphylococcus aureus* before using clindamycin for empiric therapy. For MSSA skeletal infections, oxacillin/nafcillin and cefazolin are considered equivalent. The first PIDS-IDSA guidelines for bacterial osteomyelitis were published in the *Journal of the Pediatric Infectious Diseases Society,* September 2021.[47] PIDS-IDSA acute bacterial arthritis guidelines have been completed and undergoing review as of July 2022.		
Arthritis, bacterial[47–52]	Switch to appropriate high-dose oral therapy when clinically improved, CRP decreasing (see Chapter 14).[49,53,54]	

– Newborns	See Chapter 2.	
– Infants (*Kingella kingae,* now recognized as the most common pathogen; *S aureus,* including CA-MRSA; group A streptococcus) – Children (*S aureus,* including CA-MRSA; group A streptococcus; *K kingae*) – Unimmunized or immunocompromised children (pneumococcus, *Haemophilus influenzae* type b) For Lyme disease and brucellosis, see Table 1L.	Empiric therapy: cefazolin 100 mg/kg/day IV div q8h (in locations where MRSA causes <10% of infections) ADD clindamycin 30 mg/kg/day IV div q8h (to cover CA-MRSA unless clindamycin resistance locally is >10%, then use vancomycin). Ceftaroline can be used for MSSA, MRSA, and *Kingella.* See Comments for discussion of dexamethasone adjunctive therapy. For documented CA-MRSA: clindamycin 30 mg/kg/day IV div q8h (AI) OR ceftaroline: 2 mo–<2 y, 24 mg/kg/day IV div q8h; ≥2 y, 36 mg/kg/day IV div q8h (max single dose 400 mg); >33 kg, either 400 mg/dose IV q8h or 600 mg/dose IV q12h (BI) OR vancomycin 40 mg/kg/day IV q8h (BI). For MSSA: oxacillin/nafcillin 150 mg/kg/day IV div q6h OR cefazolin 100 mg/kg/day IV div q8h (AI). For *Kingella,* BL-negative: cefazolin 100 mg/kg/day IV div q8h OR ampicillin 150 mg/kg/day IV div q6h; OR, for BL-positive, ceftriaxone 50 mg/kg/day IV, IM q24h (AII). For pen-S pneumococci or group A streptococcus: penicillin G 200,000 U/kg/day IV div q6h (BII). For pen-R pneumococci or *Haemophilus:* ceftriaxone 50–75 mg/kg/day IV, IM q24h (BII). Total therapy (IV + PO) for 14–21 days (AII).[47,51]	Dexamethasone adjunctive therapy (0.15 mg/kg/dose q6h for 4 days in one study) demonstrated significant benefit in decreasing symptoms and earlier hospital discharge (but with some "rebound" symptoms).[55,56] **NOTE:** Children with rheumatologic, postinfectious, fungal/mycobacterial infections or malignancy are also likely to improve with steroid therapy. Oral step-down therapy options: For CA-MRSA: clindamycin OR linezolid. Little data published on TMP/SMX for invasive MRSA infection. For MSSA: cephalexin OR dicloxacillin caps for older children. For *Kingella:* most penicillins or cephalosporins (but not clindamycin or linezolid).

B. SKELETAL INFECTIONS *(continued)*

Clinical Diagnosis	Therapy (evidence grade)	Comments
– Gonococcal arthritis or tenosynovitis[56–58]	Ceftriaxone 50 mg/kg IV, IM q24h (BII) for 7 days AND azithromycin 20 mg/kg PO as a single dose, OR therapy with ceftriaxone alone	Recent data from adult studies, primarily of MSM, suggest increasing azithromycin resistance, leading to recommendations to drop azithromycin from treatment for adults, with an increase in the dose of ceftriaxone.[56] However, the rate of azithromycin resistance in children is likely to still be low; therefore, we are continuing to recommend combination therapy based on the rationale in the 2015 CDC STI guidelines.[56] Cefixime 8 mg/kg/day PO as a single daily dose may not be effective due to increasing resistance. Ceftriaxone IV, IM is preferred over cefixime PO.
– Other bacteria	See Chapter 3 for preferred antibiotics.	
Osteomyelitis[47–54,59,60–63]	Step down to appropriate high-dose oral therapy when clinically improved (see Chapter 14).[47,49,51,53,62]	
– Newborns	See Chapter 2.	
– Infants and children, acute infection (usually *S aureus*, including CA-MRSA; group A streptococcus; *K kingae*[47])	Empiric therapy: cefazolin 100 mg/kg/day IV div q8h (in locations where MRSA causes <10% of bone infections), OR clindamycin 30 mg/kg/day IV div q8h (to cover CA-MRSA unless clindamycin resistance is locally >10%; then use ceftaroline or vancomycin). For CA-MRSA: clindamycin 30 mg/kg/day IV div q8h OR ceftaroline: 2 mo–<2 y, 24 mg/kg/day IV div q8h; ≥2 y, 36 mg/kg/day IV div q8h (max single dose 400 mg); >33 kg, either 400 mg/dose IV q8h or 600 mg/dose IV q12h (BI), OR vancomycin 40 mg/kg/day IV q8h (BII). For MSSA: oxacillin/nafcillin 150 mg/kg/day IV div q6h OR cefazolin 100 mg/kg/day IV div q8h (AII).	In children with open fractures secondary to trauma, add ceftazidime or cefepime for extended aerobic gram-negative bacilli activity. *Kingella* is resistant to clindamycin, vancomycin, and linezolid. The proportion of MRSA in pediatric osteomyelitis is decreasing.[64] For MSSA (BI) and *Kingella* (BIII), step-down oral therapy with cephalexin 100 mg/kg/day PO div tid. *Kingella* is usually susceptible to amoxicillin. Oral step-down therapy options for CA-MRSA include clindamycin and linezolid[65]; additional data would be helpful to support the use of TMP/SMX.[61]

	For *Kingella*, BL-negative: cefazolin 100 mg/kg/day IV div q8h OR ampicillin 150 mg/kg/day IV div q6h; OR, for BL-positive, ceftriaxone 50 mg/kg/day IV, IM q24h (AII). Total therapy (IV + PO) usually 3–4 wk for uncomplicated MSSA, but may need >4–6 wk for CA-MRSA (BII). Follow closely for clinical response to empiric therapy.	For prosthetic devices, biofilms may impair microbial eradication, requiring the addition of rifampin or other agents.[63] No prospective, controlled data on the use of antibiotic-containing beads/cement placed at surgery in the site of infection.[47]
– Acute, other organisms	See Chapter 3 for preferred antibiotics.	
– Chronic osteomyelitis (may be a complication of poorly treated acute staph osteomyelitis or the result of trauma-associated infection with multiple potential pathogens), not to be confused with chronic nonbacterial osteomyelitis/chronic recurrent multifocal osteomyelitis, which are autoinflammatory diseases	For MSSA: cephalexin 100 mg/kg/day PO div tid OR dicloxacillin caps 75–100 mg/kg/day PO div qid for ≥3–6 mo (CIII) For CA-MRSA: clindamycin, linezolid, or TMP/SMX (CIII)	Surgery to debride sequestrum is usually required for cure. For prosthetic joint infection caused by staphylococci, add rifampin (CIII).[63] Osteomyelitis associated with foreign material (spinal rods, prostheses, implanted catheters) may be difficult to cure without removal of the material, but long-term suppression may be undertaken if risks of surgery are high, until some stabilization of the healing infected bone occurs. Watch for beta-lactam–associated neutropenia with high-dose, long-term therapy and for linezolid-associated neutropenia/thrombocytopenia with long-term (>2 wk) therapy.[65]
Osteomyelitis of the foot[66] (secondary to penetrating injury to the plantar surface; *S aureus*, including CA-MRSA, with other organisms colonizing foreign bodies) Osteochondritis after a puncture wound through a shoe; *Pseudomonas aeruginosa*)	Cefepime 150 mg/kg/day IV div q8h (BIII); ADD vancomycin (enhanced Gram-positive coverage) OR gentamicin (enhanced Gram-negative coverage), pending culture results.	Surgical debridement with cultures to focus antibiotic therapy. Treatment course is based on pathogen and extent of infection and debridement.

C. EYE INFECTIONS

Clinical Diagnosis	Therapy (evidence grade)	Comments
Cellulitis, orbital[67–70] (cellulitis of the contents of the orbit; may be associated with orbital abscess; usually secondary to sinus infection; caused by respiratory tract flora and *Staphylococcus aureus,* including CA-MRSA)	Ceftriaxone 50 mg/kg/day q24h AND clindamycin 30 mg/kg/day IV div q8h (for *S aureus,* including CA-MRSA) or ceftaroline single-drug therapy: 2 mo–<2 y, 24 mg/kg/day IV div q8h; ≥2 y, 36 mg/kg/day IV div q8h (max single dose 400 mg); >33 kg, either 400 mg/dose IV q8h or 600 mg/dose IV q12h (BIII). If MSSA isolated, use oxacillin/nafcillin IV OR cefazolin IV.	Surgical drainage of significant orbital or subperiosteal abscess present by CT scan or MRI. Try medical therapy alone for small abscess (BIII).[71,72] Ampicillin/sulbactam for respiratory flora/anaerobic coverage.[72] Treatment course for 10–14 days after surgical drainage, up to 21 days. CT scan or MRI can confirm cure (BIII).
Cellulitis, periorbital[73,74] (preseptal cellulitis)		Periorbital tissues are TENDER with cellulitis. Periorbital edema with sinusitis can look identical but is NOT tender. A multidisciplinary approach with an otolaryngological, ophthalmologic, and pediatric focus is helpful.[73]
– Cellulitis associated with entry site lesion on skin (*S aureus,* including CA-MRSA; group A streptococcus) in the fully immunized child	Standard: oxacillin/nafcillin 150 mg/kg/day IV div q6h OR cefazolin 100 mg/kg/day IV div q8h (BII) CA-MRSA: clindamycin 30 mg/kg/day IV div q8h or ceftaroline: 2 mo–<2 y, 24 mg/kg/day IV div q8h; ≥2 y, 36 mg/kg/day IV div q8h (max single dose 400 mg); >33 kg, either 400 mg/dose IV q8h or 600 mg/dose IV q12h (BII)	Oral antistaphylococcal antibiotic (eg, cephalexin or clindamycin) for empiric therapy for less severe infection; treatment course for 7–10 days
– True cellulitis with no associated entry site (in febrile, unimmunized infants): pneumococcal or *Haemophilus influenzae* type b	Ceftriaxone 50 mg/kg/day q24h OR cefuroxime 150 mg/kg/day IV div q8h (AII)	Treatment course for 7–10 days; rule out meningitis if bacteremic with *H influenzae.* Alternative agents for BL-positive strains of *H influenzae:* other second-, third-, fourth-, or fifth-generation cephalosporins or amox/clav.

– Periorbital edema, not true cellulitis; non-tender erythematous swelling. Usually associated with sinusitis; sinus pathogens may *rarely* erode anteriorly, causing cellulitis.	Ceftriaxone 50 mg/kg/day q24h OR cefuroxime 150 mg/kg/day IV div q8h (BIII). For suspected *S aureus*, including CA-MRSA, can use ceftaroline instead of ceftriaxone. For chronic sinusitis, ADD clindamycin (covers anaerobes) to either ceftriaxone or ceftaroline (AIII).	For oral convalescent antibiotic therapy, see Sinusitis, acute, in Table 1D; total treatment course of 14–21 days or 7 days after resolution of symptoms.
Conjunctivitis, acute (Most conjunctivitis is caused by a virus and does not require antibiotic treatment; purulent conjunctivitis is primarily caused by *Haemophilus* and pneumococcus.)[75,76]	Polymyxin/trimethoprim ophth soln OR polymyxin/bacitracin ophth ointment OR ciprofloxacin ophth soln (BII), for 7–10 days. For neonatal infection, see Chapter 2. Steroid-containing therapy only if HSV ruled out.	Other topical antibiotics (gentamicin, tobramycin, erythromycin, besifloxacin, moxifloxacin, norfloxacin, ofloxacin, levofloxacin) may offer advantages for particular pathogens (CII). High rates of resistance to sulfacetamide.
Conjunctivitis, herpetic[77–79] (*may be associated with keratitis*) For neonatal, see Chapter 2.	1% trifluridine or 0.15% ganciclovir ophth gel (AII) AND acyclovir PO (80 mg/kg/day div qid; max daily dose: 3,200 mg/day) has been effective in limited studies (BIII). Oral valacyclovir (60 mg/kg/day div tid) has superior pharmacokinetics to oral acyclovir and can be considered for systemic treatment, as can parenteral (IV) acyclovir if extent of disease is severe (CIII).	Consultation with ophthalmologist recommended for assessment and management (eg, concomitant use of topical steroids in certain situations). Recurrences common; corneal scars may form. Long-term suppression (≥1 y) of recurrent infection with oral acyclovir 80 mg/kg/day in 3 div doses (max dose 800 mg); decisions to continue suppressive therapy should be revisited annually. The frequency of dosing may need to be increased to qid, or the drug may need to be changed to valacyclovir, if breakthrough ocular infection occurs. Potential risks must balance potential benefits to vision (BIII).
Dacryocystitis[80] (*S aureus* most often, and other skin flora)	No antibiotic usually needed; oral antibiotic therapy for more symptomatic infection, based on Gram stain and culture of pus; topical therapy as for conjunctivitis may be helpful.	Warm compresses; may require surgical probing of nasolacrimal duct.

C. EYE INFECTIONS *(continued)*

Clinical Diagnosis	Therapy (evidence grade)	Comments
Endophthalmitis[81,82]		
NOTE: This is a medical emergency. Subconjunctival/sub-tenon antibiotics are likely to be required (vancomycin/ceftazidime or clindamycin/gentamicin); steroids commonly used (except for fungal infection); requires anterior chamber or vitreous tap for microbiological diagnosis. Listed systemic antibiotics to be used in addition to ocular injections.		Refer to ophthalmologist; vitrectomy may be necessary for advanced endophthalmitis. No prospective, controlled studies.
– Empiric therapy following open globe injury	Vancomycin 40 mg/kg/day IV div q8h AND cefepime 150 mg/kg/day IV div q8h (AIII)	
– Staphylococcal	Vancomycin 40 mg/kg/day IV div q8h pending susceptibility testing; oxacillin/nafcillin 150 mg/kg/day IV div q6h if susceptible (AIII)	Consider ceftaroline for MRSA treatment, as it may penetrate the vitreous better than vancomycin.
– Pneumococcal, meningococcal, *Haemophilus*	Ceftriaxone 100 mg/kg/day IV q24h; penicillin G 250,000 U/kg/day IV div q4h if susceptible (AIII)	Treatment course for 10–14 days
– Gonococcal	Ceftriaxone 50 mg/kg q24h IV, IM AND azithromycin (AIII)	Treatment course ≥7 days
– *Pseudomonas*	Cefepime 150 mg/kg/day IV div q8h for 10–14 days (AIII)	Cefepime is preferred over ceftazidime for *Pseudomonas* based on decreased risk of development of resistance on therapy; meropenem IV and imipenem IV are alternatives (no clinical data). Very poor outcomes. Oral convalescent therapy with fluoroquinolones in the adherent child.

– *Candida*[83]	Fluconazole (25 mg/kg loading dose, then 12 mg/kg/day IV), OR voriconazole (9 mg/kg loading dose, then 8 mg/kg/day IV); for resistant strains, L-AmB (5 mg/kg/day IV). For chorioretinitis, systemic antifungals PLUS intravitreal amphotericin 5–10 mcg/0.1-mL sterile water OR voriconazole 100 mcg/0.1-mL sterile water or physiologic (normal) saline soln (AIII). Duration of therapy is at least 4–6 wk (AIII).	Echinocandins given IV may not be able to achieve adequate antifungal activity in the eye.
Hordeolum (sty) or chalazion	None (topical antibiotic unnecessary)	Warm compresses; I&D when necessary
Retinitis		
– CMV[84,85] For congenital, see Chapter 2. Predominantly in immunocompromised and transplant patients. For HIV-infected children, see https://clinicalinfo.hiv.gov/en/guidelines/pediatric-opportunistic-infection/cytomegalovirus?view=full (accessed September 21, 2022).	See Chapter 7. Ganciclovir 10 mg/kg/day IV div q12h for 2 wk (BIII); if needed, continue at 5 mg/kg/day q24h to complete 6 wk total (BIII).	Consultation with an ophthalmologist is recommended for assessment and management. Neutropenia risk increases with duration of therapy. Foscarnet IV and cidofovir IV are alternatives but demonstrate significant toxicities. Letermovir has been approved for prophylaxis of CMV in adult stem cell transplant patients but has not been studied as treatment of CMV retinitis. Oral valganciclovir has not been evaluated in HIV-infected children with CMV retinitis but is an option primarily for older children who weigh enough to receive the adult dose of valganciclovir (CIII). Intravitreal ganciclovir and combination therapy for non-responding, immunocompromised hosts; however, intravitreal injections may not be practical for most children.

D. EAR AND SINUS INFECTIONS

Clinical Diagnosis	Therapy (evidence grade)	Comments
Bullous myringitis (See Otitis media, acute, later in this table.)	Believed to be a clinical manifestation of acute bacterial otitis media	
Mastoiditis, acute (pneumococcus [less since introduction of conjugate pneumococcal vaccines], *Staphylococcus aureus,* including CA-MRSA; group A streptococcus; *Pseudomonas* in adolescents, *Haemophilus* rare)[86–88]	Ceftriaxone 50 mg/kg/day q24h AND clindamycin 40 mg/kg/day IV div q8h (BIII) For adolescents: cefepime 150 mg/kg/day IV div q8h AND clindamycin 40 mg/kg/day IV div q8h (BIII)	Consider CNS extension (meningitis); surgery as needed for mastoid and middle ear drainage. Step down to appropriate oral therapy after clinical improvement, guided by culture results. Duration of therapy not well-defined; look for evidence of mastoid osteomyelitis.
Mastoiditis, chronic (See also Otitis, chronic suppurative, below.) (anaerobes, *Pseudomonas, S aureus* [including CA-MRSA])	Antibiotics only for acute superinfections (according to culture of drainage); for *Pseudomonas:* cefepime 150 mg/kg/day IV div q8h Alternatives to enhance anaerobic coverage: meropenem 60 mg/kg/day IV div q8h, OR pip/tazo 240 mg/kg/day IV div q4–6h (BIII)	Daily cleansing of ear important; if no response to antibiotics, surgery. Be alert for CA-MRSA.
Otitis, chronic suppurative (*Pseudomonas aeruginosa; S aureus,* including CA-MRSA; and other respiratory tract/skin flora)[89]	Topical antibiotics: fluoroquinolone (ciprofloxacin, ofloxacin, besifloxacin) with or without steroid (BIII) Cleaning of canal, view of tympanic membrane, for patency; cultures important	Presumed middle ear drainage through open tympanic membrane. Avoid aminoglycoside-containing therapy given risk of ototoxicity.[90] Other topical fluoroquinolones with/without steroids available.
Otitis externa		
– Bacterial, malignant otitis externa (*P aeruginosa*)[91,92]	Cefepime 150 mg/kg/day IV div q8h (AIII)	Other antipseudomonal antibiotics should also be effective: ceftazidime IV AND tobramycin IV, OR meropenem IV or imipenem IV or pip/tazo IV. For more mild infection, ciprofloxacin PO.

– Bacterial, acute otitis externa (*P aeruginosa; S aureus,* including CA-MRSA)[91,92] Also called "swimmer's ear"	Topical antibiotics: fluoroquinolone (ciprofloxacin or ofloxacin) with steroid, OR neomycin/polymyxin B/hydrocortisone (BII) Irrigating and cleaning canal of detritus important	Wick moistened with Burow (aluminum acetate topical) soln, used for marked swelling of canal; to prevent swimmer's ear, 2% acetic acid to canal after water exposure will restore acid pH.
– Bacterial furuncle of canal (*S aureus,* including CA-MRSA)	Standard: oxacillin/nafcillin 150 mg/kg/day IV div q6h OR cefazolin 100 mg/kg/day IV div q8h (BIII) CA-MRSA: clindamycin, ceftaroline, or vancomycin (BIII)	I&D; antibiotics for cellulitis. Oral therapy for mild disease, convalescent therapy. For MSSA: cephalexin. For CA-MRSA: clindamycin, TMP/SMX, OR linezolid (BIII).
– *Candida*	Fluconazole 6–12 mg/kg/day PO qd for 5–7 days (CIII)	May occur following antibiotic therapy for bacterial external otitis; debride canal.

Otitis media, acute

NOTE: The incidence of AOM and subsequent complications has decreased substantially in the era of conjugate pneumococcal vaccines.[93] With a decrease in disease caused by pen-R pneumococci requiring alternatives to first-line therapy, very few new antibiotics have entered clinical trials within the past few years. Although the risk of antibiotic-resistant pneumococcal otitis has decreased,[94] the percentage of *Haemophilus* responsible for AOM has likely increased; therefore, some experts recommend use of amox/clav over amoxicillin as first-line therapy for well-documented AOM.[95] The most current AAP guidelines[96] and meta-analyses[97,98] suggest that the greatest benefit with therapy occurs in children with bilateral AOM who are <2 y; for other children, close observation is also an option. AAP guidelines provide an option for non-severe cases, particularly disease in older children, to provide a prescription to parents but have them fill the prescription only if the child's condition deteriorates.[96] European guidelines are similar, although somewhat more conservative.[99] Although prophylaxis is only rarely indicated, amoxicillin or other antibiotics can be given at same milligram per kilogram dose as for treatment but less frequently, qd or bid to prevent infections (if the benefits outweigh the risks of development of resistant organisms for that child).[96]

D. EAR AND SINUS INFECTIONS *(continued)*

Clinical Diagnosis	Therapy (evidence grade)	Comments
– Newborns	See Chapter 2.	
– Infants and children (pneumococcus, *Haemophilus influenzae* non–type b, *Moraxella* most common)[94,95,100]	Amox/clav (90 mg/kg/day amox component PO div bid). Amoxicillin is still a reasonable choice for empiric therapy, but failures will most likely be caused by BL-producing *Haemophilus* (or *Moraxella*). a. For *Haemophilus* strains that are BL positive: amox/clav, cefdinir, cefpodoxime, cefuroxime, ceftriaxone IM, levofloxacin. b. For pen-R pneumococci (much less common in the PCV13 era): high-dosage amoxicillin achieves greater middle ear activity than oral cephalosporins. Options include ceftriaxone IM 50 mg/kg/day q24h for 1–3 doses; OR levofloxacin 20 mg/kg/day PO div bid for children ≤5 y and 10 mg/kg PO qd for children >5 y; OR a macrolide-class antibiotic: azithromycin PO at 1 of 3 dosages: (1) 10 mg/kg on day 1, followed by 5 mg/kg qd on days 2–5; (2) 10 mg/kg qd for 3 days; or (3) 30 mg/kg once. **Caution:** Up to 40% of pneumococci are macrolide resistant.	See Chapter 18 for dosages. Current data suggest that post-PCV13, *H influenzae* is now the most common pathogen, shifting the recommendation for empiric therapy from amoxicillin to amox/clav.[95,96,100] Published data document new but uncommon emergence of penicillin resistance in pneumococci isolated in the post-PCV13 era.[101,102] We have substantial data on the safety and tolerability of high-dosage amoxicillin (90 mg/kg/day div bid) producing high serum and middle ear fluid concentrations. Because COVID-19–era isolation is associated with a decrease in pneumococcal infections overall, data on pneumococcal resistance will be important to review as post-pandemic upper respiratory tract infections increase. It is likely that we will be able to return to standard-dosage amoxicillin (45 mg/kg/day) for AOM. Tympanocentesis should be performed in children whose second-line therapy fails.

Sinusitis, acute (*H influenzae* non–type b, pneumococcus, group A streptococcus, *Moraxella*)[95,103–106]	Same antibiotic therapy as for AOM, as pathogens are similar: either amox/clav (90 mg/kg/day amox component PO div bid) or amoxicillin alone (90 mg/kg/day PO div bid).[95] Therapy of 14 days may be necessary while mucosal swelling resolves and ventilation is restored. If high-quality evidence for decreased penicillin resistance in the PCV13 era becomes available in the future, the dose of amoxicillin required for treatment may decrease.[103]	IDSA sinusitis guidelines recommend amox/clav as first-line therapy,[106] while AAP guidelines recommend amoxicillin.[104] While both represent reasonable and effective therapy, amox/clav provides activity against BL-positive strains of *H influenzae*, which are more likely to be prevalent in both sinusitis and otitis in the PCV13 era.[95] There is no controlled evidence to determine whether the use of antihistamines, decongestants, or nasal irrigation is efficacious in children with acute sinusitis.[105]

E. OROPHARYNGEAL INFECTIONS

Clinical Diagnosis	Therapy (evidence grade)	Comments
Dental abscess (mixed aerobic/anaerobic oral flora)[107,108]	Clindamycin 30 mg/kg/day PO, IV, IM div q6–8h OR penicillin G 100–200,000 U/kg/day IV div q6h and metronidazole 30–40 mg/kg/day IV div q8h (AIII)	Amox/clav PO, clindamycin PO are oral options. Metronidazole has excellent anaerobic activity but no aerobic activity. Penicillin failures reported. Other IV options include ceftriaxone and metronidazole, OR meropenem. Tooth extraction usually necessary. Erosion of abscess may occur into facial, sinusitis, deep head, and neck compartments. High-quality prospectively collected data on the value of antibiotics have not been published, particularly regarding the need for antibiotics after dental extraction.
Diphtheria pharyngitis[109]	Erythromycin 40–50 mg/kg/day PO div qid for 14 days OR penicillin G 150,000 U/kg/day IV div q6h; PLUS DAT (AIII)	DAT, a horse antiserum, is investigational and available only from the CDC Emergency Operations Center at 770/488-7100; www.cdc.gov/diphtheria/dat.html (reviewed September 9, 2022; accessed September 21, 2022).
Epiglottitis (supraglottitis; *Haemophilus influenzae* type b in an *unimmunized* child; rarely pneumococcus, *Staphylococcus aureus*)[110,111]	Ceftriaxone 50 mg/kg/day IV, IM q24h for 7–10 days	Emergency: provide airway. For suspected *S aureus* infection (causes only 5% of epiglottitis), consider adding clindamycin to ceftriaxone or using ceftaroline single-drug therapy.

Gingivostomatitis, herpetic[112–114]	Acyclovir 80 mg/kg/day PO div qid (max dose 800 mg) for 7 days (for severe disease, use IV therapy at 30 mg/kg/day div q8h) (BIII); OR for infants ≥3 mo, valacyclovir 20 mg/kg/dose PO bid (max dose 1,000 mg; instructions for preparing liquid formulation with 28-day shelf life included in package insert) (CIII).[114]	Early treatment is likely to be the most effective. Start treatment as soon as oral intake is compromised. Valacyclovir is the prodrug of acyclovir that provides improved oral bioavailability, compared with oral acyclovir. Extended duration of therapy may be needed for immunocompromised children. The oral acyclovir dose (80 mg/kg/day div into 4 equal doses) provided is safe and effective for varicella, but 75 mg/kg/day div into 5 equal doses has been studied for HSV.[113] Max daily acyclovir dose should not exceed 3,200 mg.
Lemierre syndrome (*Fusobacterium necrophorum* primarily, new reports with MRSA)[115–119] (pharyngitis with internal jugular vein septic thrombosis, postanginal sepsis, necrobacillosis)	Empiric: meropenem 60 mg/kg/day div q8h (or 120 mg/kg/day div q8h for CNS metastatic foci) (AIII) OR ceftriaxone 100 mg/kg/day q24h AND metronidazole 40 mg/kg/day div q8h or clindamycin 40 mg/kg/day div q6h (BIII). ADD empiric vancomycin if MRSA suspected if clindamycin is not in the treatment regimen.	Anecdotal reports suggest that metronidazole may be effective for apparent failures with other agents. Often requires anticoagulation. Metastatic and recurrent abscesses often develop while on active, appropriate therapy, requiring multiple debridements and prolonged antibiotic therapy. Treat until CRP and ESR are normal (AIII).
Peritonsillar cellulitis or abscess (group A streptococcus with mixed oral flora, including anaerobes, CA-MRSA)[120] See Retropharyngeal; parapharyngeal; lateral pharyngeal cellulitis or abscess later in this table.	Clindamycin 30 mg/kg/day PO, IV, IM div q8h; for preschool infants with consideration of enteric bacilli, ADD ceftriaxone 50 mg/kg/day IV q24h (BIII).	Consider I&D for larger abscess (not well-defined). Alternatives: meropenem or imipenem or pip/tazo. Amox/clav for convalescent oral therapy (BIII). No controlled, prospective data on benefits/risks of steroids.[121]

E. OROPHARYNGEAL INFECTIONS *(continued)*

Clinical Diagnosis	Therapy (evidence grade)	Comments
Pharyngitis (group A streptococcus primarily)[7,122,123]	Amoxicillin 50–75 mg/kg/day PO, qd, bid, or tid for 10 days OR penicillin V 50–75 mg/kg/day PO, qid, bid, or tid, OR benzathine penicillin 600,000 U IM for children <27 kg, 1.2 million U IM if >27 kg, as a single dose (AII) For penicillin-allergic children: erythromycin (estolate) at 20–40 mg/kg/day PO div bid to qid; OR 40 mg/kg/day PO div bid to qid for 10 days; OR azithromycin 12 mg/kg qd for 5 days[a] (AII); OR clindamycin 30 mg/kg/day PO div tid [a] This is the dose investigated and FDA approved for children since 1994, and it is higher than the standard dose for other respiratory tract infections.	Although penicillin V is the most narrow-spectrum treatment, amoxicillin displays better GI absorption than oral penicillin V; the suspension is better tolerated. These advantages should be balanced by the unnecessary increased spectrum of activity. Once-daily amoxicillin dosage: for children 50 mg/kg (max 1,000–1,200 mg).[7] A 5-day treatment course is FDA approved for azithromycin at 12 mg/kg/day for 5 days, and some oral cephalosporins have been approved (cefdinir, cefpodoxime), with rapid clinical response to treatment that can also be seen with other antibiotics; a 10-day course is preferred for the prevention of ARF, particularly areas where ARF is prevalent, as no data exist on efficacy of 5 days of therapy for prevention of ARF.[7,124,125]
Retropharyngeal; parapharyngeal; lateral pharyngeal cellulitis or abscess (mixed aerobic/anaerobic flora, now including CA-MRSA)[120,126,127]	Clindamycin 40 mg/kg/day IV div q8h AND ceftriaxone 50 mg/kg/day IV q24h	Consider I&D; possible airway compromise, mediastinitis. Alternatives: meropenem or imipenem (BIII); pip/tazo. Can step down to less broad-spectrum coverage based on cultures. Amox/clav for convalescent oral therapy (but no activity for MRSA) (BIII).
Tracheitis, bacterial (*S aureus*, including CA-MRSA; group A streptococcus; pneumococcus; *H influenzae* type b, rarely *Pseudomonas*)[128]	Clindamycin 40 mg/kg/day IV div q8h or vancomycin 40 mg/kg/day IV div q8h AND ceftriaxone 50 mg/kg/day q24h OR ceftaroline single-drug therapy: 2 mo–<2 y, 24 mg/kg/day IV div q8h; ≥2 y, 36 mg/kg/day IV div q8h (max single dose 400 mg); >33 kg, either 400 mg/dose IV q8h or 600 mg/dose IV q12h (BIII)	For susceptible *S aureus*, oxacillin/nafcillin or cefazolin May represent bacterial superinfection of viral laryngotracheobronchitis, including influenza

F. LOWER RESPIRATORY TRACT INFECTIONS

Clinical Diagnosis	Therapy (evidence grade)	Comments
Abscess, lung		
– Primary (a complication of severe, necrotizing community-acquired pneumonia caused by pneumococcus; *Staphylococcus aureus,* particularly CA-MRSA; group A streptococcus, rarely *Mycoplasma pneumoniae*)[129,130]	Empiric therapy with ceftriaxone 50–75 mg/kg/day q24h AND clindamycin 40 mg/kg/day div q8h or vancomycin 45 mg/kg/day IV div q8h for ≥14–21 days (AIII) OR (for MRSA) ceftaroline single-drug therapy: 2–<6 mo, 30 mg/kg/day IV div q8h (each dose given over 2 h); ≥6 mo, 45 mg/kg/day IV div q8h (each dose given over 2 h) (max single dose 600 mg) (BII)	For severe CA-MRSA infections, see Chapter 12. For presumed *Mycoplasma,* add a fluoroquinolone (levofloxacin) or macrolide. Bronchoscopy may be necessary if abscess fails to drain; surgical excision is rarely necessary for pneumococcus but may be important for CA-MRSA and MSSA. Focus antibiotic coverage based on culture results. For MSSA: oxacillin/nafcillin or cefazolin.
– Secondary to aspiration (ie, foul smelling; polymicrobial infection with oral aerobes and anaerobes)[131]	Clindamycin 40 mg/kg/day IV div q8h or meropenem 60 mg/kg/day IV div q8h for ≥10 days (AIII)	Alternatives: ceftriaxone AND metronidazole OR imipenem IV OR pip/tazo IV (BIII) Oral step-down therapy with clindamycin or amox/clav (BIII)
Allergic bronchopulmonary aspergillosis[132]	Prednisone 0.5 mg/kg qd for 1–2 wk and then taper (BII) for mild, acute stage illness AND (for more severe disease) voriconazole[133] 18 mg/kg/day PO div q12h load followed by 16 mg/kg/day div q12h (AIII) OR itraconazole[134] 10 mg/kg/day PO div q12h (BII). Voriconazole and itraconazole require trough concentration monitoring.	Not all allergic pulmonary disease is associated with true fungal infection. Larger steroid dosages to control inflammation may lead to tissue invasion by *Aspergillus.* Corticosteroids are the cornerstone of therapy for exacerbations, and itraconazole and voriconazole have a demonstrable corticosteroid-sparing effect.
Aspiration pneumonia (polymicrobial infection with oral aerobes and anaerobes)[131]	Clindamycin 40 mg/kg/day IV div q8h; ADD ceftriaxone 50–75 mg/kg/day q24h for additional *Haemophilus* activity OR, as a single agent, meropenem 60 mg/kg/day IV div q8h; for ≥10 days (BIII).	Alternatives: ceftriaxone AND metronidazole OR imipenem IV OR pip/tazo IV (BIII) Oral step-down therapy with clindamycin or amox/clav (BIII)

F. LOWER RESPIRATORY TRACT INFECTIONS *(continued)*

Clinical Diagnosis	Therapy (evidence grade)	Comments
Atypical pneumonia (See *Mycoplasma pneumoniae* and Legionnaires disease later in this table under Pneumonias of other established etiologies.)		
Bronchitis (bronchiolitis), acute[135]	For bronchitis/bronchiolitis in children, no antibiotic needed for most cases, as disease is usually viral	With PCR multiplex diagnosis now widely available, a nonbacterial diagnosis will allow clinicians to avoid use of antibiotics, but viral/bacterial coinfection can still occur.
Community-acquired pneumonia (See Community-acquired pneumonia: empiric therapy later in this table.)		
Cystic fibrosis: Seek advice from experts in acute and chronic management. Larger than standard dosages of beta-lactam antibiotics have been required in the past to achieve the same blood concentrations as those in children without CF, but in the current era of maximal pulmonary and nutritional support of CF, it seems that most antibiotics eliminated by the kidney can be administered at typical doses to achieve adequate blood concentrations. However, we do not know whether the concentrations of antibiotics achieved at the deep sites of infection in the CF lung are adequate, particularly with advanced CF disease. The Cystic Fibrosis Foundation posts guidelines (www.cff.org/Care/Clinical-Care-Guidelines/Respiratory-Clinical-Care-Guidelines/Pulmonary-Exacerbations-Clinical-Care-Guidelines; reviewed July 2021; accessed September 21, 2022). Dosages of beta-lactams should achieve their pharmacokinetic/pharmacodynamic goals to increase the chance of response.[136,137]		
– Acute exacerbation (*Pseudomonas aeruginosa* primarily; also *Burkholderia cepacia, Stenotrophomonas maltophilia, S aureus* [including CA-MRSA], nontuberculous mycobacteria)[138–143]	Cefepime 150–200 mg/kg/day div q8h or meropenem 120 mg/kg/day div q6h AND tobramycin 6–10 mg/kg/day IM, IV div q6–8h for treatment of acute exacerbation (AII); many alternatives: imipenem IV, ceftazidime IV, or ciprofloxacin 30 mg/kg/day PO, IV div tid May require vancomycin 60–80 mg/kg/day IV div q8h for MRSA, OR ceftaroline 45 mg/kg/day IV div q8h (each dose given over 2 h) (max single dose 600 mg) (BIII) Duration of therapy not well-defined: 10–14 days (BIII)[139]	Monitor concentrations of aminoglycosides, vancomycin. Insufficient evidence to recommend routine use of inhaled antibiotics for acute exacerbations.[144] Cultures with susceptibility will help select antibiotics, as multidrug resistance is common, but synergy testing is not well standardized.[145] Combination therapy may provide synergistic killing and delay the emergence of resistance (BIII). Attempt at early eradication of new-onset *Pseudomonas* may decrease progression of disease.[146] Failure to respond to antibacterials should prompt evaluation for appropriate drug doses and for invasive/allergic fungal disease as well as maximization of pulmonary hygiene.

– Chronic inflammation in CF: impact of inhaled antibiotics and azithromycin to minimize long-term damage to lung	Inhaled tobramycin 300 mg bid, cycling 28 days on therapy, 28 days off therapy, is effective adjunctive therapy between exacerbations, with new data suggesting a benefit of alternating inhaled tobramycin with inhaled aztreonam (AI).[147,148] Azithromycin adjunctive chronic therapy, greatest benefit for those colonized with *Pseudomonas* (AII).[149,150]	Alternative inhaled antibiotics: colistin[151] (BIII). Two newer powder preparations of inhaled tobramycin are available. Azithromycin does not decrease the benefit of improved pulmonary function with inhaled tobramycin in those with *Pseudomonas* airway colonization.[152]
Pertussis[153,154]	Azithromycin: for those ≥6 mo, 10 mg/kg/day for day 1, then 5 mg/kg/day for days 2–5; for those <6 mo, 10 mg/kg/day for 5 days; OR clarithromycin 15 mg/kg/day div bid for 7 days; or erythromycin (estolate preferable) 40 mg/kg/day PO div qid for 7–10 days (AII) Alternative: TMP/SMX 8 mg/kg/day of TMP div bid for 14 days (BIII)	Azithromycin and clarithromycin are better tolerated than erythromycin; azithromycin is preferred in young infants to reduce pyloric stenosis risk (see Chapter 2). Provide prophylaxis to family members. Unfortunately, no adjunctive therapy has been shown to be beneficial in decreasing the cough.[155]
Community-acquired pneumonia: empiric therapy for bronchopneumonia, lobar consolidation, or complicated pneumonia with pleural fluid/empyema		
– Mild to moderate "chest cold"–like illness (overwhelmingly viral, especially in preschool children)[156]	No antibiotic therapy unless epidemiologic, clinical, or laboratory reasons to suspect bacterial coinfection, or *Mycoplasma*	Broad-spectrum antibiotics may increase risk of subsequent infection with antibiotic-resistant pathogens.

F. LOWER RESPIRATORY TRACT INFECTIONS *(continued)*

Clinical Diagnosis	Therapy (evidence grade)	Comments
– Moderate to severe illness (pneumococcus; group A streptococcus; *S aureus,* including CA-MRSA; *M pneumoniae*[129,157,158]; for those with aspiration and underlying comorbidities, *Haemophilus influenzae,* non-typeable; and for unimmunized children, *H influenzae* type b)	Empiric therapy For most regions now with high PCV13 vaccine use or low pneumococcal resistance to penicillin: ampicillin 150–200 mg/kg/day div q6h. For regions with low rates of PCV13 use or high pneumococcal resistance to penicillin: ceftriaxone 50–75 mg/kg/day q24h (AI). For suspected CA-MRSA: ceftaroline: 2–<6 mo, 30 mg/kg/day IV div q8h (each dose given over 2 h); ≥6 mo, 45 mg/kg/day IV div q8h (each dose given over 2 h) (max single dose 600 mg) (BII),[158] OR vancomycin 40–60 mg/kg/day (AIII).[3] For suspected *Mycoplasma*/atypical pneumonia agents, particularly in school-aged children, ADD azithromycin 10 mg/kg IV, PO on day 1, then 5 mg/kg qd for days 2–5 of treatment (AII).	Tracheal aspirate or BAL for Gram stain/culture for severe infection in intubated children. For CA-MRSA: if vancomycin is being used rather than ceftaroline, check vancomycin serum concentrations and renal function, particularly at the higher dosage needed to achieve an AUC:MIC of 400. Alternatives to azithromycin for atypical pneumonia include erythromycin IV, PO, or clarithromycin PO, or doxycycline IV, PO for children >7 y, or levofloxacin IV, PO. Benefits of combination empiric therapy with a beta-lactam and a macrolide conflict and may apply only to certain populations.[159–161] Duration of therapy is still not well-defined in prospective, controlled trials in pediatric community-acquired pneumonia. Retrospective data with diagnosis based only on clinical examination and radiograph suggested that 10 days may be unnecessary for all children (5 days may be sufficient).[162] Empiric oral outpatient therapy for less severe illness: high-dosage amoxicillin 80–100 mg/kg/day PO div tid (NOT bid, which is used for otitis) (BIII).
– **Pleural fluid/empyema** (same pathogens as for community-associated bronchopneumonia) (Based on extent of fluid and symptoms, may benefit from chest tube drainage with fibrinolysis; rarely from video-assisted thoracoscopic surgery.)[157,139–166]	Empiric therapy: ceftriaxone 50–75 mg/kg/day q24h AND vancomycin 40–60 mg/kg/day IV div q8h (BIII) OR ceftaroline single-drug therapy: 2–<6 mo, 30 mg/kg/day IV div q8h; ≥6 mo, 45 mg/kg/day IV div q8h (each dose given over 2 h) (max single dose 600 mg) (BII)	Initial therapy based on Gram stain of empyema fluid; typically, clinical improvement is slow, with persisting but decreasing "spiking" fever for 2–3 wk. Concerns about the effectiveness of vancomycin monotherapy in influenza-associated MRSA pneumonia.[167] Combination therapy with agents added to vancomycin, or monotherapy with other agents like ceftaroline, may provide a better option.

– **Interstitial pneumonia syndrome of early infancy**	If *Chlamydia trachomatis* suspected, azithromycin 10 mg/kg on day 1, followed by 5 mg/kg/day qd days 2–5 OR erythromycin 40 mg/kg/day PO div qid for 14 days (BII)	Most often respiratory viral pathogens, CMV, or chlamydial; role of *Ureaplasma* uncertain
Pneumonia: definitive therapy for pathogens of community-acquired pneumonia		
– **Pneumococcus** (may occur with non-PCV13 serotypes)[129,157–159]	Empiric therapy For regions with high PCV13 vaccine use or low pneumococcal resistance to penicillin: ampicillin 150–200 mg/kg/day div q6h For regions with low rates of PCV13 use or high pneumococcal resistance to penicillin: ceftriaxone 50–75 mg/kg/day q24h (AI) Empiric oral outpatient therapy for less severe illness: high-dosage amoxicillin 80–100 mg/kg/day PO div tid (NOT bid, which is used for otitis)	Change to PO after improvement (decreased fever, no oxygen needed); treat until patient clinically asymptomatic and chest radiograph significantly improved (7–21 days) (BIII). No reported failures of ceftriaxone for pen-R pneumococcus; no need to add empiric vancomycin for this reason (CIII). Oral therapy for pneumococcus may also be successful with amox/clav, cefdinir, cefixime, cefpodoxime, or cefuroxime, particularly for fully pen-S strains. Levofloxacin is an alternative, particularly for those with severe allergy to beta-lactam antibiotics (BI),[168] but, due to theoretical cartilage toxicity concerns for humans, should not be first-line therapy.
– Pneumococcal, pen-S	Penicillin G 250,000–400,000 U/kg/day IV div q4–6h for 10 days (BII) OR ampicillin 150–200 mg/kg/day IV div q6h	After improvement, change to amoxicillin 50–75 mg/kg/day PO div tid OR penicillin V 50–75 mg/kg/day div qid.
– Pneumococcal, pen-R	Ceftriaxone 75 mg/kg/day q24h for 10–14 days (BIII)	Addition of vancomycin has not been required for treatment of pen-R strains. Ceftaroline is more active against pneumococcus than ceftriaxone, but with no current ceftriaxone resistance, ceftaroline is not required. For oral convalescent therapy, high-dosage amoxicillin (100–150 mg/kg/day PO div tid), clindamycin (30 mg/kg/day PO div tid), linezolid (30 mg/kg/day PO div tid), or levofloxacin PO.

F. LOWER RESPIRATORY TRACT INFECTIONS *(continued)*

Clinical Diagnosis	Therapy (evidence grade)	Comments
– ***Staphylococcus aureus*** (including CA-MRSA) is a rare (1%) cause of pediatric community-acquired pneumonia.[4,6,129,157,169,170]	For MSSA: oxacillin/nafcillin 150 mg/kg/day IV div q6h or cefazolin 100 mg/kg/day IV div q8h (AII) For suspected CA-MRSA: ceftaroline: 2–<6 mo, 30 mg/kg/day IV div q8h (each dose given over 2 h); ≥6 mo, 45 mg/kg/day IV div q8h (each dose given over 2 h) (max single dose 600 mg) (BII), OR vancomycin 40–60 mg/kg/day (AIII)[3]; may need addition of rifampin, clindamycin, or gentamicin (AIII) (See Chapter 12.)	Check vancomycin serum concentrations and renal function, particularly at the higher dosage designed to attain an AUC:MIC of 400, or serum trough concentrations of 15 mcg/mL for invasive CA-MRSA disease. For life-threatening disease, optimal therapy for CA-MRSA has not been studied and remains poorly defined: consider adding gentamicin and/or rifampin for combination therapy (CIII). Linezolid 30 mg/kg/day IV, PO div q8h is another option, more effective in adults than vancomycin for MRSA nosocomial pneumonia[171] (follow platelet and WBC counts weekly). For influenza-associated MRSA pneumonia, vancomycin monotherapy was inferior to combination therapies.[165] Do NOT use daptomycin for pneumonia. Oral convalescent therapy for MSSA: cephalexin PO; for CA-MRSA: clindamycin or linezolid PO. Total course for ≥21 days (AIII).
– **Group A streptococcus**	Penicillin G 250,000 U/kg/day IV div q4–6h for 10 days (BII)	Change to amoxicillin 75 mg/kg/day PO div tid or penicillin V 50–75 mg/kg/day div qid to tid after clinical improvement (BIII).

Pneumonia: immunosuppressed, neutropenic host		
– **Immunosuppressed, neutropenic host**[172] (*P aeruginosa,* other community-associated or nosocomial gram-negative bacilli, *S aureus,* fungi, AFB, *Pneumocystis,* viral [adenovirus, CMV, EBV, influenza, RSV, others])	Cefepime 150 mg/kg/day IV div q8h (AII), OR meropenem 60 mg/kg/day div q8h (AII) (BIII), OR pip/tazo 240–300 mg/kg/day div q6h; AND if *S aureus* (including MRSA) is suspected clinically, ADD vancomycin 40–60 mg/kg/day IV div q8h (AIII) OR ceftaroline: 2–<6 mo, 30 mg/kg/day IV div q8h; ≥6 mo, 45 mg/kg/day IV div q8h (max single dose 600 mg) (BIII).	Biopsy/BAL for histology/cultures or serum/BAL for cell-free next-generation sequencing testing helps determine need for antifungal, antiviral, antimycobacterial treatment. Antifungal therapy usually started if no response to antibiotics in 48–72 h (AmB, voriconazole, or caspofungin/micafungin—see Chapter 5). For septic patients, the addition of tobramycin will increase coverage for most gram-negative pathogens. For those with mucositis, anaerobic coverage may be needed, as provided by carbapenems and pip/tazo (or with the addition of clindamycin or metronidazole to other agents). Consider use of 2 active agents for definitive therapy for *Pseudomonas* for neutropenic hosts to assist clearing the pathogen and potentially decrease risk of resistance, but there is no evidence to support better outcomes (BIII).
Pneumonia: nosocomial (health care–associated/ventilator-associated)		
– **Nosocomial (health care–associated/ventilator-associated)** (*P aeruginosa,* gram-negative enteric bacilli [*Enterobacter, Klebsiella, Serratia, Escherichia coli*], *Acinetobacter, Stenotrophomonas,* and gram-positive organisms including CA-MRSA and *Enterococcus*)[173,174]	Commonly used regimens Meropenem 60 mg/kg/day div q8h, OR pip/tazo 240–300 mg/kg/day div q6–8h, OR cefepime 150 mg/kg/day div q8h; ± gentamicin 6.0–7.5 mg/kg/day div q8h (AIII); ADD vancomycin or ceftaroline for suspected CA-MRSA (AIII).	Empiric therapy should be institution specific, based on your hospital's nosocomial pathogens and susceptibilities. Pathogens that cause nosocomial pneumonia often have multidrug resistance. Cultures are critical. Empiric therapy also based on child's prior colonization/infection. Do not treat colonization, though. For MDR gram-negative bacilli, available IV therapy options include ceftazidime/avibactam (now FDA approved for children), tol/taz, meropenem/vaborbactam, cefiderocol, plazomicin, or colistin. Aerosol delivery of antibiotics may be required for MDR pathogens, but little high-quality controlled data are available for children.[175]

F. LOWER RESPIRATORY TRACT INFECTIONS *(continued)*

Clinical Diagnosis	Therapy (evidence grade)	Comments
Pneumonias of other established etiologies (See Chapter 3 for treatment by pathogen.)		
– *Chlamydophila pneumoniae,*[176] *Chlamydophila psittaci,* or *Chlamydia trachomatis*	Azithromycin 10 mg/kg on day 1, followed by 5 mg/kg/day qd days 2–5 or erythromycin 40 mg/kg/day PO div qid; for 14 days	Doxycycline (patients >7 y). Levofloxacin should also be effective.
– CMV (immunocompromised host)[177,178] (See chapters 2 and 7 for CMV infection in newborns and children, respectively.)	See Chapter 7. Ganciclovir IV 10 mg/kg/day IV div q12h for 2 wk (BIII); if needed, continue at 5 mg/kg/day q24h to complete 4–6 wk total (BIII).	Bone marrow transplant recipients with CMV pneumonia whose ganciclovir therapy alone fails may benefit from therapy with IV CMV hyperimmunoglobulin and ganciclovir given together (BII).[179,180] Oral valganciclovir may be used for convalescent therapy (BIII). Foscarnet for ganciclovir-resistant isolates.
– *E coli*	Ceftriaxone 50–75 mg/kg/day q24h (AII)	For cephalosporin-R strains (ESBL producers), use meropenem, imipenem, or ertapenem (AIII). Use high-dose ampicillin if susceptible.
– *Enterobacter* spp	Cefepime 100 mg/kg/day div q12h or meropenem 60 mg/kg/day div q8h; OR ceftriaxone 50–75 mg/kg/day q24h AND gentamicin 6.0–7.5 mg/kg/day IM, IV div q8h (AIII)	Addition of aminoglycoside to third-generation cephalosporins (ceftriaxone, ceftazidime) may retard the emergence of ampC-mediated constitutive high-level resistance, but concern exists for inadequate aminoglycoside concentration in airways; not an issue for ampC-stable beta-lactams (cefepime, meropenem, imipenem, or pip/tazo).
– *Francisella tularensis*[181]	Gentamicin 6.0–7.5 mg/kg/day IM, IV div q8h for ≥10 days for more severe disease (AIII); for less severe disease, ciprofloxacin or levofloxacin (AIII)	Other alternative for oral therapy for mild disease: doxycycline PO for 14–21 days (but watch for relapse). See www.cdc.gov/tularemia/clinicians/index.html (reviewed July 5, 2022; accessed September 21, 2022).

– Fungi (See Chapter 5.) Community-associated pathogens, which vary by region (eg, *Coccidioides*,[182,183] *Histoplasma*)[184,185] *Aspergillus;* mucormycosis; other mold infections in immunocompromised hosts (See Chapter 5.)	For detailed pathogen-specific recommendations, see Chapter 5. For suspected endemic fungi or mucormycosis in an *immunocompromised* host, treat empirically with a lipid AmB and not voriconazole; biopsy needed to guide therapy. Posaconazole[186] and isavuconazole[187] have in vitro activity and clinical efficacy data against some *Rhizopus* spp. For suspected invasive aspergillosis, treat with voriconazole (AI) (load 18 mg/kg/day div q12h on day 1, then continue 16 mg/kg/day div q12h).	For immunocompetent hosts, triazoles (fluconazole, itraconazole, voriconazole, posaconazole, and isavuconazole) are better tolerated than AmB and equally effective for many community-associated pathogens (see Chapter 6). For dosage, see Chapter 5. Check voriconazole trough concentrations; need to be at least >2 mcg/mL. For *Coccidioides* infection refractory to fluconazole therapy, consider increasing the dose, switching to other azoles, or switching to AmB.

F. LOWER RESPIRATORY TRACT INFECTIONS *(continued)*

Clinical Diagnosis	Therapy (evidence grade)	Comments
– Influenza virus.[188,189] – Recent seasonal influenza A and B strains continue to be resistant to adamantanes.	Empiric therapy, or documented influenza A or B Oseltamivir[189,190] (AII): <12 mo: Full-term infants 0–8 mo: 3 mg/kg/dose bid 9–11 mo: 3.5 mg/kg/dose bid ≥12 mo: ≤15 kg: 30 mg PO bid >15–23 kg: 45 mg PO bid >23–40 kg: 60 mg PO bid >40 kg: 75 mg PO bid Zanamivir inhaled (AII): for those ≥7 y, 10 mg (two 5-mg inhalations) bid Peramivir (BII): 6 mo–12 y: single IV dose of 12 mg/kg, up to 600 mg max 13–17 y: single IV dose of 600 mg Baloxavir (BI): ≥5 y: <20 kg: single dose PO of 2 mg/kg 20–79 kg: single dose PO of 40 mg ≥80 kg: single dose PO of 80 mg	Check for antiviral susceptibility each season at www.cdc.gov/flu/professionals/antivirals/index.htm (reviewed by the CDC September 8, 2022; accessed September 21, 2022). For children 12–23 mo, the unit dose of oseltamivir of 30 mg/dose may provide inadequate drug exposure. 3.5 mg/kg/dose PO bid has been studied for pharmacokinetics,[190] but sample sizes were limited. Limited data for oseltamivir in preterm neonates[189]: <38 wk of PMA (gestational plus chronologic age): 1.0 mg/kg/dose PO bid 38–40 wk of PMA: 1.5 mg/kg/dose PO bid The adamantanes (amantadine and rimantadine) had activity against influenza A before the late 1990s, but all circulating A strains of influenza have been resistant for many years. Influenza B is intrinsically resistant to adamantanes.
– *Klebsiella pneumoniae*[191,192]	Ceftriaxone 50–75 mg/kg/day IV, IM q24h (AIII); for ceftriaxone-resistant strains (ESBL strains), use meropenem 60 mg/kg/day IV div q8h (AIII) or other carbapenem.	For *K pneumoniae* that contain ESBLs, other carbapenems, pip/tazo, and fluoroquinolones are other options. Data in adults suggest that outcomes with pip/tazo are inferior to those with carbapenems.[191,192] For KPC-producing strains that are resistant to meropenem, alternatives include ceftazidime/avibactam (FDA approved for adults and children), fluoroquinolones, or colistin (BIII). See Chapter 12.

– Legionnaires disease (*Legionella pneumophila*)	Azithromycin 10 mg/kg IV, PO q24h for 5 days (AIII)	Alternatives: clarithromycin, erythromycin, ciprofloxacin, levofloxacin, doxycycline
– Mycobacteria, nontuberculous (*Mycobacterium avium* complex most common)[193]	In a normal host with pneumonia that requires therapy, 3 drugs are now recommended: azithromycin PO (or clarithromycin PO) AND ethambutol, AND rifampin, given 3 times/wk to prevent macrolide/azalide resistance. Duration of treatment is not well-defined; consider 12 mo, or 6–12 wk if susceptible. For more extensive cavitary or advanced/severe bronchiectatic disease, ADD amikacin or streptomycin (AIII).	Highly variable susceptibilities of different nontuberculous mycobacterial spp. Culture and susceptibility data are important for success. Check if immunocompromised: HIV or interferon-γ receptor deficiency. Consider consulting an ID physician.
– *Mycobacterium tuberculosis* (See Tuberculosis later in this table.)		
– *M pneumoniae*[157,194]	Azithromycin 10 mg/kg on day 1, followed by 5 mg/kg/day qd days 2–5, OR clarithromycin 15 mg/kg/day div bid for 7–14 days, OR erythromycin 40 mg/kg/day PO div qid for 14 days	*Mycoplasma* often causes self-limited infection and does not routinely require treatment (AIII). Little prospective, well-controlled data exist for treatment of documented mycoplasma pneumonia, specifically in children.[194] Doxycycline (patients >7 y) or levofloxacin. Macrolide-resistant strains have recently developed worldwide but may respond to doxycycline or levofloxacin.[195] Studies have been difficult without better diagnostic techniques, but respiratory tract PCR testing is now available to assist in early identification of possible infections.

F. LOWER RESPIRATORY TRACT INFECTIONS *(continued)*

Clinical Diagnosis	Therapy (evidence grade)	Comments
– *Paragonimus westermani*	See Chapter 9.	
– *Pneumocystis jiroveci* (formerly *carinii*)[196]; disease in immunosuppressed children and those with HIV	Severe disease: preferred regimen is TMP/SMX, 15–20 mg/kg/day of TMP IV div q8h for 3 wk (AI). Mild to moderate disease: may start with IV therapy, then after acute pneumonitis is resolving, TMP/SMX 20 mg/kg/day of TMP PO div qid for 21 days (AII). Use steroid adjunctive treatment for more severe disease (AII).	Alternatives for TMP/SMX intolerant, or clinical failure: pentamidine 3–4 mg IV qd, infused over 60–90 min (AII); TMP AND dapsone; OR primaquine AND clindamycin; OR atovaquone. Prophylaxis: TMP/SMX as 5 mg/kg/day of TMP PO, div in 2 doses, q12h, daily or 3 times/wk on consecutive days (AI); OR TMP/SMX 5 mg/kg/day of TMP PO as a single dose, qd, given 3 times/wk on consecutive days (AI); once-weekly regimens have also been successful[197]; OR dapsone 2 mg/kg (max 100 mg) PO qd, or 4 mg/kg (max 200 mg) once weekly; OR atovaquone: 30 mg/kg/day for infants 1–3 mo, 45 mg/kg/day for infants 4–24 mo, and 30 mg/kg/day for children >24 mo.
– *P aeruginosa*[198,199]	Cefepime 150 mg/kg/day IV div q8h ± tobramycin 6.0–7.5 mg/kg/day IM, IV div q8h (AII). Alternatives: meropenem 60 mg/kg/day div q8h, OR pip/tazo 240–300 mg/kg/day div q6–8h (AII) ± tobramycin (BIII).	Ciprofloxacin IV, or colistin IV for MDR strains of *Pseudomonas*[199] (See Chapter 12.)
– RSV infection (bronchiolitis, pneumonia)[200]	For immunocompromised hosts, the only FDA-approved treatment is ribavirin aerosol: 6-g vial (20 mg/mL in sterile water), by SPAG-2, over 18–20 h daily for 3–5 days, although questions remain regarding efficacy.	Treat only for severe disease, immunocompromised, severe underlying cardiopulmonary disease, as aerosol ribavirin provides only a small benefit. Airway reactivity with inhalation precludes routine use. We have not personally used inhaled ribavirin for the past several years. Palivizumab (Synagis) is not effective for treatment of an active RSV infection but cost-effective for prevention of hospitalization in high-risk patients. RSV antivirals and more potent monoclonal antibodies are currently under investigation.

Tuberculosis		
– Primary pulmonary disease[15,16,201,202]	INH 10–15 mg/kg/day (max 300 mg) PO qd for 6 mo AND rifampin 15–20 mg/kg/day (max 600 mg) PO qd for 6 mo AND PZA 30–40 mg/kg/day (max 2 g) PO qd for first 2 mo of therapy only (AII). Twice-weekly treatment, particularly with DOT, is acceptable.[15] If risk factors present for multidrug resistance, ADD ethambutol 20 mg/kg/day PO qd OR streptomycin 30 mg/kg/day IV, IM div q12h initially.	Obtain baseline LFTs. Consider monthly LFTs for at least 3 mo or as needed for symptoms. It is common to have mildly elevated liver transaminase concentrations (2–3 times normal) that do not further increase during the entire treatment interval. Children with obesity may have mild elevation when therapy is started. New recommendations on short-course (4-mo) daily therapy for children with non-severe TB may soon be made for the United States, following new World Health Organization guidelines (www.who.int/publications/i/item/9789240046764; accessed September 21, 2022). Contact TB specialist for therapy for drug-resistant TB.[201] Fluoroquinolones may play a role in treating MDR strains. Bedaquiline, in a new drug class for TB therapy, is approved for adults and children >5 y with MDR TB when used in combination therapy. Delamanid is not FDA approved as of July 2022. DOT preferred; after 2 wk of daily therapy, can change to twice-weekly dosing double dosage of INH (max 900 mg), PZA (max 2 g), and ethambutol (max 2.5 g); rifampin remains same dosage (15–20 mg/kg/day, max 600 mg) (AII). LP ± CT of head for children ≤2 y to rule out occult, concurrent CNS infection; consider testing for HIV infection (AIII). *Mycobacterium bovis* infection from unpasteurized dairy products is also called "tuberculosis" but rarely causes pulmonary disease; all strains of *M bovis* are PZA resistant. Treat 9–12 mo with INH and rifampin.

F. LOWER RESPIRATORY TRACT INFECTIONS *(continued)*

Clinical Diagnosis	Therapy (evidence grade)	Comments
– Latent TB infection[15,16,203] (skin test conversion; more recently just called "TB infection"[15] in contrast to "TB disease" for symptomatic TB infection)	Many options now INH/rifapentine: For children 2–11 y: *once-weekly* DOT for *12 wk:* INH 25 mg/kg/dose (max 900 mg), AND rifapentine: 10.0–14.0 kg: 300 mg 14.1–25.0 kg: 450 mg 25.1–32.0 kg: 600 mg 32.1–49.9 kg: 750 mg ≥50.0 kg: 900 mg (max) For children 2–11 y: INH 25 mg/kg, rounded up to nearest 50 or 100 mg (max 900 mg), AND rifapentine (See above.) Rifampin alone (all ages): 15–20 mg/kg/dose *daily* (max 600 mg) for *4 mo* INH/rifampin (all ages): INH 10–15 mg/kg/day (max 300 mg)/rifampin 15–20 mg/kg/day (max 600 mg) *daily* for *3 mo* INH 10–15 mg/kg/day (max 300 mg) PO daily for *6–9 mo (12 mo for immunocompromised patients)* (AIII); treatment with INH at 20–30 mg/kg twice weekly for *9 mo* also effective (AIII)	Obtain baseline LFTs. Consider monthly LFTs or as needed for symptoms. Stop INH/rifapentine if AST or ALT ≥5 times the ULN even in the absence of symptoms or ≥3 times the ULN in the presence of symptoms. For children <2 y: INH and rifapentine may be used, but there are less data on safety and efficacy. For exposure to known INH-resistant but rifampin-susceptible strains, use rifampin 6 mo (AIII).

– Exposed child <4 y, or immunocompromised patient (high risk for dissemination)	Prophylaxis for possible infection for 2–3 mo after last exposure with rifampin 15–20 mg/kg/dose PO qd OR INH 10–15 mg/kg PO qd; for at least 2–3 mo (AIII), with repeated skin test or interferon-γ release assay test (AIII). Also called "window prophylaxis."	Alternative regimens INH 10–15 mg/kg PO qd AND rifampin 15–20 mg/kg/dose qd (max 600 mg) for up to 3 mo. If PPD or interferon-γ release assay test remains negative at 2–3 mo and child appears well, consider stopping empiric therapy. PPD may not be reliable in immunocompromised patients. Not much data to assess reliability of interferon-γ release assays in very young infants or immunocompromised hosts, but not likely to be much better than the PPD skin test.

G. CARDIOVASCULAR INFECTIONS

Clinical Diagnosis	Therapy (evidence grade)	Comments
Bacteremia		
– Occult bacteremia/serious bacterial infection (late-onset neonatal sepsis; fever without focus), infants <1–2 mo (group B streptococcus, *Escherichia coli*, *Listeria*, pneumococcus, meningococcus)[204–209]	In general, hospitalization for late-onset neonatal sepsis in the ill-appearing infant, with cultures of blood, urine, and CSF; start ampicillin for group B streptococcus and *Listeria* at 200 mg/kg/day IV div q6h AND cefepime or ceftazidime for *E coli*/enteric bacilli; use ceftriaxone for those after the first few weeks following birth (cefotaxime no longer routinely available in the United States); higher dosages if meningitis is documented. In areas with low (<20%) ampicillin resistance in *E coli*, consider ampicillin and gentamicin (gentamicin will not cover CNS infection caused by ampicillin-resistant *E coli* when treated with ampicillin and gentamicin).	Current data document the importance of ampicillin-resistant *E coli* in bacteremia and UTI in infants <90 days.[207–209] For a nontoxic, febrile infant with good access to medical care: cultures may be obtained of blood and urine, and we are getting much closer to eliminating CSF cultures in low-risk infants. Risk scores incorporate various combinations of history (previously healthy), no skin or soft tissue infection, clinical status, urinalysis, WBC count, and procalcitonin. Infants may be discharged home without antibiotics and close follow-up if evaluation is negative (Rochester; modified Philadelphia criteria)[205–209] (BI).

G. CARDIOVASCULAR INFECTIONS *(continued)*

Clinical Diagnosis	Therapy (evidence grade)	Comments
– Occult bacteremia/serious bacterial infection (fever without focus) at age 2–3 mo to 36 mo (*Haemophilus influenzae* type b/pneumococcus in unimmunized patients; meningococcus; pneumococcus [non-vaccine strains]; increasingly *Staphylococcus aureus*)[207]	Empiric therapy: if unimmunized, febrile, mild to moderate toxic: after blood culture: ceftriaxone 50 mg/kg IM (BII). If fully immunized (*Haemophilus* and *Pneumococcus*) and nontoxic, routine *empiric* outpatient therapy for fever with antibiotics is no longer recommended, but follow closely in case of non-vaccine strain pneumococcal infection, vaccine failure, or meningococcal bacteremia (BIII).	Conjugated vaccines for *H influenzae* type b and pneumococcus have virtually eliminated occult bacteremia of infancy by these pathogens. For those who are bacteremic, oral convalescent therapy is selected by susceptibility of blood isolate, following response to IM/IV treatment, with CNS and other foci ruled out by examination ± laboratory tests ± imaging. LP is not recommended for routine evaluation of fever.[204]
– *H influenzae* type b, non-CNS infections	Ceftriaxone IM/IV OR, if BL negative, ampicillin IV, followed by oral convalescent therapy (AII)	If BL negative: amoxicillin 75–100 mg/kg/day PO div tid (AII). If positive, consider these options (but there is no data on treatment of bacteremic infection): high-dosage cefixime, ceftibuten, cefdinir PO, or levofloxacin PO (CIII).
– Meningococcus	Ceftriaxone IM/IV or penicillin G IV, followed by oral convalescent therapy (AII)	Amoxicillin 75–100 mg/kg/day PO div tid (AIII)
– Pneumococcus, non-CNS infections	Ceftriaxone IM/IV or penicillin G/ampicillin IV (if pen-S), followed by oral convalescent therapy (AII)	If pen-S or penicillin-intermediate (MIC is ≤2 or lower): amoxicillin 75–100 mg/kg/day PO div tid (AII). If pen-R (MIC is ≥4): continue ceftriaxone IM or switch to clindamycin if susceptible (CIII); linezolid or levofloxacin may also be an option (CIII).

– *S aureus*[4,6,210–213] usually associated with focal infection	MSSA: nafcillin or oxacillin/nafcillin IV 150–200 mg/kg/day div q6h ± gentamicin 6 mg/kg/day div q8h (AII). MRSA: daptomycin IV[214] 8–12 mg/kg/day q24h (BII), OR vancomycin[211] 40–60 mg/kg/day (CII) IV div q8h OR ceftaroline: 2 mo–<2 y, 24 mg/kg/day IV div q8h; ≥2 y, 36 mg/kg/day IV div q8h (max single dose 400 mg) (BIII) ± gentamicin 6 mg/kg/day div q8h ± rifampin[212] 20 mg/kg/day div q12h (AIII). Treat for 2 wk (IV + PO) from negative blood cultures unless endocarditis/endovascular thrombus is present, which may require up to 6 wk of therapy (BIII).	For persisting bacteremia caused by MRSA, consider adding gentamicin or rifampin, or changing from vancomycin (particularly for MRSA with vancomycin MIC of >2 mcg/mL) to daptomycin or ceftaroline (daptomycin will not treat pneumonia). For toxic shock syndrome, clindamycin should be added for the initial 48–72 h of therapy to decrease toxin production (linezolid may also act this way); IVIG may be added to bind circulating toxin (linezolid may also act this way); no controlled data exist for these measures. Watch for the development of metastatic foci of infection, including endocarditis. If catheter-related, remove catheter.

Endocarditis: Prospective, controlled data on therapy for endocarditis in neonates, infants, and children are quite limited, and many recommendations are extrapolated from adult studies, in which some level of evidence exists, or from other invasive bacteremia infection studies. Surgical indications: intractable heart failure; persistent infection; large mobile vegetations; peripheral embolism; and valve dehiscence, perforation, rupture, or fistula, or a large perivalvular abscess.[215–219] Consider community vs nosocomial pathogens based on recent surgeries, prior antibiotic therapy, and possible entry sites for bacteremia (skin, oropharynx and respiratory tract, GI tract). Children with congenital heart disease are more likely to have more turbulent cardiovascular blood flow, which increases risk for endovascular infection. Similar guidelines have been published for both the United States and the European Union.[216,217] Catheter-placed bovine jugular valves seem to increase risk of infection.[218,219] Immunocompromised hosts may become bacteremic with a wide range of bacteria, fungi, and mycobacteria.

G. CARDIOVASCULAR INFECTIONS *(continued)*

Clinical Diagnosis	Therapy (evidence grade)	Comments
– **Native valve**[215–217]		
– Empiric therapy for presumed endocarditis (viridans streptococci, *S aureus*, HACEK group)	Ceftriaxone IV 100 mg/kg q24h AND gentamicin IV, IM 6 mg/kg/day div q8h (AII). For more acute, severe infection, ADD vancomycin 40–60 mg/kg/day IV div q8h to cover *S aureus* (AIII) (insufficient data to recommend ceftaroline for endocarditis).	Combination (ceftriaxone + gentamicin) provides bactericidal activity against most strains of viridans streptococci, the most common pathogens in infective endocarditis. Cefepime is recommended for adults,[215] but resistance data in enteric bacilli in children suggest that ceftriaxone remains a reasonable choice. Ampicillin/sulbactam adds extended anaerobic activity that is not likely to be needed. May administer gentamicin with a qd regimen (CIII). For beta-lactam allergy, use vancomycin 45 mg/kg/day IV div q8h AND gentamicin 6 mg/kg/day IV div q8h.
– Culture-negative native valve endocarditis: treat 4–6 wk (please obtain advice from an ID specialist for an appropriate regimen that is based on likely pathogens).[215,216]		
– Viridans streptococci: follow echocardiogram for resolution of vegetation (BIII); for beta-lactam allergy: vancomycin.		
Fully susceptible to penicillin	Ceftriaxone 50 mg/kg IV, IM q24h for 4 wk OR penicillin G 200,000 U/kg/day IV div q4–6h for 4 wk (BII); OR penicillin G or ceftriaxone AND gentamicin 6 mg/kg/day IM, IV div q8h (AII) for 14 days for adults (4 wk for children per AHA guidelines due to lack of data in children)	AHA recommends higher dosage of ceftriaxone like that of penicillin non-susceptible strains, but for fully susceptible strains, standard-dose ceftriaxone provides the necessary pharmacodynamic exposure.
Relatively resistant to penicillin	Penicillin G 300,000 U/kg/day IV div q4–6h for 4 wk, or ceftriaxone 100 mg/kg IV q24h for 4 wk; AND gentamicin 6 mg/kg/day IM, IV div q8h for the first 2 wk (AIII)	Gentamicin is used for the first 2 wk for a total of 4 wk of therapy for relatively resistant strains. Vancomycin-containing regimens should use at least a 4-wk treatment course, with gentamicin used for the entire course.

– Enterococcus (dosages for native or prosthetic valve infections)		
Ampicillin-susceptible (gentamicin-S)	Ampicillin 300 mg/kg/day IV, IM div q6h or penicillin G 300,000 U/kg/day IV div q4–6h; AND gentamicin 6 mg/kg/day IV div q8h; for 4–6 wk (AII)	Combined treatment with cell wall active antibiotic plus aminoglycoside used to achieve bactericidal activity. Children are not as likely to develop renal toxicity from gentamicin as adults. For beta-lactam allergy: vancomycin. Little data exist in children for daptomycin or linezolid. For gentamicin-resistant strains, use streptomycin or other aminoglycoside if susceptible.
Ampicillin-resistant (gentamicin-S)	Vancomycin 40 mg/kg/day IV div q8h AND gentamicin 6 mg/kg/day IV div q8h; for 6 wk (AIII)	
Vancomycin-resistant (gentamicin-S)	Daptomycin IV if also ampicillin resistant (dose is age dependent; see Chapter 18 for doses) ± gentamicin 6 mg/kg/day IV div q8h; for 4–6 wk (AIII).	
– Staphylococci: *S aureus,* including CA-MRSA; *S epidermidis*[6,211] Consider continuing therapy at end of 6 wk if vegetations persist on echocardiogram. Consider septic thrombophlebitis: the risk of persisting organisms is not defined in deep venous thromboses that may be "seeded" as a result of bacteremia.	MSSA or MSSE: nafcillin or oxacillin/nafcillin 150–200 mg/kg/day IV div q6h for 4–6 wk AND gentamicin 6 mg/kg/day div q8h for first 14 days. CA-MRSA or MRSE: daptomycin IV[214] 8–12 mg/kg/day q24h (BII), OR vancomycin 40–60 mg/kg/day IV div q8h AND gentamicin for 6 wk; consider for slow response, ADD rifampin 20 mg/kg/day IV div q8–12h. Insufficient data to recommend ceftaroline routinely for MRSA endocarditis.	Surgery may be necessary in acute phase; avoid first-generation cephalosporins (conflicting data on efficacy). AHA suggests gentamicin for only the first 3–5 days for MSSA or MSSE and optional gentamicin for MRSA. Daptomycin dose is age dependent (see Chapter 18 for doses).

G. CARDIOVASCULAR INFECTIONS *(continued)*

Clinical Diagnosis	Therapy (evidence grade)	Comments
– Pneumococcus, gonococcus, group A streptococcus	Penicillin G 200,000 U/kg/day IV div q4–6h for 4 wk (BII); alternatives: ceftriaxone or vancomycin	For gonococcal endocarditis: ceftriaxone alone, 1–2 g IV q24h for >4 wk.[57] For penicillin non-susceptible strains of pneumococcus, consult with ID specialist but should be able to use high-dosage penicillin G 300,000 U/kg/day IV div q4–6h or high-dosage ceftriaxone 100 mg/kg IV q12h or q24h for 4 wk, if supported by pharmacodynamics (eg, the time that penicillin or ceftriaxone is above the MIC of the organism, during the dosing interval).
– HACEK (*Haemophilus, Aggregatibacter* [formerly *Actinobacillus*], *Cardiobacterium, Eikenella, Kingella* spp)	Usually susceptible to ceftriaxone 100 mg/kg IV q24h for 4 wk (BIII)	Some organisms will be ampicillin susceptible. Usually do not require the addition of gentamicin.
– Enteric gram-negative bacilli	Antibiotics specific to pathogen (usually ceftriaxone plus gentamicin); duration at least 6 wk (AIII)	For ESBL organisms, carbapenems or beta-lactam/BL inhibitor combinations, PLUS gentamicin, should be effective. See Chapter 12.
– *Pseudomonas aeruginosa*	Antibiotic specific to susceptibility: cefepime or meropenem PLUS tobramycin	Both cefepime and meropenem are more active against *Pseudomonas* and less likely to allow BL-resistant pathogens to emerge than ceftazidime.
– **Prosthetic valve/ material**[215,218,219]	Follow echocardiogram for resolution of vegetation. For beta-lactam allergy: vancomycin.	
– Viridans streptococci		
Fully susceptible to penicillin	Ceftriaxone 100 mg/kg IV, IM q24h for 6 wk OR penicillin G 300,000 U/kg/day IV div q4–6h for 6 wk (AII); OR penicillin G or ceftriaxone AND gentamicin 6 mg/kg/day IM, IV div q8h for first 2 wk of 6-wk course (AII)	Gentamicin is optional for the first 2 wk for a total of 6 wk of therapy for prosthetic valve/material endocarditis.

Relatively resistant to penicillin	Penicillin G 300,000 U/kg/day IV div q4–6h for 6 wk, or ceftriaxone 100 mg/kg IV q24h for 6 wk; AND gentamicin 6 mg/kg/day IM, IV div q8h for 6 wk (AIII)	Obtain the MIC of the strep spp to the antibiotic used for treatment; based on expected or measured serum antibiotic concentrations, assess pharmacodynamics (ability to achieve the desired time that penicillin [or ceftriaxone] is above the MIC of the organism, during the dosing supported by the interval). See Chapter 11. Gentamicin is used for all 6 wk of therapy for prosthetic valve/material endocarditis caused by relatively resistant strains.
– Enterococcus (See dosages earlier in this table under Native Valve.) Treatment course is at least 6 wk, particularly if vancomycin is used.[215,219]		
– Staphylococci: *S aureus*, including CA-MRSA; *S epidermidis*[6,215] Consider continuing therapy at end of 6 wk if vegetations persist on echocardiogram.	MSSA or MSSE: nafcillin or oxacillin/nafcillin 150–200 mg/kg/day IV div q6h for ≥6 wk AND gentamicin 6 mg/kg/day div q8h for first 14 days. CA-MRSA or MRSE: daptomycin IV[214] 8–12 mg/kg/day q24h (BII), OR vancomycin 40–60 mg/kg/day IV div q8h AND gentamicin for ≥6 wk; ADD rifampin 20 mg/kg/day IV div q8–12h.	Daptomycin dose is age and weight dependent (see Chapter 18 for doses).
– *Candida*[83,215,216]	AmB lipid formulation, 3–5 mg/kg q24h with/without flucytosine 100 mg/kg/day div q6h (there is more experience with AmB preparations [no comparative trials against echinocandins]), OR caspofungin 70 mg/m^2 load on day 1, then 50 mg/m^2/day or micafungin 2–4 mg/kg/day (BIII). Do not use fluconazole as initial therapy because of inferior fungistatic effect.	Poor prognosis; please obtain advice from an ID specialist. Surgery may be required to resect infected valve. Long-term suppressive therapy with fluconazole.
– Culture-negative prosthetic valve endocarditis: treat at least 6 wk.		

G. CARDIOVASCULAR INFECTIONS *(continued)*

Clinical Diagnosis	Therapy (evidence grade)	Comments
Endocarditis antibiotic prophylaxis[216,217,220]: endocarditis is rarely caused by dental/GI procedures, and antibiotic prophylaxis for procedures prevents an exceedingly small proportion of endocarditis cases; therefore, the risks of antibiotic prophylaxis outweigh the benefits. Highest-risk conditions currently recommended for prophylaxis for children undergoing procedures: (1) prosthetic heart valve (or prosthetic material used to repair a valve); (2) previous endocarditis; (3) cyanotic congenital heart disease that is unrepaired (or palliatively repaired with shunts and conduits); (4) congenital heart disease that is repaired but with defects at the site of repair adjacent to prosthetic material; (5) completely repaired congenital heart disease by using prosthetic material, for the first 6 mo after repair; or (6) cardiac transplant patients with valvulopathy. Routine prophylaxis is no longer required for children with native valve abnormalities. Assessment of recent prophylaxis guidelines does not document an increase in endocarditis.[221]		
– In highest-risk patients: dental procedures that involve manipulation of the gingival or periodontal region of teeth	Amoxicillin 50 mg/kg PO 60 min before procedure OR ampicillin or ceftriaxone or cefazolin, all at 50 mg/kg IM/IV 30–60 min before procedure	If penicillin allergy: clindamycin 20 mg/kg PO (60 min before) or IV (30 min before); OR azithromycin 15 mg/kg or clarithromycin 15 mg/kg, 60 min before (little data to support alternative regimens)
– Genitourinary and GI procedures	None	No longer recommended
Lemierre syndrome (*Fusobacterium necrophorum* primarily, new reports with MRSA)[115–119] (pharyngitis with internal jugular vein septic thrombosis, postanginal sepsis, necrobacillosis)	Empiric: meropenem 60 mg/kg/day div q8h (or 120 mg/kg/day div q8h for CNS metastatic foci) (AIII) OR ceftriaxone 100 mg/kg/day q24h AND metronidazole 40 mg/kg/day div q8h or clindamycin 40 mg/kg/day div q6h (BIII). ADD empiric vancomycin if MRSA suspected if clindamycin is not in the treatment regimen.	Anecdotal reports suggest that metronidazole may be effective for apparent failures with other agents. Often requires anticoagulation. Metastatic and recurrent abscesses often develop while on active, appropriate therapy, requiring multiple debridements and prolonged antibiotic therapy. Treat until CRP and ESR are normal (AIII).
Purulent pericarditis		
– Empiric (acute, bacterial: *S aureus* [including MRSA], group A streptococcus, pneumococcus, meningococcus; in unimmunized children, *H influenzae* type b)[222,223]	Ceftaroline: 2–<6 mo, 30 mg/kg/day IV div q8h; ≥6 mo, 45 mg/kg/day IV div q8h (max single dose 600 mg) (BIII), OR vancomycin 40 mg/kg/day IV div q8h and ceftriaxone 50–75 mg/kg/day q24h (AIII)	For presumed staph infection, ADD gentamicin (AIII). Increasingly uncommon with immunization against pneumococcus and *H influenzae* type b.[223] Pericardiocentesis is essential to establish diagnosis. Surgical drainage of pus with pericardial window or pericardiectomy is important to prevent tamponade.

– *S aureus*	For MSSA: oxacillin/nafcillin 150–200 mg/kg/day IV div q6h OR cefazolin 100 mg/kg/day IV div q8h. Treat for 2–3 wk after drainage (BIII). For CA-MRSA: continue ceftaroline or vancomycin. Treat for 3–4 wk after drainage (BIII).	Continue therapy with gentamicin; consider use of rifampin in severe cases due to tissue penetration characteristics.
– *H influenzae* type b in unimmunized children	Ceftriaxone 50 mg/kg/day q24h for 10–14 days (AIII)	Ampicillin for BL-negative strains
– Pneumococcus, meningococcus, group A streptococcus	Penicillin G 200,000 U/kg/day IV, IM div q6h for 10–14 days OR ceftriaxone 50 mg/kg qd for 10–14 days (AIII)	Ceftriaxone for penicillin non-susceptible pneumococci
– Coliform bacilli	Ceftriaxone 50–75 mg/kg/day q24h for ≥3 wk (AIII)	Alternative drugs depending on susceptibilities; for *Enterobacter, Serratia,* or *Citrobacter,* use cefepime or meropenem. For ESBL *E coli* or *Klebsiella,* use a carbapenem.
– Tuberculous[16]	INH 10–15 mg/kg/day (max 300 mg) PO, IV qd, for 6 mo AND rifampin 10–20 mg/kg/day (max 600 mg) PO qd, IV for 6 mo. ADD PZA 20–40 mg/kg/day PO qd for first 2 mo of therapy; if suspected multidrug resistance, also add ethambutol 20 mg/kg/day PO qd (AIII).	Current guidelines do not suggest a benefit from routine use of corticosteroids. However, for those at highest risk for restrictive pericarditis, steroid continues to be recommended. For children: prednisone 2 mg/kg/day for 4 wk, then 0.5 mg/kg/day for 4 wk, then 0.25 mg/kg/day for 2 wk, then 0.1 mg/kg/day for 1 wk.

H. GASTROINTESTINAL INFECTIONS (See Chapter 9 for parasitic infections.)

Clinical Diagnosis	Therapy (evidence grade)	Comments
Diarrhea/Gastroenteritis		
Note on *Escherichia coli* and diarrheal disease: Antibiotic susceptibility of *E coli* varies considerably from region to region. For mild to moderate disease, TMP/SMX may be started as initial therapy, but for more severe disease and for locations with rates of TMP/SMX resistance >10%–20%, azithromycin, an oral third-generation cephalosporin (eg, cefixime, cefdinir, ceftibuten), or ciprofloxacin should be used (AIII). Diagnostic testing by traditional cultures with antibiotic susceptibility testing is recommended for significant disease (AIII). New molecular tests (particularly multiplex PCR tests) are commercially available and quite helpful to diagnose specific pathogens but do not provide susceptibility information.		
– Empiric therapy for community-associated diarrhea in the United States (*E coli* [STEC, including O157:H7 strains, and ETEC], *Salmonella, Campylobacter,* and *Shigella* predominate; *Yersinia* and parasites cause <5%; viral pathogens are far more common, especially for children <3 y.)[224,225]	Azithromycin 10 mg/kg qd for 3 days (BII); OR ciprofloxacin 30 mg/kg/day PO div bid for 3 days; OR cefixime 8 mg/kg/day PO qd (BII). Current recommendation is to avoid treatment of Shiga toxin–containing (STEC O157:H7) strains.[224]	Alternatives: third-generation cephalosporins (eg, ceftriaxone); have been shown effective in uncomplicated *Salmonella* Typhi infections. Rifaximin is a nonabsorbable rifamycin not to be used in cases of invasive bacterial enteritis: 600 mg/day div tid for 3 days (for nonfebrile, *non-bloody* diarrhea in children ≥12 y). Retrospective data exist for treatment of O157:H7 strains to support either withholding treatment or administering it (including retrospective data on treatment with azithromycin). Antitoxins and immune globulins are under investigation.[226–229]

– Travelers diarrhea: empiric therapy (*E coli, Campylobacter, Salmonella,* and *Shigella,* plus many other pathogens, including protozoa)[230–236] The CDC provides updated advice both pre-travel and post-travel at wwwnc.cdc.gov/travel/page/clinician-information-center (reviewed March 7, 2022; accessed September 21, 2022). See 2017 guidelines from International Society of Travel Medicine: https://academic.oup.com/jtm/article/24/suppl_1/S63/3782742 (accessed September 21, 2022).[233]	For mild diarrhea, treatment is not recommended.[233] Azithromycin 10 mg/kg qd for 1–3 days (AII); OR rifaximin 200 mg PO tid for 3 days (age ≥12 y) (BIII); OR ciprofloxacin 30 mg/kg/day PO div bid for 3 days (BII).	Susceptibility patterns of *E coli, Campylobacter, Salmonella,* and *Shigella* vary widely by country, with increasing resistance to commonly used antibiotics; check the CDC and country-specific data for departing or returning travelers. Azithromycin preferable to ciprofloxacin for travelers to Southeast Asia given high prevalence of quinolone-resistant *Campylobacter.* Rifaximin, not to be used in cases of invasive bacterial enteritis. Interestingly, for adults who travel and take antibiotics (mostly fluoroquinolones), colonization with ESBL-positive *E coli* is more frequent on return home.[237] Adjunctive therapy with loperamide (antimotility) is not recommended for children <2 y and should be used only in nonfebrile, non-bloody diarrhea.[231,235,238] May shorten symptomatic illness by about 24 h.
– Travelers diarrhea: prophylaxis[230,231,233]	Prophylaxis: early self-treatment with agents listed previously is preferred over long-term prophylaxis, but may use prophylaxis for a short-term (<14 days) visit to very high-risk region: rifaximin (for children ≥12 y), azithromycin (BIII). Fluoroquinolones should not be used for prevention, due to potential cartilage toxicity.	
– *Aeromonas hydrophila*[239]	Ciprofloxacin 30 mg/kg/day PO div bid for 5 days OR cefixime 8 mg/kg/day PO qd (BIII)	Not all strains produce enterotoxins and diarrhea; role in diarrhea questioned.[239] Resistance to TMP/SMX about 10%–15%. Choose narrowest-spectrum agent based on in vitro susceptibilities.
– *Campylobacter jejuni*[240,241]	Azithromycin 10 mg/kg/day for 3 days (BII) or erythromycin 40 mg/kg/day PO div qid for 5 days (BII)	Alternatives: doxycycline or ciprofloxacin (high rate of fluoroquinolone resistance in Thailand, India, and now the United States). Single-dose azithromycin (1 g, once) is effective in adults.

H. GASTROINTESTINAL INFECTIONS (*continued*) (See Chapter 9 for parasitic infections.)

Clinical Diagnosis	Therapy (evidence grade)	Comments
– Cholera[242,243]	Azithromycin 20 mg/kg once; OR erythromycin 50 mg/kg/day PO div qid for 3 days; OR doxycycline 4.4 mg/kg/day (max 200 mg/day) PO div bid, for all ages	Ciprofloxacin or TMP/SMX (if susceptible)
– *Clostridioides* (formerly *Clostridium*) *difficile* (antibiotic-associated colitis)[244–248]	Treatment stratified by severity and recurrence. First episode: Mild to moderate illness: metronidazole 30 mg/kg/day PO div qid. Moderate to severe illness: vancomycin 40 mg/kg/day PO div qid for 7 days. Severe and complicated/systemic: vancomycin PO AND metronidazole IV; consider vancomycin enema (500 mg/100 mL physiologic [normal] saline) soln q8h until improvement).[244,245] For relapsing *C difficile* enteritis, consider pulse therapy (1 wk on/1 wk off for 3–4 cycles) or prolonged tapering therapy.	Attempt to stop antibiotics that may have represented the cause of *C difficile* infection. Vancomycin is more effective for severe infection.[244,245] Fidaxomicin approved for adults and children down to 6 mo of age.[247] Many infants and children may have asymptomatic colonization with *C difficile*.[245] Higher risk for relapse in children with multiple comorbidities. Stool transplant for failure of medical therapy in recurrent enteritis.
– *E coli*		
Enterotoxigenic (etiology of most travelers diarrhea)[231–234]	Azithromycin 10 mg/kg qd for 3 days (AII); OR ciprofloxacin 30 mg/kg/day PO div bid for 3 days (BII); OR cefixime 8 mg/kg/day PO qd for 3 days (CIII)	Most illnesses are brief and self-limited and may not require treatment. Alternatives: rifaximin 600 mg/day div tid for 3 days (for nonfebrile, non-bloody diarrhea in children ≥12 y, as rifaximin is not absorbed systemically); OR TMP/SMX. Resistance increasing worldwide; check country-specific rates.

Enterohemorrhagic (O157:H7; STEC, etiology of HUS)[224,226–229]	Current recommendations are to avoid treatment of STEC O157:H7 strains.[224] Retrospective data exist for treatment of O157:H7 strains to support either withholding treatment or administering it (including retrospective data on treatment with azithromycin).[226–229]	Animal model data suggest that some antibiotics (rifamycins) are less likely to increase toxin production than fluoroquinolones.[249] Injury to colonic mucosa may lead to invasive bacterial colitis that does require antimicrobial therapy.
– Gastritis, peptic ulcer disease (*Helicobacter pylori*)[250–252]	Triple-agent therapy in areas of low clarithromycin resistance: clarithromycin 7.5 mg/kg/dose 2–3 times each day, AND amoxicillin 40 mg/kg/dose (max 1 g) PO bid AND omeprazole 0.5 mg/kg/dose PO bid 14 days (BII), OR quadruple therapy that includes metronidazole (15 mg/kg/day div bid) added to the regimen described previously[250,252]	Resistance to clarithromycin is as high as 20% in some regions.[250,253] Current approach for empiric therapy if clarithromycin resistance may be present: high-dose triple therapy is recommended with proton pump inhibitor, amoxicillin, and metronidazole for 14 days ± bismuth to create quadruple therapy.[250] Metronidazole resistance reported.[250] Newer, fluoroquinolone-based treatment combinations used in adults with clarithromycin resistance.[251]
– Giardiasis (see Chapter 9) (*Giardia intestinalis,* formerly *lamblia*)[254]	Tinidazole[255] (for age ≥3 y) 50 mg/kg/day (max 2 g) for 1 day (BII); OR nitazoxanide PO (take with food), age 12–47 mo, 100 mg/dose bid for 3 days; age 4–11 y, 200 mg/dose bid for 3 days; age ≥12 y, 1 tab (500 mg) bid for 3 days (BII).	If therapy is unsuccessful, another course of the same agent is usually curative. Alternatives: metronidazole 20–30 mg/kg/day PO div tid for 7–10 days (BII); OR paromomycin OR albendazole (CII), OR mebendazole OR furazolidone. Prolonged or combination drug courses may be needed for immunocompromised conditions (eg, hypogammaglobulinemia). Treatment of asymptomatic carriers not usually recommended.
– Salmonellosis[256,257] (See Travelers diarrhea: prophylaxis earlier in this section of the table, and Chapter 9.)		

H. GASTROINTESTINAL INFECTIONS *(continued)* (See Chapter 9 for parasitic infections.)

Clinical Diagnosis	Therapy (evidence grade)	Comments
Non-typhoid strains[256,257]	Usually none for self-limited diarrhea in immunocompetent child (eg, diarrhea is often much improved by the time culture results are available). Treat children with persisting symptomatic infection and all infants <3 mo (greater risk for bacteremia): azithromycin 10 mg/kg PO qd for 3 days (AII); OR ceftriaxone 75 mg/kg/day IV, IM q24h for 5 days (AII); OR cefixime 20–30 mg/kg/day PO for 5–7 days (BII); OR for susceptible strains: TMP/SMX 8 mg/kg/day of TMP PO div bid for 14 days (AI).	Alternatives: ciprofloxacin 30 mg/kg/day PO div bid for 5 days (AI). Carriage of strains may be prolonged in treated children. For bacteremic infection, ceftriaxone IM/IV may be initially used until secondary sites of infection (bone/joint, liver/spleen, CNS) are ruled out, for a total of 7–10 days.[257]
Typhoid fever[258–261]	Azithromycin 20 mg/kg qd for 5 days (AII); OR ceftriaxone 75 mg/kg/day IV, IM q24h for 5 days (AII); OR cefixime 20–30 mg/kg/day PO div q12h for 14 days (BII); OR for susceptible strains: ampicillin OR TMP/SMX 8 mg/kg/day of TMP PO div bid for 14 days (AI)	Increasing cephalosporin resistance.[257,262] For newly emergent MDR strains, may require prolonged IV therapy. Amoxicillin does not achieve high colonic intraluminal concentrations or high intracellular concentrations. Alternative if susceptible: ciprofloxacin 30 mg/kg/day PO div bid for 5–7 days (AI).[260] Longer treatment courses for focal invasive disease (eg, osteomyelitis).
– Shigellosis[234,263–265]	Mild episodes do not require treatment. Azithromycin 10 mg/kg/day PO for 3 days (AII); OR ciprofloxacin 30 mg/kg/day PO div bid for 3–5 days (BII); OR cefixime[234] 8 mg/kg/day PO qd for 5 days (AII).	Alternatives for susceptible strains: TMP/SMX 8 mg/kg/day of TMP PO div bid for 5 days; OR ampicillin (*not* amoxicillin). Ceftriaxone 50 mg/kg/day IM, IV if parenteral therapy necessary, for 2–5 days. Avoid antiperistaltic drugs. Treatment for the improving child is not usually necessary to hasten recovery, but some experts would treat to decrease communicability.

– *Yersinia enterocolitica*[266–268]	Antimicrobial therapy probably not of value for mild disease in normal hosts. TMP/SMX PO, IV; OR ciprofloxacin PO, IV (BIII). Parenteral therapy for more severe infection: ceftriaxone plus gentamicin.	High rates of resistance to ampicillin. May mimic appendicitis in older children. Limited clinical data exist on oral therapy.
Intra-abdominal infection (abscess, peritonitis secondary to bowel/appendix contents)		
– Appendicitis, bowel-associated (enteric gram-negative bacilli, *Bacteroides* spp, *Enterococcus* spp, *Pseudomonas* spp)[269–274]	Source control is critical to curing this infection. Newer data suggest that stratification of cases is important to assess the effect of surgical and medical therapy on outcomes, and using just a one-size-fits-all antibiotic recommendation may not be the best approach.[269–271,275] Meropenem 60 mg/kg/day IV div q8h or imipenem 60 mg/kg/day IV div q6h; OR pip/tazo 240 mg/kg/day pip component div q6h; for 4–5 days for patients with adequate source control,[273] ≥7–10 days if suspicion of persisting intra-abdominal abscess (AII). *Pseudomonas* is found consistently in up to 30% of children,[270,273,276] providing evidence to document the need for empiric use of an antipseudomonal drug (preferably one with anaerobic activity), such as a carbapenem or pip/tazo, *unless the surgery was highly effective at drainage/source control* (gentamicin is not active in an abscess), which may explain successful outcomes in retrospective studies that did not include antipseudomonal coverage.[275,277,278]	Many other regimens may be effective. Because retrospective data are published from different centers, be aware that the patient populations, extent of disease, and surgical approach to treatment are not standardized across hospitals, so antibiotic(s) that work in institution A may not be as effective in institution B.[270,271] Options include ampicillin 150 mg/kg/day div q8h AND gentamicin 6.0–7.5 mg/kg/day IV, IM div q8h AND metronidazole 40 mg/kg/day IV div q8h; OR ceftriaxone 50 mg/kg q24h AND metronidazole 40 mg/kg/day IV div q8h. Data support IV outpatient therapy or oral step-down therapy[274,276,279] when clinically improved, particularly when oral therapy can be focused on the most prominent, invasive cultured pathogens. Publications on outcomes of antibiotic therapy regimens (IV or PO) without culture data cannot be accurately interpreted.

H. GASTROINTESTINAL INFECTIONS *(continued)* (See Chapter 9 for parasitic infections.)

Clinical Diagnosis	Therapy (evidence grade)	Comments
– Tuberculosis, abdominal (*Mycobacterium bovis,* from unpasteurized dairy products in the United States,[15,16,280,281] and, in parts of the world, as a complication of systemic TB caused by *Mycobacterium tuberculosis*)[282]	INH 10–15 mg/kg/day (max 300 mg) PO qd for 6–9 mo AND rifampin 10–20 mg/kg/day (max 600 mg) PO qd for 6–9 mo (AII). Some experts recommend routine use of ethambutol in the empiric regimen. *M bovis* is resistant to PZA. If risk factors are present for multidrug resistance (eg, poor adherence to previous therapy), ADD ethambutol 20 mg/kg/day PO qd OR a fluoroquinolone (moxifloxacin or levofloxacin).	Corticosteroids have been routinely used as adjunctive therapy to decrease morbidity from inflammation.[282,283] DOT preferred; after 2+ wk of daily therapy, can change to twice-weekly dosing double dosage of INH (max 900 mg); rifampin remains same dosage (10–20 mg/kg/day, max 600 mg) (AII). LP ± CT of head for children ≤2 y with active disease to rule out occult, concurrent CNS infection (AIII). No published prospective comparative data on a 6-mo vs 9-mo treatment course in children.
Perirectal abscess (*Bacteroides* spp, other anaerobes, enteric bacilli, and *Staphylococcus aureus* predominate.)[284]	Clindamycin 30–40 mg/kg/day IV div q8h AND ceftriaxone or gentamicin (BIII)	Surgical drainage alone may be curative. Obtaining cultures and susceptibilities is increasingly important with rising resistance to cephalosporins in community *E coli* isolates. May represent inflammatory bowel disease.
Peritonitis		
– Peritoneal dialysis indwelling catheter infection (staphylococci; enteric gram-negative bacilli; yeast)[285,286]	Antibiotic added to dialysate in concentrations approximating those attained in serum for systemic disease (eg, 4 mcg/mL for gentamicin, 25 mcg/mL for vancomycin, 125 mcg/mL for cefazolin, 25 mcg/mL for ciprofloxacin) after a larger loading dose (AII)[286]	Selection of antibiotic based on organism isolated from peritoneal fluid; systemic antibiotics if there is accompanying bacteremia/fungemia
– Primary (pneumococcus or group A streptococcus)[287]	Ceftriaxone 50 mg/kg/day q24h; if pen-S, then penicillin G 150,000 U/kg/day IV div q6h; for 7–10 days (AII)	Other antibiotics according to culture and susceptibility tests. Spontaneous pneumococcal peritonitis now infrequent in PCV13-immunized children.

I. GENITAL AND SEXUALLY TRANSMITTED INFECTIONS

Clinical Diagnosis	Therapy (evidence grade)	Comments
Consider testing for HIV and other STIs in a child with one documented STI; consider sexual abuse in prepubertal children. The most recent CDC STI treatment guidelines (2021)[57] are posted online at www.cdc.gov/std/treatment-guidelines/STI-Guidelines-2021.pdf (accessed September 21, 2022).		
Chancroid (*Haemophilus ducreyi*)[57]	Azithromycin 1 g PO as single dose OR ceftriaxone 250 mg IM as single dose	Alternative: erythromycin 1.5 g/day PO div tid for 7 days; OR ciprofloxacin 1,000 mg PO qd, div bid for 3 days
Chlamydia trachomatis (cervicitis, urethritis)[57]	Doxycycline (patients >7 y) 4.4 mg/kg/day (max 200 mg/day) PO div bid for 7 days; OR azithromycin 20 mg/kg (max 1 g) PO for 1 dose	Alternatives: erythromycin 2 g/day PO div qid for 7 days; OR levofloxacin 500 mg PO q24h for 7 days
Epididymitis (associated with positive urine cultures and STIs)[57,288]	Ceftriaxone 50 mg/kg/day q24h for 7–10 days AND (for older children) doxycycline 200 mg/day div bid for 10 days	Microbiology not well studied in children; in infants, also associated with urogenital tract anomalies. Postviral inflammation may be one etiology of epididymitis in boys.[288] Treat infants for *Staphylococcus aureus* and *Escherichia coli;* may resolve spontaneously; in STI, treat for *Chlamydia* and gonococcus.
Gonorrhea[56,57,289,290]	Antibiotic resistance is an ongoing problem, with new data suggesting the emergence of global azithromycin resistance.[56,289,290]	
– Newborns	See Chapter 2.	

I. GENITAL AND SEXUALLY TRANSMITTED INFECTIONS *(continued)*

Clinical Diagnosis	Therapy (evidence grade)	Comments
– Genital infections (uncomplicated vulvovaginitis, cervicitis, urethritis, or proctitis) and pharyngitis[56,57,289,290]	2021 CDC guidelines for uncomplicated GC[56]: ceftriaxone 25–50 mg/kg IV/IM in a single dose, not to exceed 250 mg in children ≤45 kg and not to exceed 500 mg in those >45 kg. For adults, the CDC no longer recommends azithromycin (1 g PO for 1 dose), although for most adolescents, azithromycin should still be effective. If azithromycin is not prescribed, then doxycycline 200 mg/day div q12h for 7 days should be used for possible coinfection with chlamydia.	Increased dose of ceftriaxone to reflect small decreases in documented in vitro susceptibility for GC; azithromycin no longer recommended, with 4% of strains overall with resistance, but highest resistance rates found in isolates from MSM. If ceftriaxone is not available, give gentamicin 240 mg IM as a single dose plus azithromycin 2 g PO as a single dose OR cefixime 800 mg PO as a single dose.[56] Fluoroquinolones are not recommended due to resistance.
– Conjunctivitis[57]	Ceftriaxone 1g IM for 1 dose	Lavage the eye with saline.
– Disseminated gonococcal infection[56,57]	Ceftriaxone 50 mg/kg/day IM, IV q24h (max 1 g) AND azithromycin 1 g PO for 1 dose; total course for 7 days	No studies in children: increase dosage for meningitis.
Granuloma inguinale (donovanosis; *Klebsiella* [formerly *Calymmatobacterium*] *granulomatis*)[57]	Azithromycin 1 g PO once weekly or 500 mg qd for at least 3 wk and until all lesions have completely healed	Primarily in tropical regions of India, Pacific, and Africa. Options: doxycycline 4.4 mg/kg/day div bid (max 200 mg/day) PO for at least 3 wk OR ciprofloxacin 750 mg PO bid for at least 3 wk, OR erythromycin base 500 mg PO qid for at least 3 wk OR TMP/SMX 1 double-strength (160-mg/800-mg) tab PO bid for at least 3 wk; all regimens continue until all lesions have completely healed.

Herpes simplex virus, genital infection[57,291,292]	Acyclovir 20 mg/kg/dose (max 400 mg) PO tid for 7–10 days (first episode) (AI); OR valacyclovir 20 mg/kg/dose (directions for extemporaneous suspension on package label), max 1 g PO bid for 7–10 days (first episode) (AI); OR famciclovir 250 mg PO tid for 7–10 days (AI); for more severe infection: acyclovir 15 mg/kg/day IV div q8h as 1-h infusion for 7–10 days (AII)	For recurrent episodes: treat with acyclovir PO, valacyclovir PO, or famciclovir PO, immediately when symptoms begin, for 5 days. For suppression: acyclovir 20 mg/kg/dose (max 400 mg) PO bid; OR valacyclovir 20 mg/kg/dose PO qd (max 500 mg to start, or 1 g for difficult to suppress). Prophylaxis is recommended by ACOG in pregnant women.[292]
Lymphogranuloma venereum (*C trachomatis*)[57]	Doxycycline 4.4 mg/kg/day (max 200 mg/day) PO (patients >7 y) div bid for 21 days	Alternatives: erythromycin 2 g/day PO div qid for 21 days; OR azithromycin 1 g PO once weekly for 3 wk
Pelvic inflammatory disease (*Chlamydia* or gonococcus, plus anaerobes)[57,293]	Cefoxitin 2 g IV q6h; AND doxycycline 200 mg/day PO or IV div bid; OR cefotetan 2 g IV q12h AND doxycycline 100 mg PO or IV q12h, OR clindamycin 900 mg IV q8h AND gentamicin 1.5 mg/kg IV, IM q8h until clinical improvement for 24 h, followed by doxycycline 200 mg/day PO div bid (AND clindamycin 1,800 mg/day PO div qid for tubo-ovarian abscess) to complete 14 days of therapy	Optional regimen: ceftriaxone 250 mg IM for 1 dose AND doxycycline 200 mg/day PO div bid; WITH/WITHOUT metronidazole 1 g/day PO div bid; for 14 days
Syphilis[57,294] (Test for HIV.)	Penicillin G regimens are preferred.[57]	
– Congenital	See Chapter 2.	
– Neurosyphilis (positive CSF VDRL or CSF pleocytosis with serologic diagnosis of syphilis)	Penicillin G crystalline 200–300,000 U/kg/day (max 24 million U/day) div q6h for 10–14 days (AIII)	For adults: penicillin G procaine 2.4 million U IM daily PLUS probenecid 500 mg PO qid, for 10 to 14 days OR ceftriaxone 2 g IV daily for 10 to 14 days

I. GENITAL AND SEXUALLY TRANSMITTED INFECTIONS *(continued)*

Clinical Diagnosis	Therapy (evidence grade)	Comments
– Primary, secondary	Penicillin G benzathine 50,000 U/kg (max 2.4 million U) IM as a single dose (AIII); do not use benzathine-procaine penicillin mixtures.	Follow-up serologic tests at 6, 12, and 24 mo; 15% may remain seropositive despite adequate treatment. Alternatives if penicillin-allergic: doxycycline (patients >7 y) 4.4 mg/kg/day (max 200 mg) PO div bid for 14 days, OR ceftriaxone 1 g daily for 10 days. CSF examination should be performed for children being treated for primary or secondary syphilis to rule out asymptomatic neurosyphilis. Test for HIV.
– Syphilis lasting for <1 y, without clinical symptoms (early latent syphilis)	Penicillin G benzathine 50,000 U/kg (max 2.4 million U) IM weekly for 3 doses (AIII)	Alternative if allergy to penicillin: doxycycline (patients >7 y) 4.4 mg/kg/day (max 200 mg/day) PO div bid for 14 days
– Syphilis lasting for >1 y, without clinical symptoms (late latent syphilis) or syphilis lasting for unknown duration	Penicillin G benzathine 50,000 U/kg (max 2.4 million U) IM weekly for 3 doses (AIII)	Alternative if allergy to penicillin: doxycycline (patients >7 y) 4.4 mg/kg/day (max 200 mg/day) PO div bid for 28 days. Look for neurologic, eye, and aortic complications of tertiary syphilis.
Trichomoniasis[57]	Tinidazole 50 mg/kg (max 2 g) PO for 1 dose (BII) OR metronidazole 500 mg PO bid for 7 days (preferred for women) OR metronidazole 2 g PO for 1 dose (BII)	
Urethritis, nongonococcal (See Gonorrhea earlier in this table for gonorrhea therapy.)[57,295]	Azithromycin 20 mg/kg (max 1 g) PO for 1 dose, OR doxycycline (patients >7 y) 4.4 mg/kg/day (max 200 mg/day) PO div bid for 7 days (AII)	Erythromycin, levofloxacin, or ofloxacin Increasing resistance noted in *Mycoplasma genitalium*[295]

Vaginitis[57]		
– Bacterial vaginosis[57,296]	Metronidazole 500 mg PO bid for 7 days OR metronidazole vaginal gel (0.75%) qd for 5 days, OR clindamycin vaginal cream for 7 days	Alternative: tinidazole 1 g PO qd for 5 days, OR clindamycin 300 mg PO bid for 7 days Relapse common Caused by synergy of *Gardnerella* with anaerobes
– Candidiasis, vulvovaginal[57,297]	Topical vaginal cream/tabs/suppositories (alphabetic order): butoconazole, clotrimazole, econazole, fenticonazole, miconazole, sertaconazole, terconazole, or tioconazole for 3–7 days (AI); OR fluconazole 10 mg/kg (max 150 mg) as a single dose (AII)	For uncomplicated vulvovaginal candidiasis, no topical agent is clearly superior. For severe acute *Candida* vulvovaginitis, fluconazole (max 150 mg) given q72h for a total of 2 or 3 doses. Avoid azoles during pregnancy. For recurring disease, consider 10–14 days of induction with topical agent or fluconazole, followed by fluconazole once weekly for 6 mo (AI).
– Prepubertal vaginitis[298,299]	No prospective studies	Cultures from symptomatic prepubertal girls are statistically more likely to yield *E coli*, enterococcus, coagulase-negative staphylococci, and streptococci (viridans streptococcus and group A streptococcus), but these organisms may also be present in asymptomatic girls.
– *Streptococcus*, group A[300]	Penicillin V 50–75 mg/kg/day PO div tid for 10 days	Amoxicillin 50–75 mg/kg/day PO div tid

J. CENTRAL NERVOUS SYSTEM INFECTIONS

Clinical Diagnosis	Therapy (evidence grade)	Comments
Abscess, brain (respiratory tract flora, skin flora, or bowel flora, depending on the pathogenesis of infection [direct extension or bacteremia])[301,302]	Until etiology established, use empiric therapy for presumed mixed-flora infection with origins from the respiratory tract, skin, and/or bowel, based on individual patient evaluation and risk for brain abscess (see Comments for MRSA considerations): Meropenem 120 mg/kg/day div q8h (AIII); OR nafcillin 150–200 mg/kg/day IV div q6h AND ceftriaxone 100 mg/kg/day IV q24h AND metronidazole 30 mg/kg/day IV div q8h (BIII); for 2–3 wk after successful drainage (depending on pathogen, size of abscess, and response to therapy); longer course if no surgery (3–6 wk) (BIII). Follow resolution by imaging.	Surgery for abscesses ≥2 cm in diameter. For single pathogen abscess, use a single agent in doses that will achieve effective CNS exposure. The blood-brain barrier is not intact in brain abscesses. If CA-MRSA suspected, ADD vancomycin 60 mg/kg/day IV div q8h ± rifampin 20 mg/kg/day IV div q12h, pending culture results. We have successfully treated MRSA intracranial infections with ceftaroline, but no prospective data exist. If secondary to chronic otitis, include meropenem or cefepime in regimen for anti-*Pseudomonas* activity. For enteric gram-negative bacilli, consider ESBL-producing *Escherichia coli* and *Klebsiella* that require meropenem and resist ceftriaxone.
Encephalitis[303] (may be infectious or immune-complex mediated[304])		
– Amebic (*Naegleria fowleri, Balamuthia mandrillaris*, and *Acanthamoeba*)	See Amebiasis in Chapter 9, Table 9B.	
– CMV	See Cytomegalovirus in Chapter 7, Table 7C. Not well studied in children. Consider ganciclovir 10 mg/kg/day IV div q12h; for severe immunocompromised, ADD foscarnet 180 mg/kg/day IV div q8h for 3 wk.	Follow quantitative PCR in CSF for CMV DNA. Reduce dose for renal insufficiency. Watch for neutropenia.
– Enterovirus	Supportive therapy; no antivirals currently FDA approved	Pocapavir PO is currently under investigation for enterovirus (poliovirus). As of July 2022, it is not available for compassionate use. Pleconaril has been evaluated for treatment of neonatal enteroviral sepsis syndrome.[305] As of July 2022, it is not available for compassionate use.

– EBV[306]	Not studied in a controlled comparative trial. Consider ganciclovir 10 mg/kg/day IV div q12h or acyclovir 60 mg/kg/day IV div q8h for 3 wk.	Follow quantitative PCR in CSF for EBV DNA. Efficacy of antiviral therapy not well-defined.
– HSV[307] (See Chapter 2 for neonatal infection.)	Acyclovir 60 mg/kg/day IV as 1- to 2-h infusion div q8h for 21 days for ≤4 mo; for those >4 mo, 45 mg/kg/day IV for 21 days (AIII)	Perform CSF HSV PCR near end of 21 days of therapy, and continue acyclovir until PCR negative. Safety of high-dose acyclovir (60 mg/kg/day) not well-defined beyond the neonatal period; can be used, but monitor for neurotoxicity and nephrotoxicity; FDA has approved acyclovir at this dosage for encephalitis for children up to 12 y.
– *Toxoplasma* (See Chapter 2 for neonatal congenital infection.)	See Chapter 9.	
– Arbovirus (flavivirus—Japanese encephalitis, Zika, West Nile, St Louis encephalitis, tick-borne encephalitis; togavirus—western equine encephalitis, eastern equine encephalitis; bunyavirus—La Crosse encephalitis, California encephalitis)[303,308]	Supportive therapy	Investigational only (antiviral, interferon, immune globulins). No specific antiviral agents are yet commercially available for any of the arboviruses, including Zika or West Nile.

Meningitis, bacterial, community-associated

NOTES

– Pediatric community-associated bacterial meningitis is quite uncommon in the era of conjugate vaccines. Rare cases caused by non-vaccine strains of *Pneumococcus,* or occurring in immunocompromised children, may still occur. The incidence of highly resistant pneumococci in invasive pediatric infections is so low that vancomycin is no longer needed for empiric therapy (toxicity of exposure is no longer justified). Ceftriaxone resistance is no longer a public health issue at this time.

– Dexamethasone 0.6 mg/kg/day IV div q6h for 2 days as an adjunct to antibiotic therapy decreases hearing deficits and other neurologic sequelae in adults and children (for *Haemophilus* and pneumococcus; not prospectively studied in children for meningococcus or *E coli*). The first dose of dexamethasone is given before or concurrent with the first dose of antibiotic; probably little benefit if given ≥1 h after the antibiotic.[309,310]

J. CENTRAL NERVOUS SYSTEM INFECTIONS *(continued)*

Clinical Diagnosis	Therapy (evidence grade)	Comments
– Empiric therapy[311]	Ceftriaxone 100 mg/kg/day IV q24h (AII)	Vancomycin is no longer needed for empiric treatment of possible pen-R pneumococcus given current, exceedingly high ceftriaxone susceptibility in North America.[312] The blood barrier is not competent early in the antibiotic treatment course, allowing increased penetration as culture/susceptibility results are pending. The first case of ceftriaxone treatment failure 30 y ago initially responded to our treatment with ceftriaxone.[313]
– *Haemophilus influenzae* type b[311] in unimmunized children	Ceftriaxone 100 mg/kg/day IV q24h; for 10 days (AI)	Alternative: ampicillin 200–400 mg/kg/day IV div q6h (for BL-negative strains)
– Meningococcus (*Neisseria meningitidis*)[311]	Penicillin G 250,000 U/kg/day IV div q4h; or ceftriaxone 100 mg/kg/day IV q24h, or cefotaxime 200 mg/kg/day IV div q6h; treatment course for 7 days (AI)	Meningococcal prophylaxis: rifampin 10 mg/kg PO q12h for 4 doses OR ceftriaxone 125–250 mg IM once OR ciprofloxacin 500 mg PO once (adolescents and adults)
– Neonatal	See Chapter 2.	
– Pneumococcus (*Streptococcus pneumoniae*)[311,312]	For pen-S and cephalosporin-susceptible strains: penicillin G 250,000 U/kg/day IV div q4–6h, OR ceftriaxone 100 mg/kg/day IV q24h; for 10 days (AI). For pen-R pneumococci (assuming ceftriaxone susceptibility): continue ceftriaxone IV for total course (AIII).	Some pneumococci may be resistant to penicillin but may still be susceptible to ceftriaxone and may be treated with the cephalosporin alone. For the rare ceftriaxone-resistant strain present in some parts of the world, add vancomycin to ceftriaxone (once resistance is suspected or documented) to complete a 14-day course. With the efficacy of current pneumococcal conjugate vaccines, primary bacterial meningitis is uncommon, and penicillin resistance has decreased substantially.

Meningitis, TB (*Mycobacterium tuberculosis; Mycobacterium bovis*)[15,16]	For non-immunocompromised children: INH 15 mg/kg/day PO, IV div q12–24h AND rifampin 15 mg/kg/day PO, IV div q12–24h for 12 mo AND PZA 30 mg/kg/day PO div q12–24h for first 2 mo of therapy, AND streptomycin 30 mg/kg/day IV, IM div q12h or ethionamide for first 4–8 wk of therapy; followed by INH and rifampin combination therapy to complete at least 12 mo for the total course. Streptomycin or ethionamide is used instead of ethambutol in children (primarily infants, who have this infection), due to difficulty assessing optic neuritis from ethambutol, and the lower risk for MDR strains causing infection.	*M bovis* strains are intrinsically resistant to PZA. Hyponatremia from inappropriate ADH secretion is common; ventricular drainage may be necessary for obstructive hydrocephalus. Administer corticosteroids (can use the same dexamethasone dose as for bacterial meningitis, 0.6 mg/kg/day IV div q6h) for 4 wk until neurologically stable, then taper dose for 1–3 mo to decrease neurologic complications and improve prognosis by decreasing the incidence of infarction.[314] Watch for rebound inflammation during taper; increase dose to previously effective level, then taper more slowly. For recommendations for drug-resistant strains and treatment of TB in HIV-infected patients, visit the CDC website for TB: www.cdc.gov/tb (reviewed March 17, 2022; accessed September 21, 2022).
Shunt infections: The use of antibiotic-impregnated shunts has decreased the frequency of this infection.[315] Shunt removal is usually necessary for cure, with placement of a new external ventricular drain; intraventricular injection of antibiotics should be considered in children responding poorly to systemic antibiotic therapy. Duration of therapy varies by pathogen and response to treatment.[311]		
– Empiric therapy pending Gram stain and culture[311]	Vancomycin 60 mg/kg/day IV div q8h, AND ceftriaxone 100 mg/kg/day IV q24h (AII)	If Gram stain shows only gram-positive cocci, can start with vancomycin alone. Cefepime, meropenem, or ceftazidime should be used instead of ceftriaxone if *Pseudomonas* is suspected. For ESBL-containing gram-negative bacilli, meropenem should be used as the preferred carbapenem for CNS infection.

J. CENTRAL NERVOUS SYSTEM INFECTIONS (*continued*)

Clinical Diagnosis	Therapy (evidence grade)	Comments
– *Staphylococcus epidermidis* or *Staphylococcus aureus*[311]	Vancomycin (for *S epidermidis* and CA-MRSA) 60 mg/kg/day IV div q8h; OR nafcillin (if organisms susceptible) 150–200 mg/kg/day AND rifampin; for 10–14 days (AIII)	For children who cannot tolerate vancomycin, ceftaroline has anecdotally been successful in our hands and others': ceftaroline[316]: 2–<6 mo, 30 mg/kg/day IV div q8h (each dose given over 2 h); ≥6 mo, 45 mg/kg/day IV div q8h (each dose given over 2 h) (max single dose 600 mg) (BIII). Linezolid, daptomycin, and TMP/SMX are other untested options.
– Gram-negative bacilli[311]	Empiric therapy with meropenem 120 mg/kg/day IV div q8h OR cefepime 150 mg/kg/day IV div q8h (AIII) For *E coli* (without ESBLs): ceftriaxone 100 mg/kg/day IV q12h for at least 10–14 days, preferably 21 days	Remove shunt. Select appropriate therapy based on in vitro susceptibilities. Meropenem, ceftriaxone, cefotaxime, and cefepime have all been studied in pediatric meningitis. Systemic gentamicin as combination therapy is not routinely recommended with carbapenems and cefepime. Intrathecal therapy with aminoglycosides not routinely necessary with highly active beta-lactam therapy and shunt removal. See Chapter 12.

K. URINARY TRACT INFECTIONS

Clinical Diagnosis	Therapy (evidence grade)	Comments
NOTE: Antibiotic susceptibility profiles of *Escherichia coli,* the most common cause of UTI, vary considerably. Please check your local microbiology laboratory for susceptibilities from urinary tract isolates in your clinic (community-acquired) and your hospital (potentially nosocomially acquired). For mild disease, TMP/SMX may be started as initial empiric therapy if local susceptibility is ≥80%, and up to a 20% failure rate is acceptable. Amoxicillin resistance in most communities is >50%. For moderate to severe disease (possible pyelonephritis), obtain cultures and begin an oral second- or third-generation cephalosporin (cefuroxime, cefaclor, cefprozil, cefixime, ceftibuten, cefdinir, cefpodoxime), ciprofloxacin PO, or ceftriaxone IM. Antibiotic susceptibility testing will help direct your therapy to the narrowest-spectrum agent.		
Cystitis, acute (*E coli*)[317–319]	For mild to moderate disease: TMP/SMX 8 mg/kg/day of TMP PO div bid for 3 days (see NOTE above about resistance to TMP/SMX), OR cephalexin 50–75 mg/kg/day div q8–12h. In children, for moderate to severe disease, it is often difficult to distinguish between upper tract and lower tract infections: cefixime 8 mg/kg/day PO qd; OR ceftriaxone 50 mg/kg IM q24h for 3–5 days (with normal anatomy) (BII); follow-up culture after 36–48 h of treatment ONLY if still symptomatic.	Alternative: amoxicillin 30 mg/kg/day PO div tid OR amox/clav PO if susceptible (BII); ciprofloxacin 20–30 mg/kg/day PO div bid for suspected or documented resistant (including ESBL-producing) organisms.[320] Gentamicin is another option with excellent activity against community strains of *E coli,* but it is only IM or IV and is nephrotoxic. End-of-therapy cultures are not routinely recommended.
Nephronia, lobar *E coli* and other enteric rods (also called "focal bacterial nephritis")[321,322]	Ceftriaxone 50 mg/kg/day IV, IM q24h. Duration depends on resolution of renal cellulitis vs development of abscess (10–21 days) (AIII). For ESBL-positive *E coli,* carbapenems and fluoroquinolones are often active agents.	Nephronia, a complication of pyelonephritis, is an invasive, consolidative parenchymal infection; it can evolve into renal abscess. Step-down therapy with oral cephalosporins once cellulitis/abscess has initially responded to therapy.

K. URINARY TRACT INFECTIONS *(continued)*

Clinical Diagnosis	Therapy (evidence grade)	Comments
Pyelonephritis, acute (*E coli*)[192,317,319,320,323–327]	Ceftriaxone 50 mg/kg/day IV, IM q24h OR gentamicin 5–6 mg/kg/day IV, IM q24h (yes, qd). For documented or suspected ceftriaxone-resistant ESBL-positive strains, use meropenem IV, imipenem IV, or ertapenem IV[192,324,325]; OR gentamicin IV/IM, pip/tazo, OR tol/taz. Switch to oral therapy following clinical response (BII). If organism resistant to amoxicillin and TMP/SMX, use an oral first-, second-, or third-generation cephalosporin (BII); if cephalosporin-R or for *Pseudomonas,* can use ciprofloxacin PO 30 mg/kg/day div q12h (up to 40 mg/kg/day)[320] (BIII); for 7–14 days total (depending on response to therapy). See Chapter 12.	For mild to moderate infection, shorter courses and oral therapy are likely to be as effective as IV/IM therapy for a standard duration of 10–14 days, for susceptible strains, down to 3 mo of age.[324,326] In children, it is often difficult to distinguish between upper tract and lower tract infections. If bacteremia documented and infant <2–3 mo, rule out meningitis and treat 14 days IV + PO (AIII). Aminoglycosides at any dose are more nephrotoxic than beta-lactams but represent effective therapy (AI). Once-daily dosing of gentamicin is preferred to tid.[323] The duration of treatment is a function of the extent of infection (with potential renal abscess formation in severe pyelonephritis); no prospective data collection has addressed the extent of infection at the time of diagnosis. Early renal cellulitis should respond to 5–7 days of therapy; renal abscesses may take 14+ days to resolve.[324]
Recurrent UTI, prophylaxis[317,318,328–331]	Only for those with grade III–V reflux or with recurrent febrile UTI: TMP/SMX 2 mg/kg/dose of TMP PO qd OR nitrofurantoin 1–2 mg/kg PO qd at bedtime; more rapid resistance may develop by using beta-lactams (BII).	Prophylaxis is not recommended for patients with grade I–II reflux and no evidence of renal damage (although the RIVUR study[330] included these children, and they may also benefit), but early treatment of new infection is recommended for these children. *Resistance eventually develops to every antibiotic;* follow resistance patterns for each patient. The use of periodic urine cultures is controversial, as there are no comparative data to guide management of asymptomatic bacteriuria in a child at high risk for recurrent UTI. Although one can prevent febrile UTIs, it is not clear that one can prevent renal scar formation.[332]

L. MISCELLANEOUS SYSTEMIC INFECTIONS

Clinical Diagnosis	Therapy (evidence grade)	Comments
Actinomycosis[333–335]	Penicillin G 250,000 U/kg/day IV div q6h, OR ampicillin 150 mg/kg/day IV div q8h until improved (often up to 6 wk for extensive infection); then long-term convalescent therapy with penicillin V 100 mg/kg/day (up to 4 g/day) PO for 6–12 mo (AII)	Surgery with debridement as indicated. Alternatives: amoxicillin, doxycycline for children >7 y clarithromycin, erythromycin; ceftriaxone IM/IV, or meropenem IV.
Anaplasmosis[336,337] (human granulocytotropic anaplasmosis, *Anaplasma phagocytophilum*)	Doxycycline 4.4 mg/kg/day IV, PO (max 200 mg/day) div bid for 7–10 days (regardless of age) (AIII)	No contraindication for doxycycline treatment in ANY age-group. For mild disease, consider rifampin 20 mg/kg/day PO div bid for 7–10 days (BIII).
Anthrax, sepsis/pneumonia, community vs bioterror exposure (inhalation, cutaneous, GI, meningoencephalitis)[17]	For community-associated anthrax infection, amoxicillin 75 mg/kg/day div q8h OR doxycycline for children >7 y For bioterror-associated exposure (regardless of age): ciprofloxacin 20–30 mg/kg/day IV div q12h, OR levofloxacin 16 mg/kg/day IV div q12h not to exceed 250 mg/dose (AIII); OR doxycycline 4.4 mg/kg/day PO (max 200 mg/day) div bid (regardless of age)	For invasive infection after bioterror exposure, 2 or 3 antibiotics may be required.[17] For oral step-down therapy, can use oral ciprofloxacin or doxycycline; if susceptible, can use penicillin, amoxicillin, or clindamycin. May require long-term postexposure prophylaxis after bioterror event.
Appendicitis (See Appendicitis, bowel-associated, in Table 1H under Intra-abdominal infection.)		
Brucellosis[338,339]	Doxycycline 4.4 mg/kg/day PO (max 200 mg/day) div bid (for children >7 y) AND rifampin (15–20 mg/kg/day div q12h) (BIII); OR for children <8 y: TMP/SMX 10 mg/kg/day of TMP IV, PO div q12h AND rifampin 15–20 mg/kg/day div q12h (BIII); for at least 6 wk	Combination therapy with rifampin will decrease the risk of relapse. For more serious infections, ADD gentamicin 6.0–7.5 mg/kg/day IV, IM div q8h for the first 1–2 wk of therapy to further decrease risk of relapse (BIII), particularly for endocarditis, osteomyelitis, or meningitis. Prolonged treatment for 4–6 mo and surgical debridement may be necessary for deep infections (AIII).

L. MISCELLANEOUS SYSTEMIC INFECTIONS *(continued)*

Clinical Diagnosis	Therapy (evidence grade)	Comments
Cat-scratch disease (*Bartonella henselae*)[340–342]	Supportive care for adenopathy (I&D of infected lymph node); azithromycin 12 mg/kg/day PO qd for 5 days shortens the duration of adenopathy (AIII). No prospective data exist for invasive CSD: gentamicin (for 14 days) AND TMP/SMX AND rifampin for hepatosplenic disease and osteomyelitis (AIII). For CNS infection, use ceftriaxone AND gentamicin ± TMP/SMX (AIII).	This dosage of azithromycin has been documented to be safe and effective for strep pharyngitis and may offer greater deep tissue exposure than the dosage studied by Bass et al[8] and used for otitis media. Alternatives: ciprofloxacin, doxycycline.
Chickenpox/shingles (varicella-zoster virus)	See Varicella-zoster virus in Chapter 7, Table 7C.	
COVID-19 (acute SARS-CoV-2 infection)	See Coronavirus (SARS-CoV-2) in Chapter 7, Table 7C.	

COVID-19 MIS-C/PIMS-TS (postinfection inflammatory syndrome). Please consult with a pediatric rheumatologist/ immunologist for current recommendations.	Based on the CDC case definition, a SARS-CoV-2 diagnosis must *first* be made (see Comments). Recommendations from the American College of Rheumatology (see Comments); grading based on consensus, as low (L), moderate (M), and high (H). High-dose IVIG (typically 1–2 g/kg) may be considered (M/H). Low- to moderate-dose glucocorticoids may be considered (M/H). Anakinra may be considered for treatment of MIS-C refractory to IVIG and glucocorticoids or in patients with contraindications to these treatments (M/H). Consultation with a pediatric rheumatologist is advised. Low-dose aspirin (3–5 mg/kg/day; max 81 mg/day) should be used (M). Patients with MIS-C and documented thrombosis or an ejection fraction <35% should receive therapeutic anticoagulation with enoxaparin.	Treatment recommendations from the "American College of Rheumatology Clinical Guidance for Multisystem Inflammatory Syndrome in Children Associated With SARS-CoV-2 and Hyperinflammation in Pediatric COVID-19: Version 1" (https://onlinelibrary.wiley.com/doi/abs/10.1002/art.41454; published July 23, 2020; accessed September 21, 2022) CDC case definition: an individual aged <21 y presenting with fever, laboratory evidence of inflammation, and evidence of clinically severe illness requiring hospitalization, with multisystem (>2) organ involvement (cardiac, renal, respiratory, hematologic, GI, dermatologic, or neurologic); *AND* no alternative plausible diagnoses; *AND* positive for current or recent SARS-CoV-2 infection by RT-PCR, serology, or antigen test; or COVID-19 exposure within the 4 wk before the onset of symptoms (www.cdc.gov/mis; reviewed June 25, 2021; accessed September 21, 2022)
Ehrlichiosis (human monocytic ehrlichiosis, caused by *Ehrlichia chaffeensis,* and *Ehrlichia ewingii*)[336,337,343,344]	Doxycycline 4.4 mg/kg/day IV, PO div bid (max 100 mg/dose) for 7–10 days (regardless of age) (AIII)	For mild disease, consider rifampin 20 mg/kg/day PO div bid (max 300 mg/dose) for 7–10 days (BIII).

L. MISCELLANEOUS SYSTEMIC INFECTIONS *(continued)*

Clinical Diagnosis	Therapy (evidence grade)	Comments
Febrile, neutropenic patient (empiric therapy for invasive infection: *Pseudomonas,* enteric gram-negative bacilli, staphylococci, streptococci, yeast, fungi)[345–348]	Cefepime 150 mg/kg/day div q8h (AI); OR meropenem 60 mg/kg/day div q8h (AII); OR pip/tazo (300 mg/kg/day pip component div q8h for infants/children >9 mo; 240 mg/kg/day div q8h for infants 2–9 mo), OR ceftazidime 150 mg/kg/day IV div q8h AND tobramycin 6 mg/kg/day IV q8h (AII). ADD vancomycin 40 mg/kg/day IV div q8h if MRSA or coagulation-negative staph infection suspected (eg, central catheter infection) (AIII). ADD metronidazole to ceftazidime or cefepime if colitis, head/neck space infection, or other deep anaerobic infection suspected (AIII).	Alternatives: other anti-*Pseudomonas* beta-lactams (imipenem) AND antistaphylococcal antibiotics, including ceftaroline for MRSA. If no response in 3–4 days and no alternative etiology demonstrated, begin additional empiric therapy with antifungals (BII)[345,347]; dosages and formulations outlined in Chapter 5. Increasingly resistant pathogens (ESBL *Escherichia coli* and KPC *Klebsiella*) will require alternative empiric therapy if MDR organisms are colonizing the patient or present on the child's hospital unit. For low-risk patients with negative cultures and close follow-up, alternative management strategies have been explored: oral therapy with amox/clav and ciprofloxacin may be used, with cautious discontinuation of antibiotics (even in those without marrow recovery).[345,349]
HIV infection	See Chapter 7.	
Infant botulism[350]	Botulism immune globulin for infants (BabyBIG) 50 mg/kg IV for 1 dose (AI); BabyBIG can be obtained from the California Department of Public Health at www.infantbotulism.org, through your state health department.	See www.infantbotulism.org for information for physicians and parents. Website organized by the California Department of Public Health (accessed September 21, 2022). Aminoglycosides should be avoided because they potentiate the neuromuscular effect of botulinum toxin.

Kawasaki syndrome[351–354]	No antibiotics; IVIG 2 g/kg as single dose (AI); may need to repeat dose in up to 15% of children for persisting fever that lasts 24 h after completion of the IVIG infusion (AII). Corticosteroids as primary adjunctive therapy in the acute phase of Kawasaki syndrome can be associated with reduced coronary artery abnormalities, reduced inflammatory markers, and shorter duration of hospital stay when compared to no corticosteroids.[352] Consult an ID physician or a pediatric cardiologist. Adjunctive therapy with corticosteroids for those at high risk for the development of aneurysms.[352,353]	Aspirin 80–100 mg/kg/day div qid in acute febrile phase; once afebrile for 24–48 h, aspirin may no longer add benefit. Role of corticosteroids, infliximab, etanercept, calcineurin inhibitors, and antithrombotic therapy, as well as methotrexate, for IVIG-resistant Kawasaki syndrome is under investigation, and some interventions are likely to improve outcome in severe cases.[353,354] Infliximab may decrease acute symptoms in patients whose IVIG fails to respond but may not decrease the risk for coronary artery abnormalities.[355] Similar findings were noted with another tumor necrosis factor inhibitor, etanercept, in the overall population, although subsets of children within the study may have benefited.[354,356]
Leprosy (Hansen disease)[357]	Dapsone 1 mg/kg/day PO qd AND rifampin 10 mg/kg/day PO qd; ADD (for multibacillary disease) clofazimine 1 mg/kg/day PO qd; for 12 mo for paucibacillary disease; for 24 mo for multibacillary disease (AII).	Consult Health Resources and Services Administration National Hansen's Disease (Leprosy) Program at www.hrsa.gov/hansens-disease (reviewed June 2021; accessed September 21, 2022) for advice about treatment and free antibiotics: 800/642-2477.
Leptospirosis[358,359]	Penicillin G 250,000 U/kg/day IV div q6h, OR ceftriaxone 50 mg/kg/day IV, IM q24h; for 7 days (BII) For mild disease in all age-groups, doxycycline (>7 y) 4.4 mg/kg/day (max 200 mg/day) PO div bid for 7–10 days (BII)	Alternative: for those with mild disease, intolerant of doxycycline, azithromycin 20 mg/kg on day 1, 10 mg/kg on days 2 and 3, or amoxicillin
Lyme disease (*Borrelia burgdorferi*)[360,361]	Neurologic evaluation, including LP, if there is clinical suspicion of CNS involvement	

L. MISCELLANEOUS SYSTEMIC INFECTIONS *(continued)*

Clinical Diagnosis	Therapy (evidence grade)	Comments
– Early localized disease (erythema migrans, single or multiple) (any age)	Doxycycline 4.4 mg/kg/day (max 200 mg/day) PO div bid for 10 days for all ages (AII) OR amoxicillin 50 mg/kg/day (max 1.5 g/day) PO div tid for 14 days (AII)	Alternative: cefuroxime, 30 mg/kg/day (max 1,000 mg/day) PO, in 2 div doses for 14 days OR azithromycin 10 mg/kg/day PO qd for 7 days
– Arthritis (no CNS disease)	Oral therapy as outlined in early localized disease but for 28 days (AIII)	Persistent or recurrent joint swelling after treatment: repeat a 4-wk course of oral antibiotics or give ceftriaxone 50–75 mg/kg IV q24h for 14–28 days. For persisting arthritis after 2 defined antibiotic treatment courses, use symptomatic therapy.
– Isolated facial (Bell) palsy	Doxycycline as outlined in early localized disease, for 14 days (AIII); efficacy of amoxicillin unknown	LP is not routinely required unless CNS symptoms develop. Treatment to prevent late sequelae; will not provide a quick response for palsy.
– Carditis	Oral therapy as outlined in early localized disease, for 14 days (range 14–21 days) OR ceftriaxone 50–75 mg/kg IV q24h for 14 days (range 14–21 days) (AIII)	
– Neuroborreliosis	Doxycycline 4.4 mg/kg/day (max 200 mg/day) PO div bid for 14–21 days (AII) OR ceftriaxone 50–75 mg/kg IV q24h OR penicillin G 300,000 U/kg/day IV div q4h; for 14–21 days (AIII)	
Melioidosis (*Burkholderia pseudomallei*)[362,363]	Acute sepsis: meropenem 75 mg/kg/day div q8h; OR ceftazidime 150 mg/kg/day IV div q8h; followed by TMP/SMX (10 mg/kg/day of TMP) PO div bid for 3–6 mo	Alternative convalescent therapy: amox/clav (90 mg/kg/day of amox div tid, not bid) for children ≤7 y, or doxycycline for children >7 y; for 20 wk (AII)

Mycobacteria, nontuberculous[9,11,12,193]		
– Adenitis in normal host (See Adenitis entries in Table 1A.)	Excision usually curative (BII); azithromycin PO OR clarithromycin PO for 6–12 wk (with or without rifampin or ethambutol) if susceptible (BII)	Antibiotic susceptibility patterns are quite variable; cultures should guide therapy; medical therapy is 60%–70% effective. Data suggest that toxicity of antimicrobials may not be worth the small clinical benefit. For more resistant organisms, other antibiotics may be active, including TMP/SMX, fluoroquinolones, doxycycline, or, for parenteral therapy, amikacin, meropenem, or cefoxitin. See Chapter 3 for specific mycobacterial pathogens.
– Pneumonia or disseminated infection in compromised hosts (HIV, interferon-γ receptor deficiency, CF)[11,193,364,365]	The more severe the infection, the more aggressive the treatment: usually treated with 3 or 4 active drugs (eg, clarithromycin OR azithromycin, AND ethambutol, AND amikacin, cefoxitin, or meropenem). Also test for ciprofloxacin, TMP/SMX, rifampin, linezolid, clofazimine, and doxycycline (BII).	Outcomes particularly poor for *Mycobacterium abscessus*.[365,366] See Chapter 18 for dosages; cultures are essential, as the susceptibility patterns of nontuberculous mycobacteria are varied.
Nocardiosis (*Nocardia asteroides* and *Nocardia brasiliensis*)[367,368]	TMP/SMX 8 mg/kg/day of TMP div bid or sulfisoxazole 120–150 mg/kg/day PO div qid for ≥6–12 wk. For severe infection, particularly in immunocompromised hosts, IN ADDITION to TMP/SMX, use amikacin 15–20 mg/kg/day IM, IV div q8h OR imipenem or meropenem (not ertapenem) (AIII). For susceptible strains, ceftriaxone.	Wide spectrum of disease, from skin lesions to brain abscess. Surgery when indicated. Alternatives: doxycycline (for children >7 y), amox/clav, or linezolid. Immunocompromised children may require months of therapy.
Plague (*Yersinia pestis*)[369–371]	Gentamicin 7.5 mg/kg/day IV div q8h (AII) OR doxycycline 4.4 mg/kg/day (max 200 mg/day) PO div bid OR ciprofloxacin 30 mg/kg/day PO div bid. Gentamicin is poorly active in abscesses; consider alternatives for bubonic plague.	A complete listing of treatment options and doses for children is provided on the CDC website (www.cdc.gov/plague/healthcare/clinicians.html; reviewed February 25, 2022; accessed September 21, 2022).

L. MISCELLANEOUS SYSTEMIC INFECTIONS *(continued)*

Clinical Diagnosis	Therapy (evidence grade)	Comments
Q fever (*Coxiella burnetii*)[372,373]	Acute stage: doxycycline 4.4 mg/kg/day (max 200 mg/day) PO div bid for 14 days (AII) for children of any age. Endocarditis and chronic disease (ongoing symptoms for 6–12 mo): doxycycline for children >7 y AND hydroxychloroquine for 18–36 mo (AIII). Seek advice from pediatric ID specialist for children ≤7 y: may require TMP/SMX 8–10 mg/kg/day of TMP div q12h with doxycycline; OR levofloxacin with rifampin for 18 mo.	Follow doxycycline and hydroxychloroquine serum concentrations during endocarditis/chronic disease therapy. CNS: use fluoroquinolone (no prospective data) (BIII). Clarithromycin may be an alternative based on limited data (CIII).
Rocky Mountain spotted fever (fever, petechial rash with centripetal spread; *Rickettsia rickettsii*)[374,375]	Doxycycline 4.4 mg/kg/day (max 200 mg/day) PO div bid for 7–10 days (AI) for children of any age	Start empiric therapy early.
Tetanus (*Clostridium tetani*)[376,377]	Metronidazole 30 mg/kg/day IV, PO div q8h OR penicillin G 100,000 U/kg/day IV div q6h for 10–14 days; AND TIG 500 U IM (AII)	Wound debridement essential; may infiltrate wound with a portion of TIG dose, but not well studied; IVIG may provide antibody to toxin if TIG not available. Immunize with Td or Tdap. See Chapter 15 for prophylaxis recommendations.

Toxic shock syndrome (toxin-producing strains of *Staphylococcus aureus* [including MRSA] or group A streptococcus)[3,6,7,378,379]	Empiric: oxacillin/nafcillin 150 mg/kg/day IV div q6h AND vancomycin 45 mg/kg/day IV div q8h (to cover MRSA) AND clindamycin 30–40 mg/kg/day div q8h for 7–10 days (AIII)	Clindamycin added for the initial 48–72 h of therapy to decrease toxin production. Ceftaroline is an option for MRSA treatment, particularly with renal injury from shock and vancomycin (BIII). IVIG may provide additional benefit by binding circulating toxin (CIII). For MSSA: oxacillin/nafcillin AND clindamycin ± gentamicin. For CA-MRSA: ceftaroline (or vancomycin) AND clindamycin ± gentamicin. For group A streptococcus: penicillin G AND clindamycin.
Tularemia (*Francisella tularensis*)[181,380]	Gentamicin 6.0–7.5 mg/kg/day IM, IV div q8h; for 10–14 days (AII) Alternative for mild disease: ciprofloxacin (for 10 days)	Doxycycline as an alternative, although relapse rates may be higher than with other antibiotics. See www.cdc.gov/tularemia/clinicians/index.html (reviewed July 5, 2022; accessed September 21, 2022).

2. Antimicrobial Therapy for Neonates

NOTES

- Prospectively collected neonatal antimicrobial pharmacokinetic, safety, and efficacy data continue to become available, thanks in large part to federal legislation (especially the US Food and Drug Administration [FDA] Safety and Innovation Act of 2012 that mandates neonatal studies). In situations of inadequate data, suggested doses in this chapter are based on efficacy, safety, and pharmacological data from older children or adults. These may not account for the effect of developmental changes (effect of ontogeny) on drug metabolism and, hence, are not optimal, particularly for the unstable preterm neonate.[1]
- For those drugs with an intramuscular (IM) route, an assumption is being made that the IM absorption in neonates is like that in older children or adults in whom that route has been better studied. The IM and intravenous (IV) routes are not equivalent. The IM route is reasonable as post-initial IV therapy in hemodynamically stable neonates with difficult-to-maintain IV access whose infection has been microbiologically controlled and who are clinically recovering.

  Oral convalescent therapy for neonatal infections has not been well studied but may be used cautiously in non–life-threatening infections in adherent families with ready access to medical care.[2,3]
- **Substitution for cefotaxime in neonates and very young infants:** Since 2018, US pharmaceutical companies have discontinued manufacturing and marketing cefotaxime. The FDA is allowing temporary importation of cefotaxime from a Canadian distributor (877/404-3338). For centers without cefotaxime readily available, we are recommending the following 3 agents as substitutes:

  Cefepime has been available for more than 20 years, with many pediatric studies published, including neonatal ones. The original manufacturer did not seek approval from the FDA for neonates and infants younger than 2 months, so the FDA has not evaluated data or approved cefepime for neonates. Both cefepime and ceftazidime have activity against gram-negative bacilli, including *Pseudomonas aeruginosa,* and both would be expected to penetrate neonatal cerebrospinal fluid to treat meningitis. Cefepime is more active in vitro against enteric bacilli (*Escherichia coli*) and *Pseudomonas* than ceftazidime and is stable against ampC beta-lactamase often expressed by *Enterobacter, Serratia,* and *Citrobacter.* Cefepime is stable to many, but not all, extended-spectrum beta-lactamases (ESBLs), although it is routinely reported as resistant to ESBL-containing gram-negative bacteria. Cefepime also has more in vitro activity than ceftazidime against some gram-positive bacteria such as group B streptococci and methicillin-susceptible *Staphylococcus aureus.* There are no meaningful differences in the safety profiles or therapeutic monitoring of cefepime and ceftazidime.[4]

Ceftazidime has been in clinical use longer than cefepime, also has evidence supporting use in neonates, and is approved by the FDA for neonates.

Ceftriaxone is FDA approved for neonates with the following 2 caveats:

1. *Neonates with hyperbilirubinemia should not be treated with ceftriaxone* due to the potential for ceftriaxone to displace albumin-bound bilirubin, creating more free bilirubin that can diffuse into the brain and increase the risk for kernicterus. Our recommendation is to avoid ceftriaxone in any at-risk neonates with hyperbilirubinemia, particularly those who are unstable or acidotic and particularly preterm neonates and infants up to a postmenstrual age of 41 weeks (gestational + chronologic age).[5] Full-term neonates and infants with total bilirubin concentrations less than 10 mg/dL and falling (usually older than 1 week) may be considered for treatment, but no prospective data exist to support this bilirubin cutoff.[6]
2. Ceftriaxone is *contraindicated in neonates younger than 28 days if they require concomitant treatment with calcium-containing IV solutions.* Neonates should not receive IV ceftriaxone while receiving IV calcium-containing products, including parenteral nutrition, by the same or different infusion lines. Fatal reactions with ceftriaxone-calcium precipitates in lungs and kidneys in neonates have occurred. There are no data on interactions between IV ceftriaxone and oral calcium-containing products or between IM ceftriaxone and IV or oral calcium-containing products.[7]

- **Abbreviations:** 3TC, lamivudine; ABLC, lipid complex amphotericin; ABR, auditory brainstem response; ALT, alanine transaminase; AmB, amphotericin B; AmB-D, amphotericin B deoxycholate; amox/clav, amoxicillin/clavulanate; AOM, acute otitis media; AUC, area under the curve; bid, twice daily; BPD, bronchopulmonary dysplasia; BSA, body surface area; CBC, complete blood cell count; CDC, Centers for Disease Control and Prevention; CLD, chronic lung disease; CMV, cytomegalovirus; CNS, central nervous system; CRO, carbapenem-resistant organism; CSF, cerebrospinal fluid; CT, computed tomography; div, divided; ECMO, extracorporeal membrane oxygenation; ESBL, extended-spectrum beta-lactamase; FDA, US Food and Drug Administration; GA, gestational age; GBS, group B streptococcus; G-CSF, granulocyte colony-stimulating factor; GNR, gram-negative rods (bacilli); HSV, herpes simplex virus; IAI, intra-abdominal infection; ID, infectious disease; IM, intramuscular; IUGR, intrauterine growth restriction; IV, intravenous; IVIG, intravenous immune globulin; L-AmB, liposomal amphotericin B; max, maximum; MIC, minimal inhibitory concentration; MRSA, methicillin-resistant *Staphylococcus aureus;* MSSA, methicillin-susceptible *S aureus;* NDM, New Delhi metallo-beta-lactamase; NEC, necrotizing enterocolitis; NICU, neonatal intensive care unit; NVP, nevirapine; PCR, polymerase chain reaction; pip/tazo, piperacillin/tazobactam; PMA, postmenstrual age; PNA, postnatal age; PO, orally; q, every; RAL, raltegravir; RSV, respiratory syncytial virus; SCr, serum creatinine; spp, species; tab, tablet; tid, 3 times daily; TIG, tetanus immune globulin; TMP/SMX, trimethoprim/sulfamethoxazole; UCSF, University of California, San Francisco; UTI, urinary tract infection; VCUG, voiding cystourethrogram; VDRL, Venereal Disease Research Laboratories; VIM, Verona integron-encoded metallo-beta-lactamase; ZDV, zidovudine.

A. RECOMMENDED THERAPY FOR SELECT NEONATAL CONDITIONS

Condition	Therapy (evidence grade) *See tables 2B–2D for neonatal dosages.*	Comments
Conjunctivitis		
– Chlamydial[8–11]	Azithromycin 10 mg/kg/day PO for 1 day, then 5 mg/kg/day PO for 4 days (AII), or erythromycin ethylsuccinate PO for 10–14 days (AII)	Macrolides PO preferred to topical eye drops to prevent development of pneumonia; association of erythromycin and pyloric stenosis in young neonates.[12] Alternative: 3-day course of higher-dose azithromycin at 10 mg/kg/dose once daily, although safety not well-defined in neonates (CIII). Oral sulfonamides may be used after the immediate neonatal period for infants who do not tolerate erythromycin.
– Gonococcal[13–17]	Ceftriaxone 25–50 mg/kg (max 250 mg) IV, IM once (AIII)	For adults, ceftriaxone in higher doses is now recommended as single-agent therapy. Ceftriaxone should be used for neonates with no risk for hyperbilirubinemia[5] or IV calcium-drug interactions.[7] Cefotaxime or cefepime is preferred for neonates with hyperbilirubinemia[5] and those with risk for calcium-drug interactions (see Notes). Saline irrigation of eyes. Evaluate for chlamydial infection if maternal chlamydial infection not excluded. All neonates born to mothers with untreated gonococcal infection (regardless of symptoms) require therapy. Cefixime and ciprofloxacin not recommended for maternal empiric therapy.
– *Staphylococcus aureus*[18–20]	Topical therapy is sufficient for mild *S aureus* cases (AII), but oral or IV therapy may be considered for moderate to severe conjunctivitis. MSSA: oxacillin/nafcillin IV or cefazolin (for non-CNS infections) IM, IV for 7 days. MRSA: vancomycin IV or ceftaroline IV.	Aminoglycoside ophthalmic drops or ointment, polymyxin/trimethoprim drops No prospective data for MRSA conjunctivitis (BIII) Cephalexin PO for mild to moderate disease caused by MSSA Increased *S aureus* resistance with ciprofloxacin/levofloxacin ophthalmic formulations (AII)

– *Pseudomonas aeruginosa*[21–23]	Ceftazidime IM, IV AND tobramycin IM, IV for 7–10 days (alternatives: meropenem, cefepime, pip/tazo) (BIII)	Aminoglycoside or polymyxin B–containing ophthalmic drops or ointment as adjunctive therapy
– Other gram-negative	Aminoglycoside or polymyxin B–containing ophthalmic drops or ointment if mild (AII) Systemic therapy if moderate to severe or unresponsive to topical therapy (AIII)	Duration of therapy dependent on clinical course and may be as short as 5 days if clinically resolved
Cytomegalovirus		
– Congenital[24–28]	For moderately to severely symptomatic neonates with congenital CMV disease: oral valganciclovir at 16 mg/kg/dose bid for 6 mo[27] (AI); IV ganciclovir at 6 mg/kg/dose q12h can be used for some of or all the first 6 wk of therapy if oral therapy not advised but provides no added benefit over oral valganciclovir (AII).[29] An "induction period" starting with IV ganciclovir is not recommended if oral valganciclovir can be tolerated.	Benefit for hearing loss and neurodevelopmental outcomes (AI). Treatment recommended for neonates with moderate to severe symptomatic congenital CMV disease, with or without CNS involvement. If used, treatment of congenital CMV must start within the first month after birth. Treatment is not routinely recommended for "mildly symptomatic" neonates congenitally infected with CMV (eg, only 1 or perhaps 2 manifestations of congenital CMV infection, which are mild in scope [eg, isolated IUGR, mild hepatomegaly] or transient and mild in nature [eg, a single platelet count of 80,000 µL or an ALT of 130 U/L, with these numbers serving only as examples]), as the risks of treatment may not be balanced by benefits in mild disease.[28] This includes neonates who are asymptomatic except for sensorineural hearing loss. Treatment for asymptomatic neonates congenitally infected with CMV should not be given. Neutropenia develops in 20% (oral valganciclovir) to 68% (IV ganciclovir) of neonates receiving long-term therapy (responds to G-CSF or temporary discontinuation of therapy). CMV-IVIG not recommended for infants.

A. RECOMMENDED THERAPY FOR SELECT NEONATAL CONDITIONS *(continued)*

Condition	Therapy (evidence grade) ***See tables 2B–2D for neonatal dosages.***	Comments
– Perinatally or postnatally acquired[26]	Ganciclovir 10 mg/kg/day IV div q12h for 14–21 days (AIII)	Antiviral treatment has not been studied in this population but can be considered in patients with acute, severe visceral (end-organ) disease, such as pneumonitis, hepatitis, encephalitis, NEC, or persistent thrombocytopenia. If such patients are treated with parenteral ganciclovir, a reasonable approach is to treat for 2 wk and then reassess responsiveness to therapy. If clinical and laboratory data suggest benefit of treatment, an additional 1 wk of parenteral ganciclovir can be considered if symptoms and signs have not fully resolved. Oral valganciclovir is not recommended in these more severe disease manifestations. Observe for possible relapse after completion of therapy (AIII).
Fungal infections (See also Chapter 5.)		
– Candidiasis[30–39]	**Treatment** AmB-D (1 mg/kg/day) is recommended therapy (AII). Fluconazole (25 mg/kg on day 1, then 12 mg/kg q24h) is an alternative if patient has not been on fluconazole prophylaxis (AII).[40] For treatment of neonates and young infants (<120 days) receiving ECMO, fluconazole loading dose is 35 mg/kg on day 1, then 12 mg/kg q24h (BII).[41] Lipid formulation AmB is an alternative but carries a theoretical risk of decreasing urinary tract penetration, compared with AmB-D (CIII).[42]	Neonates have high risk for urinary tract and CNS infections, problematic for echinocandins with poor penetration at those sites; therefore, AmB-D is preferred, followed by fluconazole. Echinocandins are discouraged, despite their fungicidal activity. Infants with invasive candidiasis should be evaluated for other sites of infection: CSF analysis, echocardiogram, abdominal ultrasound to include bladder, retinal eye examination (AIII). CT or ultrasound imaging of genitourinary tract, liver, and spleen should be performed if blood culture results are persistently positive (AIII). Meningoencephalitis in the neonate occurs at a higher rate than in older children/adults. Central venous catheter removal strongly recommended. Infected CNS devices, including ventriculostomy drains and shunts, should be removed, if possible. Length of therapy dependent on disease (BIII), usually 2 wk after all clearance.

Duration of therapy for candidemia without obvious metastatic complications is for 2 wk after documented clearance and resolution of symptoms (therefore, generally 3 wk total). **Prophylaxis** In nurseries with high rates of candidiasis (>10%),[43] IV or oral fluconazole prophylaxis (AI) (3–6 mg/kg twice weekly for 6 wk) in high-risk neonates (birth weight <1,000 g) is recommended. Oral nystatin, 100,000 U tid for 6 wk, is an alternative to fluconazole in neonates with birth weights <1,500 g if availability or resistance precludes fluconazole use (CII). Prophylaxis of neonates and children receiving ECMO: fluconazole 12 mg/kg on day 1, followed by 6 mg/kg/day (BII).	Antifungal susceptibility testing is suggested with persistent disease. *Candida krusei* is inherently resistant to fluconazole; *Candida parapsilosis* may be less susceptible to echinocandins; there is increasing resistance of *Candida glabrata* to fluconazole and echinocandins. No proven benefit for combination antifungal therapy in candidiasis. Change from AmB or fluconazole to echinocandin if cultures persistently positive (BIII) despite source control. Although fluconazole prophylaxis has been shown to reduce colonization, it has not reduced mortality.[33] Echinocandins should be used with caution and generally limited to salvage therapy or situations in which resistance or toxicity precludes use of AmB-D or fluconazole (CIII). Role of flucytosine in neonates with meningitis is questionable and not routinely recommended due to toxicity concerns. The addition of flucytosine (100 mg/kg/day div q6h) may be considered as salvage therapy in patients who have not had a clinical response to initial AmB therapy, but adverse effects are frequent (CIII). Serum flucytosine concentrations should be obtained after 3–5 days to achieve a 2-h post-dose peak <100 mcg/mL (ideally 30–80 mcg/mL) to prevent neutropenia. See Skin and soft tissues later in this table for management of congenital cutaneous candidiasis.

A. RECOMMENDED THERAPY FOR SELECT NEONATAL CONDITIONS *(continued)*

Condition	Therapy (evidence grade) ***See tables 2B–2D for neonatal dosages.***	Comments
– Aspergillosis (usually cutaneous infection with systemic dissemination)[27,44–46]	Voriconazole dosing never studied in neonates but likely initial dosing same or higher as pediatric ≥2 y: 18 mg/kg/day IV div q12h for a loading dose on the first day, then 16 mg/kg/day IV div q12h as a maintenance dose. Continued dosing is guided by monitoring of trough serum concentrations (AII). When stable, may switch from voriconazole IV to voriconazole PO 18 mg/kg/day div bid (AII). Unlike in adults, oral bioavailability in children is about only 60%. Oral bioavailability in neonates has never been studied. Trough monitoring is crucial after switch.[26] Alternatives for primary therapy when voriconazole cannot be administered: L-AmB 5 mg/kg/day (AII). ABLC is another alternative. Echinocandin primary monotherapy should not be used for treating invasive aspergillosis (CII). AmB-D should be used only in resource-limited settings in which no alternative agent is available (AII).	Aggressive antifungal therapy and early debridement of skin lesions, which are a common manifestation in neonatal aspergillosis (AIII). Voriconazole is preferred primary antifungal therapy for all clinical forms of aspergillosis (AI). Early initiation of therapy in patients with strong suspicion of disease is important while a diagnostic evaluation is conducted. Therapeutic voriconazole trough serum concentrations of 2–5 mg/L are important for success. It is critical to monitor trough concentrations to guide therapy due to high inter-patient variability.[28] Low voriconazole concentrations are a leading cause of clinical failure. Neonatal and infant voriconazole dosing is not well-defined, but doses required to achieve therapeutic troughs are generally higher than in children >2 y (AIII).[47] Limited experience with posaconazole and no experience with isavuconazole in neonates.[48] Total treatment course is for a minimum of 6–12 wk, largely dependent on the degree and duration of immunosuppression and evidence of disease improvement. Salvage antifungal therapy options after failed primary therapy include a change of antifungal class (using L-AmB or an echinocandin), a switch to posaconazole (trough concentrations >1 mcg/mL [see Chapter 18 for pediatric dosing]), or use of combination antifungal therapy. Combination therapy with voriconazole + an echinocandin may be considered in select patients. In vitro data suggest some synergy with 2 (but not 3) drug combinations: an azole + an echinocandin is the most well studied. If combination therapy is used, this is likely best done initially when voriconazole trough concentrations may not yet be therapeutic.

		Routine susceptibility testing is not recommended but is suggested for patients who are suspected of having an azole-resistant isolate or who are unresponsive to therapy. Azole-resistant *Aspergillus fumigatus* is increasing. If local epidemiology suggests >10% azole resistance, initial empiric therapy should be voriconazole + echinocandin OR + L-AmB, and subsequent therapy guided based on antifungal susceptibilities.[49] Micafungin likely has equal efficacy to caspofungin against aspergillosis.[31]
Gastrointestinal infections		
– NEC or peritonitis secondary to bowel rupture[50–54]	Ampicillin IV AND gentamicin AND metronidazole IV for ≥10 days (AII). Clindamycin may be used in place of metronidazole (AII). Alternatives: meropenem (AI); pip/tazo ± gentamicin (AII). ADD fluconazole if known to have gastrointestinal colonization with susceptible *Candida* spp (BIII).	Surgical drainage (AII). Definitive antibiotic therapy based on blood-culture results (aerobic, anaerobic, and fungal); meropenem for ESBL-positive GNR or cefepime for ampC-positive (inducible cephalosporinase) GNR. Vancomycin rather than ampicillin if MRSA prevalent. *Bacteroides* colonization may occur as early as the first week after birth (AIII). Duration of therapy dependent on clinical response and risk for persisting IAI abscess (AIII). Probiotics may prevent NEC in preterm neonates, but the optimal strain(s), dose, duration, safety, and target subgroups are not fully known.[55,56]
– *Salmonella* (non-Typhi and Typhi)[57]	Ampicillin IM, IV (if susceptible) OR ceftriaxone or cefepime IM, IV for 7–10 days (AII)	Observe for focal complications (eg, meningitis, arthritis) (AIII). TMP/SMX for focal gastrointestinal infection and low risk for unconjugated hyperbilirubinemia due to interaction between sulfa and bilirubin-albumin binding.

A. RECOMMENDED THERAPY FOR SELECT NEONATAL CONDITIONS *(continued)*

Condition	Therapy (evidence grade) *See tables 2B–2D for neonatal dosages.*	Comments
Herpes simplex infection		
– CNS and disseminated disease[58–60]	Acyclovir 60 mg/kg/day div q8h IV for 21 days (AII). ALT may help identify early disseminated infection.	If CNS involvement, perform CSF HSV PCR near end of 21 days of therapy and continue IV acyclovir until PCR negative. Monitor early in treatment of acute kidney injury, particularly in sicker infants and those receiving additional nephrotoxins.[61] Infuse over 1 h and maintain adequate infant hydration to decrease risk for crystal nephropathy. Involve ophthalmologist when acute ocular HSV disease suspected. If present, ADD topical 1% trifluridine or 0.15% ganciclovir ophthalmic gel (AII) (see Chapter 18 for pediatric dosing). Acyclovir PO (300 mg/m^2/dose tid) suppression for 6 mo recommended following parenteral therapy (AI).[62] Observe for possible relapse after completion of therapy (BII).[63] Monitor for neutropenia. Different IV acyclovir dosages have been modeled,[64] but no clinical data are available in humans to support them. Use foscarnet for acyclovir-resistant disease (see Chapter 18 for pediatric dosing).
– Skin, eye, or mouth disease[58–60]	Acyclovir 60 mg/kg/day div q8h IV for 14 days (AII). Obtain CSF PCR for HSV to assess for CNS infection.	

HIV prophylaxis following perinatal exposure[65,66]		
– Prophylaxis following low-risk exposure (mother who had HIV infection before pregnancy, received antiretroviral therapy during pregnancy, and sustained viral suppression within 4 wk of delivery)	ZDV for the first 4 wk of age (AI). GA ≥35 wk: ZDV 8 mg/kg/day PO div q12h OR 6 mg/kg/day IV div q8h. GA 30–34 wk: ZDV 4 mg/kg/day PO (OR 3 mg/kg/day IV) div q12h. Increase at 2 wk of age to 6 mg/kg/day PO (OR 4.5 mg/kg/day IV) div q12h. GA ≤29 wk: ZDV 4 mg/kg/day PO (OR 3 mg/kg/day IV) div q12h. Increase at 4 wk of age to 6 mg/kg/day PO (OR 4.5 mg/kg/day IV) div q12h. The preventive ZDV doses listed for neonates are also treatment doses for infants with diagnosed HIV infection. Treatment of HIV-infected neonates should be considered only with expert consultation.	For detailed information: https://clinicalinfo.hiv.gov/en/guidelines/perinatal/whats-new-guidelines (accessed September 26, 2022). UCSF Clinician Consultation Center (888/448-8765) provides free clinical consultation. Start prevention therapy as soon after delivery as possible but by 6–8 h of age for best effectiveness (AII). Monitor CBC at birth and 4 wk (AII). Perform HIV-1 DNA PCR or RNA assays at 14–21 days, 1–2 mo, and 4–6 mo (AI). Initiate TMP/SMX prophylaxis for pneumocystis pneumonia at 6 wk of age if HIV infection not yet excluded (AII). TMP/SMX dosing is 2.5–5 mg/kg/dose of TMP component PO q12h.

A. RECOMMENDED THERAPY FOR SELECT NEONATAL CONDITIONS *(continued)*

Condition	Therapy (evidence grade) ***See tables 2B–2D for neonatal dosages.***	Comments
– Prophylaxis following higher-risk perinatal exposure (mother who had primary HIV infection during pregnancy OR who was not treated before delivery OR who was treated but did not achieve viral suppression within 4 wk of delivery, especially if delivery was vaginal)	Presumptive HIV treatment (BII): ZDV and 3TC for 6 wk AND EITHER NVP or RAL **ZDV dosing** as above; in infants ≥35 wk of gestation, the dosage should be increased to 12 mg/kg/day PO div q12 once the infant is >4 wk of age. **3TC dosing (≥32 wk of gestation at birth):** Birth–4 wk: 4 mg/kg/day PO div q12h. >4 wk: 8 mg/kg/day PO div q12h. **NVP dosing:** **≥37 wk of gestation at birth:** Birth–4 wk: NVP 12 mg/kg/day PO div q12h. >4 wk: NVP 400 mg/m²/day of BSA PO div q12h; make this dose increase only for infants with confirmed HIV infection. **≥34–<37 wk of gestation at birth:** Birth–1 wk: NVP 8 mg/kg/day PO div q12h. 1–4 wk: NVP 12 mg/kg/day PO div q12h. >4 wk: NVP 400 mg/m²/day of BSA PO div q12h; make this dose increase only for infants with confirmed HIV infection. **RAL dosing:** **≥37 wk of gestation at birth and ≥2,000 g in weight:** Birth–1 wk: once-daily dosing at about 1.5 mg/kg/dose. 2–<3 kg: 0.4 mL (4 mg) once daily. 3–<4 kg: 0.5 mL (5 mg) once daily. 4–<5 kg: 0.7 mL (7 mg) once daily.	Delivery management of women with HIV who are receiving antiretroviral therapy and have viral loads between 20 and 999 copies/mL varies. Data do not show a clear benefit to IV ZDV and cesarean delivery for these women. Decisions about the addition of NVP, 3TC, or RAL for infants born to these mothers should be made in consultation with a pediatric ID specialist. NVP dosing and safety not established for infants whose birth weight <1,500 g. The HIV Guidelines Committee recommends using "treatment" antiretroviral regimens for high-risk, exposed neonates in an attempt to preclude infection or to increase the chance of HIV remission or cure. This was initially stimulated by the experience of a baby from Mississippi: high-risk neonate treated within the first 2 days after birth with subsequent infection documentation; off therapy at 18 mo of age without evidence of circulating virus until 4 y of age, at which point HIV became detectable.[67] Clinical trials are ongoing to study these issues further. When empiric treatment is used for high-risk infants and HIV infection is subsequently excluded, NVP, 3TC, and/or RAL can be discontinued and ZDV can be continued for 6 wk total. If HIV infection is confirmed, see Chapter 7 for treatment recommendations. Consider consultation with a pediatric ID specialist, especially when considering use of RAL (CIII). If the mother has taken RAL within 2–24 h before delivery, the neonate's first dose of RAL should be delayed until 24–48 h after birth; other antiretroviral drugs should be started as soon as possible.

	1–4 wk: bid dosing at about 3 mg/kg/dose. 2–<3 kg: 0.8 mL (8 mg) bid. 3–<4 kg: 1 mL (10 mg) bid. 4–<5 kg: 1.5 mL (15 mg) bid. 4–6 wk: bid dosing at about 6 mg/kg/dose. 3–<4 kg: 2.5 mL (25 mg) bid. 4–<6 kg: 3 mL (30 mg) bid. 6–<8 kg: 4 mL (40 mg) bid.	
Influenza A and B viruses[68–71]		
Treatment	Oseltamivir: Preterm, <38 wk of PMA: 1 mg/kg/dose PO bid Preterm, 38–40 wk of PMA: 1.5 mg/kg/dose PO bid Preterm, >40 wk of PMA: 3 mg/kg/dose PO bid[69] Full-term, birth–8 mo: 3 mg/kg/dose PO bid[69,72]	Oseltamivir chemoprophylaxis is not recommended for infants <3 mo unless the situation is judged critical because of limited safety and efficacy data in this age-group. Parenteral peramivir is approved in the United States for use in children ≥2 y; no pharmacokinetic or safety data exist in neonates.[73] Oral baloxavir is approved in the United States for use in persons ≥12 y; no pharmacokinetic or safety data exist in neonates.[74]
Omphalitis and funisitis		
– Empiric therapy for omphalitis and necrotizing funisitis; direct therapy against coliform bacilli, *S aureus* (consider MRSA), and anaerobes[75–77]	Cefepime OR gentamicin, AND clindamycin for ≥10 days (AII)	Appropriate wound management for infected cord and necrotic tissue (AIII). Need to culture to direct therapy. Alternatives for coliform coverage if resistance likely: cefepime, meropenem. For suspect MRSA: ADD ceftaroline or vancomycin. Alternative for combined MSSA and anaerobic coverage: pip/tazo.
– Group A or B streptococcus[78]	Penicillin G IV for ≥7–14 days (shorter course for superficial funisitis without invasive infection) (AII)	Group A streptococcus usually causes "wet cord" without pus and with minimal erythema; single dose of penicillin benzathine IM adequate. Consultation with pediatric ID specialist recommended for necrotizing fasciitis (AII).

A. RECOMMENDED THERAPY FOR SELECT NEONATAL CONDITIONS *(continued)*

Condition	Therapy (evidence grade) ***See tables 2B–2D for neonatal dosages.***	Comments
– *S aureus*[77]	MSSA: oxacillin/nafcillin IV, IM for ≥5–7 days (shorter course for superficial funisitis without invasive infection) (AIII) MRSA: vancomycin (AIII) or ceftaroline (BII)	Assess for bacteremia and other focus of infection. Alternatives for MRSA: clindamycin (if susceptible) (BIII) or linezolid (CIII).
– *Clostridium* spp[79]	Clindamycin OR penicillin G IV for ≥10 days, with additional agents based on culture results (AII)	Crepitation and rapidly spreading cellulitis around umbilicus Mixed infection with other gram-positive and gram-negative bacteria common
Osteomyelitis, suppurative arthritis[79–82] Obtain cultures (aerobic; fungal if NICU) of bone or joint fluid before antibiotic therapy. Duration of therapy dependent on causative organism and normalization of erythrocyte sedimentation rate and C-reactive protein; minimum for osteomyelitis 3 wk and arthritis therapy 2–3 wk if no organism identified (AIII). Surgical drainage of pus (AIII); physical therapy may be needed (BIII).		
– Empiric therapy	Nafcillin/oxacillin IV (or vancomycin or ceftaroline if MRSA is a concern) AND cefepime OR gentamicin IV, IM (AIII)	Alternatives for MRSA: clindamycin (if susceptible) or linezolid
– Coliform bacteria (eg, *Escherichia coli, Klebsiella* spp, *Enterobacter* spp)	For *E coli* and *Klebsiella:* cefepime OR ceftazidime OR ampicillin (if susceptible) (AIII) For *Enterobacter, Serratia,* or *Citrobacter:* cefepime OR ceftazidime AND gentamicin IV, IM (AIII)	Meropenem for ESBL-producing coliforms (AIII). Gentamicin if abscesses can be drained.
– Gonococcal arthritis and tenosynovitis[14–17]	Ceftriaxone IV, IM AND azithromycin 10 mg/kg PO q24h for 5 days (AIII)	Ceftriaxone no longer recommended as single-agent therapy due to increasing cephalosporin resistance; therefore, addition of azithromycin recommended (no data in neonates; azithromycin dose is that recommended for pertussis). Cefotaxime or cefepime is preferred for neonates with hyperbilirubinemia and those with risk for calcium-drug interactions (see Notes).

– *S aureus*	MSSA: oxacillin/nafcillin IV (AII) MRSA: vancomycin IV (AIII) OR ceftaroline IV (BII)	Alternative for MSSA: cefazolin (AIII). Alternatives for MRSA: clindamycin (if susceptible) (BIII) or linezolid (CIII). Addition of rifampin if persistently positive cultures.
– Group B streptococcus	Ampicillin or penicillin G IV (AII)	
– *Haemophilus influenzae*	Ampicillin IV OR cefepime/ceftazidime IV, IM if ampicillin resistant	Start with IV therapy and switch to oral therapy when clinically stable. Amox/clav PO OR amoxicillin PO if susceptible (AIII).
Otitis media[83] No controlled treatment trials in neonates; if no response, obtain middle ear fluid for culture.		
– Empiric therapy[84]	Cefepime/ceftazidime OR oxacillin/nafcillin AND gentamicin	Start with IV therapy and switch to amox/clav PO when clinically stable (AIII).
– *E coli* (therapy for other coliforms based on susceptibility testing)	Cefepime/ceftazidime	Start with IV therapy and switch to oral therapy when clinically stable. In addition to pneumococcus and *Haemophilus,* coliforms and *S aureus* may also cause AOM in neonates (AIII). For ESBL-producing strains, use meropenem (AII). Amox/clav if susceptible (AIII).
– *S aureus*	MSSA: oxacillin/nafcillin IV (AII) MRSA: vancomycin IV (AIII) OR ceftaroline IV (BII)	Start with IV therapy and switch to oral therapy when clinically stable. MSSA: cephalexin PO for 10 days or cloxacillin PO (AIII). Alternatives for MRSA: clindamycin (if susceptible) (BIII) or linezolid (CIII).
– Group A or B streptococcus	Penicillin G or ampicillin IV, IM	Start with IV therapy and switch to oral therapy when clinically stable. Amoxicillin 30–40 mg/kg/day PO div q8h for 10 days.
Parotitis, suppurative[85]	Oxacillin/nafcillin IV AND gentamicin IV, IM for 10 days; consider vancomycin if MRSA suspected (AIII).	Usually staphylococcal but occasionally coliform. Antimicrobial regimen without incision/drainage is adequate in >75% of cases.[86]

A. RECOMMENDED THERAPY FOR SELECT NEONATAL CONDITIONS *(continued)*

Condition	Therapy (evidence grade) ***See tables 2B–2D for neonatal dosages.***	Comments
Pulmonary infections		
– Empiric therapy for the neonate with early onset of pulmonary infiltrates (within the first 48–72 h after birth)	Ampicillin IV, IM AND gentamicin or ceftazidime/cefepime for 7–10 days; consider treating low-risk neonates for <7 days (see Comments).	For neonates with no additional risk factors for bacterial infection (eg, maternal chorioamnionitis) who (1) have negative blood cultures, (2) have no need for >8 h of oxygen, and (3) are asymptomatic at 48 h into therapy, 4 days may be sufficient therapy, based on babies with clinical pneumonia, none of whom had positive cultures.[87]
– Aspiration pneumonia[88]	Ampicillin IV, IM AND gentamicin IV, IM for 7–10 days (AIII)	Early-onset neonatal pneumonia may represent aspiration of amniotic fluid, particularly if fluid is not sterile. Mild aspiration episodes may not require antibiotic therapy.
– *Chlamydia trachomatis*[89]	Azithromycin PO, IV q24h for 5 days OR erythromycin ethylsuccinate PO for 14 days (AII)	Association of erythromycin and azithromycin with pyloric stenosis in infants treated <6 wk of age[90]
– *Mycoplasma hominis*[91,92]	Clindamycin PO, IV for 10 days (resistant to macrolides)	Pathogenic role in pneumonia not well-defined and clinical efficacy unknown; no association with BPD (BIII)
– Pertussis[93]	Azithromycin 10 mg/kg PO, IV q24h for 5 days OR erythromycin ethylsuccinate PO for 14 days (AII)	Association of erythromycin and azithromycin with pyloric stenosis in infants treated <6 wk of age[90] Alternatives: for >1 mo of age, clarithromycin for 7 days; for >2 mo of age, TMP/SMX for 14 days
– *P aeruginosa*[94]	Cefepime IV, IM for 10–14 days (AIII)	Alternatives: ceftazidime AND tobramycin, meropenem, OR pip/tazo AND tobramycin

– Respiratory syncytial virus[95]	Treatment (see Comments). Prophylaxis: palivizumab (a monoclonal antibody) 15 mg/kg IM monthly (max 5 doses) for the following high-risk infants (AI): In first year after birth, palivizumab prophylaxis is recommended for infants born before 29 wk 0 days' gestation. Palivizumab prophylaxis is not recommended for otherwise healthy infants born at ≥29 wk 0 days' gestation. In first year after birth, palivizumab prophylaxis is recommended for preterm infants with CLD of prematurity, defined as birth at <32 wk 0 days' gestation and a requirement for >21% oxygen for at least 28 days after birth or at 36 wk of PMA. Clinicians may administer palivizumab prophylaxis in the first year after birth to certain infants with hemodynamically significant heart disease.	Aerosol ribavirin (6-g vial to make 20-mg/mL solution in sterile water), aerosolized over 18–20 h daily for 3–5 days (BII), provides little benefit and should be considered for use only in life-threatening RSV infection. Difficulties in administration, complications with airway reactivity, concern for potential toxicities to health care professionals, and lack of definitive evidence of benefit preclude routine use. Palivizumab does not provide benefit in the treatment of an active RSV infection. Palivizumab prophylaxis may be considered for children <24 mo who will be profoundly immunocompromised during the RSV season. Palivizumab prophylaxis is not recommended in the second year after birth except for children who required at least 28 days of supplemental oxygen after birth and who continue to require medical support (supplemental oxygen, chronic corticosteroid therapy, or diuretic therapy) during the 6-mo period before the start of the second RSV season. Monthly prophylaxis should be discontinued in any child who experiences a breakthrough RSV hospitalization. Children with pulmonary abnormality or neuromuscular disease that impairs the ability to clear secretions from the upper airways may be considered for prophylaxis in the first year after birth. Insufficient data are available to recommend palivizumab prophylaxis for children with cystic fibrosis or Down syndrome. The burden of RSV disease and costs associated with transport from remote locations may result in a broader use of palivizumab for RSV prevention in Alaska Native populations and possibly in select other American Indian populations.[96,97] Palivizumab prophylaxis is not recommended for prevention of health care–associated RSV disease. In neonates, 2 monoclonal antibodies against RSV are in phase 3 clinical trials but are not yet approved, so stay tuned: we may have new options beyond palivizumab by 2023. RSV antivirals are currently investigational for neonates and young infants.

A. RECOMMENDED THERAPY FOR SELECT NEONATAL CONDITIONS *(continued)*

Condition	Therapy (evidence grade) ***See tables 2B–2D for neonatal dosages.***	Comments
– SARS-CoV-2 (COVID-19)	Remdesivir (AII) 5 mg/kg on day 1, followed by 2.5 mg/kg/day for up to 10 days	Must be ≥28 days of age and ≥3 kg, with positive result on SARS-CoV-2 viral testing. Consider corticosteroids. Remdesivir for preterm infants not FDA approved or covered by Emergency Use Authorization; consultation with pediatric ID specialist recommended.
– *S aureus*[20,98–100]	MSSA: oxacillin/nafcillin IV (AIII). MRSA: ceftaroline IV (BIII) OR vancomycin IV (BII). Duration of therapy depends on extent of disease (pneumonia vs pulmonary abscesses vs empyema) and should be individualized with therapy up to ≥21 days.	Alternative for MSSA: cefazolin IV Alternatives for MRSA: clindamycin (if susceptible) (BIII) or linezolid (CIII) Addition of rifampin or linezolid if persistently positive cultures (AIII) Thoracostomy drainage of empyema
– Group B streptococcus[101,102]	Penicillin G IV OR ampicillin IV, IM for 10 days (AIII)	For serious infections, ADD gentamicin for synergy until clinically improved. No prospective, randomized data on the efficacy of a 7-day treatment course.
– *Ureaplasma* spp (*urealyticum* or *parvum*)[103]	Azithromycin[104] IV 20 mg/kg once daily for 3 days (BII)[105]	Pathogenic role of *Ureaplasma* not well-defined and BPD prophylaxis not currently recommended. Clinical trials are ongoing.[106] If only the nasogastric route is available, 10 mg/kg PO q12h × 6 can be trialed instead of 20 mg/kg to improve gastrointestinal tolerability, but the absorption has not been evaluated and this approach may not achieve the same concentrations as IV. Many *Ureaplasma* spp resistant to erythromycin. Association of erythromycin and pyloric stenosis in young infants.

Sepsis and meningitis[100,107,108] Duration of therapy: 10 days for sepsis without a focus (AIII); minimum of 21 days for gram-negative meningitis (or at least 14 days after CSF is sterile) and 14–21 days for GBS meningitis and other gram-positive bacteria (AIII). There are no prospective, controlled studies on 5- or 7-day courses for mild or presumed sepsis.		
– Initial therapy, organism unknown	Ampicillin IV AND a second agent, either cefepime/ceftazidime IV or gentamicin IV, IM (AII)	Gentamicin preferred over cephalosporins for empiric therapy for sepsis when meningitis has been ruled out. Cephalosporin preferred if meningitis suspected or cannot be excluded clinically or by lumbar puncture (AIII). For locations with a high rate (≥10%) of ESBL-producing *E coli*, and in which meningitis is suspected, empiric therapy with meropenem is preferred over cephalosporins. Initial empiric therapy for nosocomial infection should be based on each hospital's pathogens and susceptibilities. **Essential:** Always narrow antibiotic coverage once susceptibility data are available.
– *Bacteroides fragilis*	Metronidazole or meropenem IV, IM (AIII)	Alternative: clindamycin, but increasing resistance reported
– CRO[109]	Ceftazidime/avibactam IV 40 mg/kg q8h (see Chapter 18) (BIII)	Combination options: amikacin, colistin IV 2.5 mg/kg q12h.[110] ADD aztreonam if metallo-beta-lactamase producing (such as NDM or VIM, not currently prevalent in NICUs in the United States). Alternative: high-dose meropenem if CRO with MIC 4–8 mg/L. Consultation with ID specialist strongly recommended to assist with drug selection, monitoring, and acquisition of investigational agents if needed for emergency use (eg, meropenem/vaborbactam, imipenem/relebactam, fosfomycin, plazomicin).
– *Enterococcus* spp	Ampicillin IV, IM AND gentamicin IV, IM (AIII); for ampicillin-resistant organisms: vancomycin AND gentamicin IV (AIII)	Gentamicin needed with ampicillin or vancomycin for bactericidal activity; continue until clinical and microbiological response documented (AIII). For vancomycin-resistant enterococci that are also ampicillin resistant: linezolid (AIII).

A. RECOMMENDED THERAPY FOR SELECT NEONATAL CONDITIONS *(continued)*

Condition	Therapy (evidence grade) *See tables 2B–2D for neonatal dosages.*	Comments
– Enterovirus	Supportive therapy; no antivirals currently FDA approved	Pocapavir PO is currently under investigation for enterovirus (poliovirus). See Chapter 7. Pleconaril PO is currently under consideration for submission to FDA for approval for treatment of neonatal enteroviral sepsis syndrome.[111] As of May 2022, it is not available for compassionate use.
– *E coli*[107,108]	Cefepime/ceftazidime IV or gentamicin IV, IM (AII)	Cephalosporin preferred if meningitis suspected or cannot be excluded by lumbar puncture (AIII) For locations with a high rate (≥10%) of ESBL-producing *E coli*, and in which meningitis is suspected, empiric therapy with meropenem preferred over cephalosporins
– Group A or viridans streptococcus	Penicillin G or ampicillin IV (AII)	Penicillin resistance increasingly reported for *Staphylococcus mitis* isolates; alternatives: vancomycin or linezolid
– Group B streptococcus[101]	Penicillin G or ampicillin IV AND gentamicin IV, IM (AI)	Continue gentamicin until clinical and microbiological response documented (AIII). Duration of therapy: 10 days for bacteremia/sepsis (AII); minimum of 14 days for meningitis (AII).
– *Listeria monocytogenes*[112]	Ampicillin IV, IM AND gentamicin IV, IM (AIII)	Gentamicin is synergistic in vitro with ampicillin. Continue until clinical and microbiological response documented (AIII).
– *Neisseria gonorrhoeae*[113]	Ceftriaxone OR cefepime OR ceftazidime IV (AI)	Duration of therapy: 7 days for bacteremia/sepsis (AII), 10–14 days if meningitis is suspected or confirmed (BII). See Gonococcal earlier in this table under Conjunctivitis for recommendations.
– *Neisseria meningitidis*	Ceftriaxone OR cefepime OR ceftazidime IV (AI)	Duration of therapy: 7 days for bacteremia/sepsis (AII), 10–14 days if meningitis is suspected or confirmed (BII)

– *P aeruginosa*	Cefepime IV, IM OR ceftazidime IV, IM AND tobramycin IV, IM (AIII)	Meropenem is a suitable alternative (AIII). Pip/tazo should not be used for CNS infection.
– *Staphylococcus epidermidis* (or any coagulase-negative staphylococci)	Vancomycin IV (AIII)	Oxacillin/nafcillin and cefazolin are alternatives for methicillin-susceptible strains. Cefazolin does not enter CNS. Add rifampin if cultures persistently positive.[114] Alternatives: linezolid, ceftaroline.
– *S aureus*[20,98–100,115–117]	MSSA: oxacillin/nafcillin IV, IM or cefazolin IV, IM (AII) MRSA: vancomycin IV or ceftaroline IV (AIII)	Alternatives for MRSA: clindamycin (if susceptible), linezolid
Skin and soft tissues		
– Breast abscess[118]	Oxacillin/nafcillin IV, IM (for MSSA) OR vancomycin IV or ceftaroline IV (for MRSA). ADD cefepime/ceftazidime OR gentamicin if GNR seen on Gram stain (AIII).	Gram stain of expressed pus guides empiric therapy; vancomycin or ceftaroline if MRSA prevalent in community; other alternatives: clindamycin, linezolid; may need surgical drainage to minimize damage to breast tissue. Treatment duration individualized until clinical findings have completely resolved (AIII).
– Congenital cutaneous candidiasis[119]	AmB for 14 days, or 10 days if CSF culture negative (AII) Alternative: fluconazole if *Candida albicans* or other *Candida* spp with known fluconazole susceptibility	Treat promptly with full IV treatment dose, not prophylactic dosing or topical therapy. Diagnostic workup includes aerobic cultures of skin lesions, blood, and CSF. Pathology examination of placenta and umbilical cord if possible.
– Erysipelas (and other group A streptococcal infections)	Penicillin G IV for 5–7 days, followed by oral therapy (if bacteremia not present) to complete a 10-day course (AIII)	Alternative: ampicillin. GBS may produce similar cellulitis or nodular lesions.
– Impetigo neonatorum	MSSA: oxacillin/nafcillin IV, IM OR cephalexin (AIII) MRSA: vancomycin IV or ceftaroline IV for 5 days (AIII)	Systemic antibiotic therapy not usually required for superficial impetigo; local chlorhexidine cleansing may help with or without topical mupirocin (MRSA) or bacitracin (MSSA). Alternatives for MRSA: clindamycin IV, PO or linezolid IV, PO.

A. RECOMMENDED THERAPY FOR SELECT NEONATAL CONDITIONS *(continued)*

Condition	Therapy (evidence grade) *See tables 2B–2D for neonatal dosages.*	Comments
– *S aureus*[20,98,100,120]	MSSA: oxacillin/nafcillin IV, IM (AII) MRSA: ceftaroline IV (AIII) or vancomycin IV	Surgical drainage may be required. MRSA may cause necrotizing fasciitis. Alternatives for MRSA: clindamycin (if susceptible) IV, linezolid IV. Convalescent oral therapy if infection responds quickly to IV therapy.
– Group B streptococcus[101]	Penicillin G IV OR ampicillin IV, IM	Usually no pus formed Treatment duration dependent on extent of infection, 7–14 days
Syphilis, congenital (<1 mo of age)[121] When availability of penicillin is compromised, contact CDC. Evaluation and treatment do not depend on mother's HIV status. Obtain follow-up serology q2–3mo until nontreponemal test nonreactive or decreased 4-fold.		
– Proven or highly probable disease: (1) abnormal physical examination; (2) serum quantitative nontreponemal serologic titer 4-fold higher than mother's titer; or (3) positive dark field or fluorescent antibody test of body fluid(s)	Aqueous penicillin G 50,000 U/kg/dose q12h (day after birth 1–7), q8h (>7 days) IV OR procaine penicillin G 50,000 U/kg IM q24h for 10 days (AII)	Evaluation to determine type and duration of therapy: CSF analysis (VDRL, cell count, protein), CBC, and platelet count. Other tests, as clinically indicated, including long-bone radiography, chest radiography, liver function tests, cranial ultrasonography, ophthalmologic examination, and hearing test (ABR). If CSF positive, repeat spinal tap with CSF VDRL at 6 mo and, if abnormal, re-treat. If >1 day of therapy is missed, entire course is restarted.

– Normal physical examination, serum quantitative nontreponemal serologic titer ≤ maternal titer, and maternal treatment was (1) none, inadequate, or undocumented; (2) erythromycin, azithromycin, or other non-penicillin regimen; or (3) <4 wk before delivery.	Evaluation abnormal or not done completely: aqueous penicillin G 50,000 U/kg/dose q12h (day after birth 1–7), q8h (>7 days) IV OR procaine penicillin G 50,000 U/kg IM q24h for 10 days (AII) Evaluation normal: aqueous penicillin G 50,000 U/kg/dose q12h (day after birth 1–7), q8h (>7 days) IV OR procaine penicillin G 50,000 U/kg IM q24h for 10 days; OR penicillin G benzathine 50,000 U/kg/dose IM in a single dose (AIII)	Evaluation: CSF analysis, CBC with platelet count, long-bone radiographs. If >1 day of therapy is missed, entire course is restarted. Reliable follow-up important if only a single dose of penicillin benzathine given.
– Normal physical examination, serum quantitative nontreponemal serologic titer ≤ maternal titer, mother treated adequately during pregnancy and >4 wk before delivery; no evidence of reinfection or relapse in mother	Penicillin G benzathine 50,000 U/kg/dose IM in a single dose (AIII)	No evaluation required. Some experts would not treat but provide close serologic follow-up.

A. RECOMMENDED THERAPY FOR SELECT NEONATAL CONDITIONS *(continued)*

Condition	Therapy (evidence grade) ***See tables 2B–2D for neonatal dosages.***	Comments
– Normal physical examination, serum quantitative nontreponemal serologic titer ≤ maternal titer, mother treated adequately before pregnancy	No treatment	No evaluation required. Some experts would treat with penicillin G benzathine 50,000 U/kg as a single IM injection, particularly if follow-up is uncertain.
Syphilis, congenital (>1 mo of age)[121]	Aqueous penicillin G crystalline 200,000–300,000 U/kg/day IV div q4–6h for 10 days (AII)	Evaluation to determine type and duration of therapy: CSF analysis (VDRL, cell count, protein), CBC, and platelet count. Other tests as clinically indicated, including long-bone radiography, chest radiography, liver function tests, neuroimaging, ophthalmologic examination, and hearing evaluation. If there are no clinical manifestations of disease, CSF examination is normal, and CSF VDRL test result is nonreactive, some specialists would treat with up to 3 weekly doses of penicillin G benzathine 50,000 U/kg IM. Some experts would provide a single dose of penicillin G benzathine 50,000 U/kg IM after 10 days of parenteral treatment, but value of this additional therapy is not well-documented.
Tetanus neonatorum[122]	Metronidazole IV, PO (alternative: penicillin G IV) for 10–14 days (AIII) Human TIG 3,000–6,000 U IM for 1 dose (AIII)	Wound cleaning and debridement vital; IVIG (200–400 mg/kg) is an alternative if TIG not available; equine tetanus antitoxin not available in the United States but is alternative to TIG.
Toxoplasmosis, congenital[123,124]	Sulfadiazine 100 mg/kg/day PO div q12h AND pyrimethamine 2 mg/kg PO daily for 2 days (loading dose), then 1 mg/kg PO q24h for 2–6 mo, then 3 times weekly (M-W-F) up to 1 y (AII) Folinic acid (leucovorin) 10 mg 3 times weekly (AII)	Corticosteroids (1 mg/kg/day div q12h) if active chorioretinitis or CSF protein >1 g/dL (AIII). Round sulfadiazine dose to 125 or 250 mg (¼ or ½ of 500-mg tab); round pyrimethamine dose to 6.25 or 12.5 mg (¼ or ½ of 25-mg tab). OK to crush tabs to give with feeding. Start sulfadiazine after neonatal jaundice has resolved. Therapy is effective against only active trophozoites, not cysts.

Urinary tract infection[125]

No prophylaxis for grades 1–3 reflux.[126,127]

In neonates with reflux, prophylaxis reduces recurrences but increases likelihood of recurrences being due to resistant organisms. Prophylaxis does not affect renal scarring.[126]

– Initial therapy, organism unknown	Ampicillin AND gentamicin; OR ampicillin AND cefepime/ceftazidime, pending culture and susceptibility test results, for 7–10 days	Renal ultrasound and VCUG indicated after first UTI to identify abnormalities of urinary tract Oral therapy acceptable once neonate asymptomatic and culture sterile
– Coliform bacteria (eg, *E coli, Klebsiella, Enterobacter, Serratia*)	Cefepime/ceftazidime IV, IM OR, in absence of renal or perinephric abscess, gentamicin IV, IM for 7–10 days (AII)	Ampicillin or cefazolin used for susceptible organisms
– *Enterococcus*	Ampicillin IV, IM for 7 days for cystitis, may need 10–14 days for pyelonephritis, add gentamicin until cultures are sterile (AIII); for ampicillin resistance, use vancomycin, add gentamicin until cultures are sterile.	Aminoglycoside needed with ampicillin or vancomycin for synergistic bactericidal activity (assuming organisms are susceptible to an aminoglycoside)
– *P aeruginosa*	Cefepime IV, IM, OR ceftazidime IV, IM OR, in absence of renal or perinephric abscess, tobramycin IV, IM for 7–10 days (AIII)	Meropenem is an alternative.
– *Candida* spp[35–37]	See Candidiasis earlier in this table under Fungal infections.	

B. ANTIMICROBIAL DOSAGES FOR NEONATES—Lead author Jason Sauberan, assisted by the editors and John Van Den Anker

Antimicrobial	Route	Dosages (mg/kg/day) and Intervals of Administration				
		Chronologic Age ≤28 days				Chronologic Age 29–60 days
		Body Weight ≤2,000 g		Body Weight >2,000 g		
		0–7 days old	8–28 days old	0–7 days old	8–28 days old	
NOTE: This table contains empiric dosage recommendations for each agent listed. See Table 2A for more details of dosages for specific pathogens in specific tissue sites and for information on anti-influenza and antiretroviral drug dosages.						
Acyclovir (treatment of acute disease)	IV	60 div q8h	60 div q8h	60 div q8h	60 div q8h	60 div q8h
Acyclovir (suppression following treatment of acute disease)	PO	—	900/m²/day div q8h	—	900/m²/day div q8h	900/m²/day div q8h
Only IV acyclovir should be used for the treatment of acute neonatal HSV disease. Oral suppression therapy for a duration of 6 mo after completion of initial IV treatment.						
Amoxicillin	PO	—	75 div q12h	100 div q12h	100 div q12h	100 div q12h
Amoxicillin/clavulanate[a]	PO	—	—	30 div q12h	30 div q12h	30 div q12h
Amphotericin B						
– Deoxycholate	IV	1 q24h	1 q24h	1 q24h	1 q24h	1 q24h
– Lipid complex	IV	5 q24h	5 q24h	5 q24h	5 q24h	5 q24h
– Liposomal	IV	5 q24h	5 q24h	5 q24h	5 q24h	5 q24h
Ampicillin	IV, IM	100 div q12h	150 div q12h	150 div q8h	150 div q8h	200 div q6h
Ampicillin (GBS meningitis)	IV	300 div q8h	300 div q6h	300 div q8h	300 div q6h	300 div q6h
Anidulafungin[b]	IV	1.5 q24h	1.5 q24h	1.5 q24h	1.5 q24h	1.5 q24h
Azithromycin[c]	IV, PO	10 q24h	10 q24h	10 q24h	10 q24h	10 q24h

Aztreonam	IV, IM	60 div q12h	90 div q8h[d]	90 div q8h	120 div q6h	120 div q6h
Cefazolin (Enterobacterales)[e]	IV, IM	50 div q12h	75 div q8h	100 div q12h	150 div q8h	100–150 div q6–8h
Cefazolin (MSSA)	IV, IM	50 div q12h	50 div q12h	75 div q8h	75 div q8h	75 div q8h
Cefepime	IV, IM	60 div q12h	60 div q12h	100 div q12h	100 div q12h	150 div q8h[f]
Cefotaxime	IV, IM	100 div q12h	150 div q8h	100 div q12h	150 div q6h	200 div q6h
Ceftaroline	IV, IM	12 div q12h[g]	18 div q8h[g]	18 div q8h	18 div q8h	18 div q8h
Ceftazidime	IV, IM	100 div q12h	150 div q8h[d]	100 div q12h	150 div q8h	150 div q8h
Ceftriaxone[h]	IV, IM	—	—	50 q24h	50 q24h	50 q24h
Ciprofloxacin	IV	15 div q12h	15 div q12h	25 div q12h	25 div q12h	25 div q12h
Clindamycin	IV, IM, PO	15 div q8h	15 div q8h	21 div q8h	27 div q8h	30 div q8h
Daptomycin (Potential neurotoxicity; use cautiously if no other options.)	IV	12 div q12h	12 div q12h	12 div q12h	12 div q12h	12 div q12h
Erythromycin	IV, PO	40 div q6h	40 div q6h	40 div q6h	40 div q6h	40 div q6h
Fluconazole						
– Treatment[i]	IV, PO	12 q24h	12 q24h	12 q24h	12 q24h	12 q24h
– Prophylaxis	IV, PO	6 mg/kg/dose twice weekly	6 mg/kg/dose twice weekly	6 mg/kg/dose twice weekly	6 mg/kg/dose twice weekly	6 mg/kg/dose twice weekly
Flucytosine[j]	PO	75 div q8h	100 div q6h[d]	100 div q6h	100 div q6h	100 div q6h
Ganciclovir	IV	12 div q12h	12 div q12h	12 div q12h	12 div q12h	12 div q12h
Linezolid	IV, PO	20 div q12h	30 div q8h	30 div q8h	30 div q8h	30 div q8h

B. ANTIMICROBIAL DOSAGES FOR NEONATES *(continued)*—Lead author Jason Sauberan, assisted by the editors and John Van Den Anker

Antimicrobial	Route	Dosages (mg/kg/day) and Intervals of Administration				
		Chronologic Age ≤28 days				Chronologic Age 29–60 days
		Body Weight ≤2,000 g		Body Weight >2,000 g		
		0–7 days old	8–28 days old	0–7 days old	8–28 days old	
Meropenem						
– Sepsis, IAI[k]	IV	40 div q12h	60 div q8h[k]	60 div q8h	90 div q8h[k]	90 div q8h
– Meningitis – CRO with MIC 4–8 mg/L	IV	80 div q12h	120 div q8h[k]	120 div q8h	120 div q8h	120 div q8h
Metronidazole[l]	IV, PO	15 div q12h	15 div q12h	22.5 div q8h	30 div q8h	30 div q8h
Micafungin	IV	10 q24h	10 q24h	10 q24h	10 q24h	10 q24h
Nafcillin,[m] oxacillin[m]	IV, IM	50 div q12h	75 div q8h[d]	75 div q8h	100 div q6h	150 div q6h
Penicillin G benzathine	IM	50,000 U	50,000 U	50,000 U	50,000 U	50,000 U
Penicillin G crystalline (GBS sepsis, congenital syphilis)	IV	100,000 U div q12h	150,000 U div q8h	100,000 U div q12h	150,000 U div q8h	200,000 U div q6h
Penicillin G crystalline (GBS meningitis)	IV	450,000 U div q8h	500,000 U div q6h	450,000 U div q8h	500,000 U div q6h	500,000 U div q6h
Penicillin G procaine	IM	50,000 U q24h	50,000 U q24h	50,000 U q24h	50,000 U q24h	50,000 U q24h
Piperacillin/tazobactam	IV	300 div q8h	320 div q6h[n]	320 div q6h	320 div q6h	320 div q6h
Rifampin[o]	IV, PO	10 q24h	10 q24h	10 q24h	10 q24h	10 q24h
Valganciclovir	PO	Insufficient data	Insufficient data	32 div q12h	32 div q12h	32 div q12h
Voriconazole[p]	IV	12 div q12h	12 div q12h	12 div q12h	12 div q12h	16 div q12h

Zidovudine	IV	3 div q12h[q]	3 div q12h[q]	6 div q12h	6 div q12h	See HIV prophylaxis in Table 2A.
	PO	4 div q12h[q]	4 div q12h[q]	8 div q12h	8 div q12h	See HIV prophylaxis in Table 2A.

[a] For susceptible *H influenzae* infections. Higher dosing 75 mg/kg/day div q8h needed for IV to oral step-down treatment of susceptible *E coli.* May use 25- or 50-mg/mL formulation.

[b] Loading dose 3 mg/kg followed 24 h later by maintenance dose listed.

[c] See Table 2A for pathogen-specific dosing.

[d] Use 0–7 days old dosing until 14 days old if birth weight <1,000 g.

[e] If isolate MIC <8 mg/L and no CNS focus.

[f] Infusion over 3 h, or 200 mg/kg/day div q6h, to treat organisms with MIC 8 mg/L.

[g] Serum concentration monitoring recommended by high-performance liquid chromatography assay (available commercially) to avoid excessive exposure, although no specific toxicity is associated with this cephalosporin. Goal exposure is a concentration > MIC (usually 0.5 or 1 mg/L) at 60% of the dosing interval post-dose.

[h] Usually avoided in neonates. Can be considered for transitioning to outpatient treatment of GBS bacteremia in well-appearing neonates with low risk for hyperbilirubinemia. Contraindicated if concomitant IV calcium (see Notes at beginning of chapter).

[i] Loading dose 25 mg/kg followed 24 h later by maintenance dose listed.

[j] Desired serum concentrations peak 60–80 mg/L, trough 5–10 mg/L to achieve time-above-MIC of >40% for invasive candidiasis (trough 10–20 mg/L acceptable for *Cryptococcus*). Dose range 50–100 mg/kg/day. Always use in combination with other agents; be alert to development of resistance. Time-above-MIC of >40% is target for invasive candidiasis.

[k] Adjust dosage after 14 days of age instead of after 7 days of age.

[l] Loading dose 15 mg/kg.

[m] Double the dose for meningitis.

[n] When PMA reaches >30 wk.

[o] May require 15 mg/kg q24h after 14 days of age at any weight to clear persistent *Staphylococcus* bacteremia. Monitor potential toxicities with platelet count and liver function testing.

[p] Adjust dose to target trough 2–5 mg/L (see Aspergillosis in Table 2A under Fungal Infections).

[q] Starting dose if GA <35 wk 0 days and PNA ≤14 days. See HIV prophylaxis in Table 2A for ZDV dosage after 2 wk of age and for NVP and 3TC recommendations.

C. AMINOGLYCOSIDES

		Empiric Dosage (mg/kg/dose) by Gestational and Postnatal Ages					
		<30 wk		30–34 wk[a]		≥35 wk[a]	
Medication	**Route**	**0–14 days**	**>14 days**	**0–10 days**	**>10 days**	**0–7 days**	**>7 days**
Amikacin[b]	IV, IM	15 q48h	15 q36h	15 q36h	15 q24h	15 q24h	17.5 q24h
Gentamicin[c]	IV, IM	5 q48h	5 q36h	5 q36h	5 q24h	4 q24h	5 q24h
Tobramycin[c]	IV, IM	5 q48h	5 q36h	5 q36h	5 q24h	4 q24h	5 q24h

[a] If >60 days of age, see Chapter 18.

[b] Desired serum or plasma concentrations: 20–35 mg/L or 10 × MIC (peak), <7 mg/L (trough).

[c] Desired serum or plasma concentrations: 6–12 mg/L or 10 × MIC (peak), <2 mg/L (trough). A 7.5 mg/kg dose q48h, or q36h if ≥30 wk of GA and >7 days' PNA, more likely to achieve desired concentrations if pathogen MIC = 1 mg/L.[128]

D. VANCOMYCIN[a]

Empiric Dosage by Gestational Age and SCr
Begin with a 20 mg/kg loading dose.

≤28 wk of GA			>28 wk of GA		
SCr (mg/dL)	**Dose (mg/kg)**	**Frequency**	**SCr (mg/dL)**	**Dose (mg/kg)**	**Frequency**
<0.5	15	q12h	<0.7	15	q12h
0.5–0.7	20	q24h	0.7–0.9	20	q24h
0.8–1.0	15	q24h	1.0–1.2	15	q24h
1.1–1.4	10	q24h	1.3–1.6	10	q24h
>1.4	15	q48h	>1.6	15	q48h

[a] SCr concentrations normally fluctuate and are partly influenced by transplacental maternal creatinine in the first week after birth. Cautious use of creatinine-based dosing strategy with frequent reassessment of renal function and vancomycin serum concentrations is recommended in neonates ≤7 days old. Desired serum concentrations: a 24-h AUC:MIC of at least 400 mg·h/L is recommended based on adult studies of invasive MRSA infections. The AUC is best calculated from 2 concentrations (ie, peak and trough) rather than 1 trough serum concentration. When AUC calculation is not feasible, a trough concentration ≥10 mg/L is very highly likely (>90%) to achieve the goal AUC target in neonates when the MIC is 1 mg/L. However, troughs as low as 7 mg/L can still achieve an AUC ≥400 in some preterm neonates due to their slower clearance. Thus, AUC is preferred over trough monitoring to prevent unnecessary overexposure. For centers where invasive MRSA infection is relatively common or where MRSA with MIC of 1 mg/L is common, an online dosing tool is available that may improve the likelihood of empirically achieving AUC ≥400, compared with Table 2D (https://connect.insight-rx.com/neovanco; accessed September 26, 2022). If >60 days of age, see Chapter 18.

E. Use of Antimicrobials During Pregnancy or Breastfeeding

The use of antimicrobials during pregnancy and lactation should balance benefit to the mother with the risk for fetal and neonatal toxicity (including anatomic anomalies with fetal exposure). A number of factors determine the degree of transfer of antibiotics across the placenta: lipid solubility, degree of ionization, molecular weight, protein binding, placental maturation, and placental and fetal blood flow. The Pregnancy and Lactation Labeling Rule of 2014 began replacing the traditional A to X risk categories with narrative summaries of risks associated with the use of a drug during pregnancy and lactation for the mother, the fetus, and the breastfeeding newborn/infant/child. The risk categories from A to X were felt to be too simplistic. This transition was completed in 2020. Risks are now all clearly noted, and for drugs with high fetal risk, black box warnings are included (eg, ribavirin).[129] Fetal serum antibiotic concentrations (or cord blood concentrations) following maternal administration have not been systematically studied, but new pharmacokinetic models of transplacental drug transfer and fetal metabolism have recently been developed to provide some insight into fetal drug exposure.[130–132] The following commonly used drugs appear to achieve fetal concentrations that are equal to or only slightly less than those in the mother: penicillin G, amoxicillin, ampicillin, sulfonamides, trimethoprim, tetracyclines, and oseltamivir. The aminoglycoside concentrations in fetal serum are 20% to 50% of those in maternal serum. Cephalosporins, carbapenems, nafcillin, oxacillin, clindamycin, and vancomycin penetrate poorly (10%–30%), and fetal concentrations of erythromycin and azithromycin are less than 10% of those in the mother.

The most current updated information on the pharmacokinetics and safety of antimicrobials and other agents in human milk can be found at the National Library of Medicine LactMed website (www.ncbi.nlm.nih.gov/books/NBK501922; accessed September 26, 2022).[133]

In general, neonatal exposure to antimicrobials in human milk is minimal or insignificant. Aminoglycosides, beta-lactams, ciprofloxacin, clindamycin, macrolides, fluconazole, and agents for tuberculosis are considered safe for the mother to take during breastfeeding.[134,135] The most commonly reported neonatal side effect of maternal antimicrobial use during breastfeeding is increased stool output.[136] Clinicians should recommend that mothers alert their pediatric health care professional if stool output changes occur. Maternal treatment with sulfa-containing antibiotics should be approached with caution in the breastfed infant who is jaundiced or ill.

3. Preferred Therapy for Specific Bacterial and Mycobacterial Pathogens

NOTES

- For fungal, viral, and parasitic infections, see chapters 5, 7, and 9, respectively.
- Limitations of space do not permit listing of all possible alternative antimicrobials.
- Again this year, cefotaxime, a third-generation cephalosporin approved by the US Food and Drug Administration for children more than 3 decades ago, is not given as an option for therapy for pathogens, as it is not routinely available in the United States. Ceftriaxone has a virtually identical antibacterial spectrum of activity to cefotaxime; cefepime is very similar in gram-positive activity but adds *Pseudomonas aeruginosa* (and some enhanced activity for *Enterobacter*, *Serratia*, and *Citrobacter*) to the gram-negative activity of cefotaxime; ceftazidime adds *Pseudomonas* activity but loses gram-positive activity, compared with cefotaxime. Cefepime,[1] ceftazidime,[2] and, of course, ceftriaxone have been documented to be effective in pediatric meningitis clinical trials.
- **Abbreviations:** amox/clav, amoxicillin/clavulanate (Augmentin); amp/sul, ampicillin/sulbactam; bid, twice daily; CA-MRSA, community-associated methicillin-resistant *Staphylococcus aureus;* CAZ/AVI, ceftazidime/avibactam; CDC, Centers for Disease Control and Prevention; CNS, central nervous system; div, divided; ESBL, extended-spectrum beta-lactamase; FDA, US Food and Drug Administration; HACEK, *Haemophilus aphrophilus, Actinobacillus actinomycetemcomitans, Cardiobacterium hominis, Eikenella corrodens,* and *Kingella* spp; HRSA, Health Resources and Services Administration; IM, intramuscular; INH, isoniazid; IV, intravenous; IVIG, intravenous immunoglobulin; KPC, *Klebsiella pneumoniae* carbapenemase; MDR, multidrug resistant; mero/vabor, meropenem/vaborbactam; MIC, minimal inhibitory concentration; MRSA, methicillin-resistant *S aureus;* MSSA, methicillin-susceptible *S aureus;* NARMS, National Antimicrobial Resistance Monitoring System for Enteric Bacteria; NDM, New Delhi metallo-beta-lactamase; PCV13, pneumococcal 13-valent conjugate vaccine; pen-S, penicillin-susceptible; pip/tazo, piperacillin/tazobactam; PO, oral; PZA, pyrazinamide; spp, species; tid, 3 times daily; TIG, tetanus immune globulin; TMP/SMX, trimethoprim/sulfamethoxazole; UTI, urinary tract infection.

A. COMMON BACTERIAL PATHOGENS AND USUAL PATTERN OF SUSCEPTIBILITY TO ANTIBIOTICS (GRAM POSITIVE)

	Commonly Used Antibiotics (One Agent per Class Listed) (scale — to ++ defined in footnote)			
	Penicillin	**Ampicillin/ Amoxicillin**	**Amoxicillin/ Clavulanate**	**Methicillin/ Oxacillin**
Enterococcus faecalis[a]	++	++	+	—
Enterococcus faecium[a]	++	++	+	—
Nocardia spp[b]	—	—	±	—
Staphylococcus, coagulase negative	—	—	—	±
Staphylococcus aureus, methicillin-resistant	—	—	—	—
Staphylococcus aureus, methicillin-susceptible	—	—	—	++
Streptococcus pneumoniae	++	++	++	+
Streptococcus pyogenes	++	++	++	++

NOTE: ++ = preferred; **+** = acceptable; **±** = possibly effective (see text for further discussion); **—** = unlikely to be effective.

[a] Need to add gentamicin or other aminoglycoside to ampicillin/penicillin or vancomycin for in vitro bactericidal activity.

[b] *Nocardia* is usually susceptible to TMP/SMX, carbapenems (meropenem), and amikacin.

Commonly Used Antibiotics (One Agent per Class Listed) (scale — to ++ defined in footnote)					
Cefazolin/ Cephalexin	Vancomycin	Clindamycin	Linezolid	Daptomycin	Ceftaroline
–	+	–	+	+	–
–	+	–	+	+	–
–	–	–	+	–	–
±	++	+	++	++	++
–	++	++	++	++	++
++	++	+	++	++	++
++	+	+	++	+	++
++	+	++	+	++	++

B. COMMON BACTERIAL PATHOGENS AND USUAL PATTERN OF SUSCEPTIBILITY TO ANTIBIOTICS (GRAM NEGATIVE)[a]

	Commonly Used Antibiotics (One Agent per Class Listed) (scale — to ++ defined in footnote)					
	Ampicillin/ Amoxicillin	**Amoxicillin/ Clavulanate**	**Cefazolin/ Cephalexin**	**Cefuroxime**	**Ceftriaxone**	**Ceftazidime/ Avibactam**
Acinetobacter spp	—	—	—	—	+	+
Citrobacter spp	—	—	—	+	+	++
Enterobacter spp[b]	—	—	—	±	+	++
Escherichia coli[c]	+	+	+	++[d]	++[d]	++
Haemophilus influenzae[f]	+	++	+	++	++	++
Klebsiella spp[c]	—	—	+	++	++	++
Neisseria meningitidis	++	++		+	++	+
Pseudomonas aeruginosa	—	—	—	—	—	++
Salmonella, non-typhoid spp	+	++			++	++
Serratia spp[b]	—	—	—	±	+	++
Shigella spp	+	++	+	+	++	++
Stenotrophomonas maltophilia	—	—	—	—	—	+

NOTE: **++** = preferred; **+** = acceptable; **±** = possibly effective (see text for further discussion); **—** = unlikely to be effective; [blank cell] = untested.

[a] CDC (NARMS) statistics for each state, by year, are found for many enteric pathogens on the CDC website at https://wwwn.cdc.gov/narmsnow and are also provided by the SENTRY surveillance system (JMI Laboratories); we also use current pediatric hospital antibiograms from the editors' hospitals to assess pediatric trends. When sufficient data are available, pediatric community isolate susceptibility data are used. Nosocomial resistance patterns may be quite different, usually with increased resistance, particularly in adults; please check your local/regional hospital antibiogram for your local susceptibility patterns.

[b] AmpC will be constitutively produced in low frequency in every population of organisms and will be selected out during therapy with 3rd-generation cephalosporins if used as single-agent therapy.

[c] Rare carbapenem-resistant isolates in pediatrics (KPC, NDM strains).

[d] Will be resistant to virtually all current cephalosporins if ESBL producing.

[e] Follow the MIC, not the report for susceptible (S), intermediate (I), or resistant (R), as some ESBL producers will have low MICs and can be effectively treated with higher dosages.

[f] Will be resistant to ampicillin/amoxicillin if beta-lactamase producing.

Commonly Used Antibiotics (One Agent per Class Listed) (scale — to ++ defined in footnote)						
Ceftazidime	Cefepime	Meropenem/ Imipenem	Piperacillin/ Tazobactam	TMP/SMX	Ciprofloxacin	Gentamicin
+	+	+	+	+	+	—
+	++	++	+	++	++	+
+	++	++	+	++	++	+
++[d]	++[e]	++	++	+	++	+
++	++	++	++	++	++	±
++	++[e]	++	++	++	++	++
+	++	++	++		+	
+	++	++	++	—	++	+
++	++	++	++	++	++	+
+	++	++	+	++	++	++
++	++	++	++	±	++	
+	±	—	±	++	+	—

C. COMMON BACTERIAL PATHOGENS AND USUAL PATTERN OF SUSCEPTIBILITY TO ANTIBIOTICS (ANAEROBES)

	Commonly Used Antibiotics (One Agent per Class Listed) (scale — to ++ defined in footnote)				
	Penicillin	**Ampicillin/ Amoxicillin**	**Amoxicillin/ Clavulanate**	**Cefazolin**	**Cefoxitin**
Anaerobic streptococci	++	++	++	++	++
Bacteroides fragilis	±	±	++	—	+
Clostridia (eg, *tetani, perfringens*)	++	++	++		+
Clostridium difficile	—	—	—		—

NOTE: ++ = preferred; + = acceptable; ± = possibly effective (see text for further discussion); — = unlikely to be effective; [blank cell] = untested.

Commonly Used Antibiotics (One Agent per Class Listed) (scale — to ++ defined in footnote)					
Ceftriaxone/ Cefepime	**Meropenem/ Imipenem**	**Piperacillin/ Tazobactam**	**Metronidazole**	**Clindamycin**	**Vancomycin**
++	++	++	++	++	++
–	++	++	++	+	
±	++	++	++	+	++
–	++		++	–	++

D. PREFERRED THERAPY FOR SPECIFIC BACTERIAL AND MYCOBACTERIAL PATHOGENS

Organism	Clinical Illness	Drug of Choice (evidence grade)	Alternatives
Acinetobacter baumannii[3–7]	Sepsis, meningitis, nosocomial pneumonia, wound infection	Cefepime; meropenem (BIII) or other carbapenem	Use culture results to guide therapy. Consult an infectious disease specialist for highly MDR strains, as there are multiple mechanisms of resistance, with no single antibiotic that is routinely effective against all strains. Possible options: ceftazidime ± avibactam, amp/sul, pip/tazo, TMP/SMX, ciprofloxacin, tigecycline/eravacycline, colistin/polymyxin B/cefiderocol. Cefiderocol is currently under active pediatric investigation. Watch for emergence of resistance *during* therapy, including to colistin. Consider combination therapy for life-threatening infection.[7] Inhaled colistin for pneumonia caused by MDR strains (BIII).
Actinomyces israelii[8,9]	Actinomycosis (cervicofacial, thoracic, abdominal)	Penicillin G; ampicillin (CIII)	Amoxicillin, doxycycline, clindamycin, ceftriaxone, meropenem, pip/tazo, linezolid
Aeromonas hydrophila[10]	Diarrhea	Ciprofloxacin (CIII)	TMP/SMX, ceftriaxone, cefepime
	Sepsis, cellulitis, necrotizing fasciitis	Cefepime (BIII); ciprofloxacin (BIII)	Meropenem, TMP/SMX

Aggregatibacter (formerly *Actinobacillus*) *actinomycetemcomitans*[11]	Periodontitis, abscesses (including brain), endocarditis	Ceftriaxone (CIII)	Ampicillin/amoxicillin for beta-lactamase–negative strains, or amox/clav, doxycycline, TMP/SMX, ciprofloxacin
Aggregatibacter (formerly *Haemophilus*) *aphrophilus*[12]	Sepsis, endocarditis, abscesses (including brain)	Ceftriaxone (AII); OR ampicillin (if beta-lactamase negative) AND gentamicin (BII)	Ciprofloxacin, amox/clav (for strains resistant to ampicillin) One of the HACEK organisms that cause endocarditis
Anaplasma (formerly *Ehrlichia*) *phagocytophilum*[13,14]	Human granulocytic anaplasmosis	Doxycycline (all ages) (AII)	Rifampin, levofloxacin
Arcanobacterium haemolyticum[15]	Pharyngitis, cellulitis, Lemierre syndrome	Azithromycin; penicillin (BIII)	Erythromycin, amoxicillin, ceftriaxone, clindamycin, vancomycin
Bacillus anthracis[16]	Anthrax (cutaneous, gastrointestinal, inhalational, meningoencephalitis)	Ciprofloxacin (regardless of age) (AIII). For invasive systemic infection, use combination therapy. Wild-type strains are likely to be susceptible to penicillin.	Doxycycline, amoxicillin, levofloxacin, clindamycin, penicillin G, vancomycin, meropenem. Bioterror strains may be antibiotic resistant.
Bacillus cereus or *subtilis*[17,18]	Sepsis; toxin-mediated gastroenteritis	Vancomycin (BIII)	Clindamycin, ciprofloxacin, linezolid, daptomycin
Bacteroides fragilis[19,20]	Peritonitis, sepsis, abscesses	Metronidazole (AI)	Meropenem or imipenem (AI); pip/tazo (AI); amox/clav (BII). Recent surveillance suggests resistance of up to 25%–50% globally for clindamycin.
Bacteroides, other spp[19,20]	Pneumonia, sepsis, abscesses	Metronidazole (BII)	Meropenem or imipenem; penicillin G or ampicillin if beta-lactamase negative

D. PREFERRED THERAPY FOR SPECIFIC BACTERIAL AND MYCOBACTERIAL PATHOGENS *(continued)*

Organism	Clinical Illness	Drug of Choice (evidence grade)	Alternatives
Bartonella henselae[21,22]	Cat-scratch disease	Azithromycin for lymph node disease (BII); gentamicin AND TMP/SMX AND rifampin for hepatosplenic disease and osteomyelitis (BIII). For CNS infection, use ceftriaxone AND gentamicin ± TMP/SMX (BIII).	Ciprofloxacin, doxycycline
Bartonella quintana[22,23]	Bacillary angiomatosis, peliosis hepatis, endocarditis	Gentamicin plus rifampin, OR doxycycline plus rifampin (BIII); erythromycin; ciprofloxacin (BIII)	Azithromycin, doxycycline
Bordetella pertussis, parapertussis[24,25]	Pertussis	Azithromycin (AIII); erythromycin (BII)	Clarithromycin, TMP/SMX, ciprofloxacin (in vitro data)
Borrelia burgdorferi, Lyme disease[26,27]	Treatment based on stage of infection (See Lyme disease in Chapter 1, Table 1L.)	Doxycycline for all ages (AII); amoxicillin or cefuroxime can be used in children ≤7 y (AIII); ceftriaxone IV for CNS/meningitis (AII).	Azithromycin. A single course of doxycycline is not associated with detectable tooth staining in children.
Borrelia hermsii, turicatae, parkeri; tick-borne relapsing fever[28,29]	Relapsing fever	Doxycycline for all ages (AIII)	Penicillin or erythromycin in children intolerant of doxycycline (BIII). A single course of doxycycline is not associated with detectable tooth staining in children.
Borrelia recurrentis, louse-borne relapsing fever[28,29]	Relapsing fever	Single-dose doxycycline for all ages (AIII)	Penicillin or erythromycin in children intolerant of doxycycline (BIII). Amoxicillin; ceftriaxone. A single course of doxycycline is not associated with detectable tooth staining in children.

Brucella spp[30–32]	Brucellosis (See Chapter 1.)	Doxycycline AND rifampin (BIII); OR, for children ≤7 y: TMP/SMX AND rifampin (BIII)	For serious infection: doxycycline AND gentamicin AND rifampin; or TMP/SMX AND gentamicin AND rifampin (AIII). May require extended therapy (months).
Burkholderia cepacia complex[33–36]	Pneumonia, sepsis in immunocompromised children; pneumonia in children with cystic fibrosis[36]	Meropenem (BIII); for severe disease, consider combination therapy with TMP/SMX or levofloxacin (AIII).	Ceftolozane/tazobactam, doxycycline, minocycline, ceftazidime, CAZ/AVI, pip/tazo, ciprofloxacin, TMP/SMX. Aerosolized antibiotics may provide higher concentrations in lung.
Burkholderia pseudomallei[37–39]	Melioidosis	Meropenem (AIII) or ceftazidime (BIII), followed by prolonged TMP/SMX for 12 wk (AII)	TMP/SMX, doxycycline, or amox/clav for chronic disease
Campylobacter fetus[40–42]	Sepsis, meningitis in the neonate	Meropenem (BIII)	Ampicillin, gentamicin, erythromycin, ciprofloxacin
Campylobacter jejuni[42,43]	Diarrhea	Azithromycin (BII); erythromycin (BII)	Amox/clav, doxycycline, ciprofloxacin (very high rates of ciprofloxacin-resistant strains in Thailand, Hong Kong, and Spain)
Capnocytophaga canimorsus[44,45]	Sepsis after dog bite (increased risk with asplenia)	Pip/tazo OR meropenem; amox/clav (BIII)	Clindamycin, linezolid, penicillin G, imipenem, ciprofloxacin, ceftriaxone
Capnocytophaga ochracea[46,47]	Neonatal sepsis, abscesses	Ampicillin, ceftriaxone (BIII); amox/clav (BIII)	Meropenem, pip/tazo, ciprofloxacin
Cellulosimicrobium (formerly *Oerskovia*) *cellulans*[48]	Wound infection; catheter infection	Vancomycin ± rifampin (AIII)	Linezolid; resistant to beta-lactams, macrolides, clindamycin, aminoglycosides

D. PREFERRED THERAPY FOR SPECIFIC BACTERIAL AND MYCOBACTERIAL PATHOGENS *(continued)*

Organism	Clinical Illness	Drug of Choice (evidence grade)	Alternatives
Chlamydia trachomatis[49–51]	Lymphogranuloma venereum	Doxycycline (AII)	Azithromycin, erythromycin
	Urethritis, cervicitis	Doxycycline (AII)	Azithromycin, erythromycin, ofloxacin
	Inclusion conjunctivitis of newborn	Azithromycin (AIII)	Erythromycin
	Pneumonia of infancy	Azithromycin (AIII)	Erythromycin, ampicillin
	Trachoma	Azithromycin (AI)	Doxycycline, erythromycin
Chlamydophila (formerly *Chlamydia*) *pneumoniae*[49,50,52]	Pneumonia	Azithromycin (AII); erythromycin (AII)	Doxycycline, levofloxacin
Chlamydophila (formerly *Chlamydia*) *psittaci*[53]	Psittacosis	Doxycycline (AII) for >7 y; azithromycin (AIII) OR erythromycin (AIII) for ≤7 y	Levofloxacin
Chromobacterium violaceum[54–56]	Sepsis, pneumonia, abscesses	Meropenem ± ciprofloxacin depending on severity of the disease (AIII)	Susceptibility is variable. Other options may include TMP/SMX, cefepime, amikacin, imipenem, ceftriaxone, ceftazidime, and pip/tazo.
Citrobacter koseri (formerly *diversus*) and *freundii*[57,58]	Meningitis, sepsis	Cefepime should be active against most ampC beta-lactamase–expressing strains; meropenem will be active against both ampC and ESBL-expressing strains.	Ciprofloxacin, pip/tazo, ceftriaxone AND gentamicin, TMP/SMX, colistin Carbapenem-resistant strains now reported; may be susceptible to CAZ/AVI, mero/vabor, imipenem/relebactam, or cefiderocol[5,57]

Clostridioides (formerly *Clostridium*) *difficile*[59–61]	Antibiotic-associated colitis (See *Clostridioides difficile* in Chapter 1, Table 1H.)	Treatment stratified by severity and recurrence First episode Mild to moderate illness: metronidazole PO Moderate to severe illness: vancomycin PO or fidaxomicin PO[62] Severe and complicated/systemic: vancomycin PO AND metronidazole IV	Stop the predisposing antimicrobial therapy, if possible. For relapsing *C difficile* enteritis, consider pulse therapy with vancomycin (1 wk on/1 wk off for 3–4 cycles) or prolonged tapering therapy. No pediatric data on fecal transplant for recurrent disease.
Clostridium botulinum[63–65]	Botulism: foodborne; wound; potentially bioterror related	Botulism antitoxin heptavalent (equine) types A–G FDA approved in 2013 (www.fda.gov/vaccines-blood-biologics/approved-blood-products/bat-botulism-antitoxin-heptavalent-b-c-d-e-f-g-equine; accessed September 27, 2022). No antibiotic treatment except for wound botulism when treatment for vegetative organisms can be provided after antitoxin administered (no controlled data).	For more information, call your state health department or the CDC clinical emergency botulism service, 770/488-7100 (www.cdc.gov/botulism/health-professional.html; accessed September 27, 2022). For bioterror public exposure, treatment recommendations will be emergently posted on the CDC website.
	Infant botulism	Human botulism immune globulin for infants (BabyBIG) (AII) No antibiotic treatment	BabyBIG available nationally from the California Department of Public Health at 510/231-7600 (www.infantbotulism.org; accessed September 27, 2022)

D. PREFERRED THERAPY FOR SPECIFIC BACTERIAL AND MYCOBACTERIAL PATHOGENS *(continued)*

Organism	Clinical Illness	Drug of Choice (evidence grade)	Alternatives
Clostridium perfringens[66,67]	Gas gangrene/necrotizing fasciitis/sepsis (also caused by *Clostridium sordellii, septicum, novyi*) Food poisoning	Penicillin G AND clindamycin for invasive infection (BII); no antimicrobials indicated for foodborne illness. The clindamycin is recommended by some experts to inhibit toxin production.	Meropenem, metronidazole, clindamycin monotherapy No defined benefit of hyperbaric oxygen over aggressive surgery/antibiotic therapy
Clostridium tetani[68–70]	Tetanus	TIG 500 U (previously 3,000–6,000 U) IM, with part injected directly into the wound (IVIG at 200–400 mg/kg if TIG not available) Metronidazole (AIII) OR penicillin G (BIII)	Prophylaxis for contaminated wounds: 250 U IM for those with <3 tetanus immunizations. Start/continue immunization for tetanus. Alternative antibiotics: meropenem; doxycycline, clindamycin.
Corynebacterium diphtheriae[71]	Diphtheria	Diphtheria equine antitoxin (available through the CDC under an investigational protocol [www.cdc.gov/diphtheria/dat.html; accessed September 27, 2022) AND erythromycin or penicillin G (AIII)	Antitoxin from the CDC Emergency Operations Center, 770/488-7100; protocol: www.cdc.gov/diphtheria/downloads/protocol.pdf (version 10.0; June 9, 2022) (accessed September 27, 2022)
Corynebacterium jeikeium[72,73]	Sepsis, endocarditis, nosocomial infections	Vancomycin (AIII)	Daptomycin (emerging resistance reported), tigecycline, linezolid
Corynebacterium minutissimum[74,75]	Erythrasma; bacteremia in compromised hosts	Erythromycin or clindamycin PO for erythrasma (BIII); OR, for bacteremia,[75] vancomycin OR penicillin IV (BIII)	Topical 1% clindamycin for cutaneous infection; meropenem, penicillin/ampicillin, ciprofloxacin

Coxiella burnetii[76,77]	Q fever (See Q fever in Chapter 1, Table 1L.)	Acute infection: doxycycline (all ages) (AII) Chronic infection or endocarditis (course not well-defined): doxycycline for children >7 y AND hydroxychloroquine for 18–36 mo	Alternative for acute infection: TMP/SMX Alternative for chronic infection: TMP/SMX AND doxycycline (BII); OR levofloxacin AND rifampin
Cutibacterium (formerly *Propionibacterium*) *acnes*[78,79]	In addition to acne, invasive infection: sepsis, postoperative wound/shunt infection	Penicillin G (AIII); vancomycin (AIII)	Ceftriaxone, doxycycline, clindamycin, linezolid, daptomycin Resistant to metronidazole
Ehrlichia chaffeensis,[14,80] *muris*[80,81]	Human monocytic ehrlichiosis	Doxycycline (all ages) (AII)	Rifampin
Ehrlichia ewingii[14,80]	*E ewingii* ehrlichiosis	Doxycycline (all ages) (AII)	Rifampin
Eikenella corrodens[82,83]	Human bite wounds; abscesses, meningitis, endocarditis	Amox/clav PO; ceftriaxone; meropenem/imipenem For beta-lactamase–negative strains: ampicillin; penicillin G (BIII)	Pip/tazo, amp/sul, ciprofloxacin Resistant to clindamycin, cephalexin, erythromycin
Elizabethkingia (formerly *Chryseobacterium*) *meningoseptica*[84,85]	Sepsis, meningitis (particularly in neonates)	Levofloxacin; TMP/SMX (BIII)	Pip/tazo, minocycline Add rifampin to another active drug.
Enterobacter spp[5,57,58,86–89]	Sepsis, pneumonia, wound infection, UTI	Cefepime; meropenem; pip/tazo (BII)	CAZ/AVI, ertapenem, imipenem, ceftriaxone AND gentamicin, TMP/SMX, ciprofloxacin Newly emerging carbapenem-resistant strains worldwide[89]

D. PREFERRED THERAPY FOR SPECIFIC BACTERIAL AND MYCOBACTERIAL PATHOGENS *(continued)*

Organism	Clinical Illness	Drug of Choice (evidence grade)	Alternatives
Enterococcus spp[90–92]	Endocarditis, UTI, intra-abdominal abscess	Ampicillin AND gentamicin (AI), OR vancomycin AND gentamicin (for ampicillin-resistant strains); bactericidal activity present only with combination Ampicillin AND ceftriaxone in combination also effective[92,93]	For strains resistant to gentamicin on synergy testing, use streptomycin or other active aminoglycoside for invasive infections. For vancomycin-resistant strains that are also ampicillin resistant: daptomycin OR linezolid.[91,92]
Erysipelothrix rhusiopathiae[94]	Cellulitis (erysipeloid), sepsis, abscesses, endocarditis	Invasive infection: ampicillin (BIII); penicillin G; ceftriaxone, meropenem (BIII) Cutaneous infection: penicillin V; amoxicillin; cephalexin; clindamycin	Resistance to penicillin reported. Ciprofloxacin, erythromycin. Resistant to vancomycin, daptomycin, TMP/SMX.
Escherichia coli (See Chapter 1 for specific infection entities and references.) *Increasing resistance to 3rd-generation cephalosporins due to ESBLs and to carbapenems due to carbapenemases (KPC)*[4,5,88,89] (See Chapter 12.)	UTI, community acquired, not hospital acquired	A 1st-, 2nd-, or 3rd-generation cephalosporin PO, IM as empiric therapy (BI)	Amoxicillin; TMP/SMX if susceptible. Ciprofloxacin if resistant to other options. For hospital-acquired UTI, review hospital antibiogram for best empiric choices.
	Travelers diarrhea	Azithromycin (AII)	Rifaximin (for nonfebrile, non-bloody diarrhea for children >11 y); cefixime
	Sepsis, pneumonia, hospital-acquired UTI	A 2nd-, 3rd-, or 4th-generation cephalosporin IV (BI)	For ESBL-producing strains: cefepime or meropenem (AIII) or other carbapenem; pip/tazo and ciprofloxacin if resistant to other antibiotics For KPC-producing strains: CAZ/AVI

	Meningitis	Ceftriaxone or cefepime (AIII)	For ESBL-producing strains: meropenem (AIII)
Francisella tularensis[95,96]	Tularemia	Gentamicin (AII) for invasive disease	Convalescent PO therapy, or treatment of mild disease with doxycycline, ciprofloxacin. Resistant to beta-lactam antibiotics.
Fusobacterium spp[97–99]	Sepsis, soft tissue infection, Lemierre syndrome	Metronidazole (AIII); meropenem; clindamycin (BIII)	Penicillin G, pip/tazo. Combinations often used for Lemierre syndrome. Anticoagulation for ongoing thromboembolic complications.
Gardnerella vaginalis[51,100]	Bacterial vaginosis	Metronidazole (BII)	Tinidazole, clindamycin, metronidazole gel, clindamycin cream/gel
Haemophilus ducreyi[51]	Chancroid	Azithromycin (AIII); ceftriaxone (BIII)	Erythromycin, ciprofloxacin

D. PREFERRED THERAPY FOR SPECIFIC BACTERIAL AND MYCOBACTERIAL PATHOGENS *(continued)*

Organism	Clinical Illness	Drug of Choice (evidence grade)	Alternatives
Haemophilus influenzae[101]	Nonencapsulated strains: upper respiratory tract infections	Beta-lactamase negative: ampicillin IV (AI); amoxicillin PO (AI) Beta-lactamase positive: ceftriaxone IV, IM (AI); amox/clav (AI) OR 2nd- or 3rd-generation cephalosporins PO (AI)	Levofloxacin, azithromycin, TMP/SMX
	Type b strains in unimmunized children: meningitis, arthritis, cellulitis, epiglottitis, pneumonia	Beta-lactamase negative: ampicillin IV (AI); amoxicillin PO (AI) Beta-lactamase positive: ceftriaxone IV, IM (AI) or cefepime IV; amox/clav (AI) OR 2nd- or 3rd-generation cephalosporins PO (AI)	Other regimens: meropenem IV, levofloxacin IV Full IV course (10 days) for meningitis, but PO step-down therapy well-documented after response to treatment of non-CNS infections Levofloxacin PO as step-down therapy for beta-lactamase–positive strains
Helicobacter pylori[102–104]	Gastritis, peptic ulcer	Triple-agent therapy: clarithromycin (susceptible strains) AND amoxicillin AND omeprazole (AII); ADD metronidazole for suspected resistance to clarithromycin.	For clarithromycin/metronidazole resistance, tetracycline for children >7 y. Other regimens include bismuth in addition to other proton pump inhibitors.
Kingella kingae[105,106]	Osteomyelitis, arthritis	Ampicillin; penicillin G (AII)	Ceftriaxone, TMP/SMX, cefuroxime, ceftaroline, ciprofloxacin. Resistant to clindamycin, vancomycin, linezolid.

Klebsiella spp (*Klebsiella pneumoniae, oxytoca*)[88,89,107–110] *Increasing resistance to 3rd-generation cephalosporins (ESBLs) and carbapenems (KPC), as well as to colistin* (See Chapter 12.)	UTI	A 2nd- or 3rd-generation cephalosporin (AII)	Use most narrow spectrum agent active against pathogen: TMP/SMX, ciprofloxacin, gentamicin. ESBL producers should be treated with a carbapenem (meropenem, ertapenem, imipenem), but KPC (carbapenemase)-containing bacteria may require ciprofloxacin, CAZ/AVI, colistin.[108,109]
	Sepsis, pneumonia, meningitis, hospital-acquired infection	Ceftriaxone; cefepime (AIII) For carbapenem-resistant KPC strains: CAZ/AVI, mero/vabor, or imipenem/relebactam. For carbapenem-resistant NDM strains, use aztreonam AND CAZ/AVI.	Carbapenem or ciprofloxacin if resistant to other routine antibiotics Meningitis caused by ESBL producer: meropenem if susceptible KPC (carbapenemase) producers: ciprofloxacin, colistin, OR CAZ/AVI (approved by FDA for children in 2019 and active against current strains of KPC[108–110])
Klebsiella granulomatis[51]	Granuloma inguinale	Azithromycin (AII)	Doxycycline, TMP/SMX, ciprofloxacin
Legionella spp[111]	Legionnaires disease	Azithromycin (AI) OR levofloxacin (AII)	Erythromycin, clarithromycin, TMP/SMX, doxycycline
Leptospira spp[112]	Leptospirosis	Penicillin G IV (AII); ceftriaxone IV (AII)	PO therapy: amoxicillin, doxycycline, azithromycin

D. PREFERRED THERAPY FOR SPECIFIC BACTERIAL AND MYCOBACTERIAL PATHOGENS *(continued)*

Organism	Clinical Illness	Drug of Choice (evidence grade)	Alternatives
Leuconostoc[113]	Bacteremia	Penicillin G (AIII); ampicillin (BIII)	Clindamycin, erythromycin, doxycycline (uniformly resistant to vancomycin)
Listeria monocytogenes[114]	Sepsis, meningitis in compromised host; neonatal sepsis	Ampicillin (ADD gentamicin for severe infection, compromised hosts [new retrospective data in adults suggest no benefit from added gentamicin].)[115] (AII)	Ampicillin AND TMP/SMX; ampicillin AND linezolid; levofloxacin
Moraxella catarrhalis[116]	Otitis, sinusitis, bronchitis	Amox/clav (AI)	TMP/SMX; a 2nd- or 3rd-generation cephalosporin
Morganella morganii[57,58,87,117,118]	UTI, neonatal sepsis, wound infection	Cefepime (AIII); meropenem (AIII); levofloxacin (BIII)	Intrinsically resistant to penicillin/ampicillin and colistin. Pip/tazo, ceftriaxone AND gentamicin, ciprofloxacin, TMP/SMX. Has intrinsic inducible ampC beta-lactamase; 3rd-generation cephalosporins may be selected for resistance. New carbapenem-resistant strains with metallo-beta-lactamases that will require aztreonam AND CAZ/AVI now reported in Asia.

Mycobacterium abscessus[119–124] *3 subspecies now identified*	Skin and soft tissue infections; pneumonia in cystic fibrosis	For localized skin/soft tissue: clarithromycin or azithromycin (with or without rifampin or ethambutol if susceptible) (AIII). For pneumonia: Initial phase for severe disease (3 drugs are now recommended): clarithromycin or azithromycin AND amikacin IV AND cefoxitin or imipenem IV. Continuation phase: nebulized amikacin AND azithromycin AND 1–3 of the following antibiotics guided by drug susceptibility results and patient tolerance: clofazimine, linezolid PO, minocycline PO, moxifloxacin PO, TMP/SMX PO.[123] For less severe disease: azithromycin PO (or clarithromycin PO); ADD ethambutol, AND rifampin, given 3 times weekly to prevent macrolide/azalide resistance.	Consider consulting an infectious disease physician. Should test for susceptibility to all possible antibiotic options listed as well as cefoxitin. May need pulmonary resection. Initial intensive phase of therapy followed by months of "maintenance" therapy.

D. PREFERRED THERAPY FOR SPECIFIC BACTERIAL AND MYCOBACTERIAL PATHOGENS *(continued)*

Organism	Clinical Illness	Drug of Choice (evidence grade)	Alternatives
Mycobacterium avium complex[119,124,125]	Cervical adenitis	Clarithromycin (AII); azithromycin (AII)	Surgical excision is more likely than sole medical therapy to lead to cure. May increase cure rate with addition of rifampin or ethambutol.
	Pneumonia	For pneumonia, ADD rifampin AND ethambutol AND, for severe disease, amikacin (AIII).[123]	Depending on susceptibilities and severity of the illness, ADD amikacin ± ciprofloxacin.
	Disseminated disease in competent host, or disease in immunocompromised host	Clarithromycin or azithromycin AND ethambutol AND rifampin (AIII), AND, for severe disease, amikacin	Depending on susceptibilities and severity of the illness, ADD additional agents.
Mycobacterium bovis[126–128]	Tuberculosis (historically not differentiated from *Mycobacterium tuberculosis* infection; causes adenitis, abdominal tuberculosis, meningitis)	INH AND rifampin (AII); ADD ethambutol for suspected resistance (AIII).	*M bovis* is always resistant to PZA. Consider ADDING streptomycin for severe infection.
Mycobacterium chelonae[119,129]	Abscesses; catheter infection	Clarithromycin or azithromycin (AIII); ADD amikacin for invasive disease, ± meropenem if susceptible (AIII).	Also test for susceptibility to tigecycline, TMP/SMX, doxycycline, tobramycin, imipenem (more active than meropenem),[129] moxifloxacin, linezolid.
Mycobacterium fortuitum complex[118,119,124,125,129]	Skin and soft tissue infections; catheter infection	Amikacin AND cefoxitin ± levofloxacin (AIII)	Also test for susceptibility to clarithromycin, imipenem, tigecycline, minocycline, sulfonamides, doxycycline, linezolid.

Mycobacterium leprae[130]	Leprosy	Dapsone AND rifampin for paucibacillary (1–5 patches) (AII). ADD clofazimine for lepromatous, multibacillary (>5 patches) disease (AII).	Consult HRSA (National Hansen's Disease [Leprosy] Program) at www.hrsa.gov/hansens-disease for advice about treatment and free antibiotics: 800/642-2477 (reviewed June 2021; accessed September 27, 2022).
Mycobacterium marinum/balnei[119,131]	Papules, pustules, abscesses (swimming pool granuloma)	Clarithromycin ± ethambutol (AIII)	TMP/SMX AND rifampin; ethambutol AND rifampin, doxycycline ± 1 or 2 additional antibiotics Surgical debridement
Mycobacterium tuberculosis[126,132] (See Tuberculosis in Chapter 1, Table 1F, for detailed recommendations for active infection, latent infection, and exposures in high-risk children.)	Tuberculosis (pneumonia; meningitis; cervical adenitis; mesenteric adenitis; osteomyelitis)	For active infection in children without risk factors for resistance: INH AND rifampin AND PZA (AI); ADD ethambutol for suspected resistance. For latent infection: INH AND rifapentine once weekly for 12 wk (AII) OR rifampin daily for 4 mo, OR INH/rifampin combination *daily* (all ages) for 3 mo OR INH daily or biweekly for 9 mo (AII).	Add streptomycin for severe infection. For MDR tuberculosis, bedaquiline is FDA approved for adults and for children ≥5 y. The 3-drug PO combination of pretomanid, bedaquiline, and linezolid has orphan drug approval for MDR tuberculosis in adults, to be taken together for 26 wk. Corticosteroids should be added to regimens for meningitis, mesenteric adenitis, and endobronchial infection (AIII).
Mycoplasma hominis[133,134]	Neonatal infection including meningitis/ventriculitis; nongonococcal urethritis	Neonates: doxycycline; moxifloxacin Urethritis: clindamycin (AIII)	Usually erythromycin resistant

D. PREFERRED THERAPY FOR SPECIFIC BACTERIAL AND MYCOBACTERIAL PATHOGENS *(continued)*

Organism	Clinical Illness	Drug of Choice (evidence grade)	Alternatives
Mycoplasma pneumoniae[135,136]	Pneumonia	Azithromycin (AI); erythromycin (BI); macrolide resistance emerging worldwide[137]	Doxycycline and fluoroquinolones are usually active against macrolide-susceptible and macrolide-resistant strains.
Neisseria gonorrhoeae[51,138]	Gonorrhea; arthritis	Formerly, ceftriaxone AND azithromycin or doxycycline (AIII), but in 2020, due to increasing resistance to azithromycin (4% in adults), only ceftriaxone is now routinely recommended.	PO cefixime as single-drug therapy is no longer routinely recommended due to increasing resistance but can be used when ceftriaxone cannot.[138] Spectinomycin IM
Neisseria meningitidis[139,140]	Sepsis, meningitis	Ceftriaxone (AI)	Penicillin G or ampicillin if susceptible with amoxicillin step-down therapy for non-CNS infection
			For prophylaxis following exposure: rifampin or ciprofloxacin (ciprofloxacin-resistant strains have now been reported). Azithromycin may be less effective.
Nocardia asteroides or *brasiliensis*[141,142]	Pneumonia with abscess, cutaneous cellulitis/abscess, brain abscess	TMP/SMX (AII); sulfisoxazole (BII); for severe infection, ADD imipenem or meropenem AND amikacin (AII).	Linezolid, ceftriaxone, clarithromycin, minocycline, levofloxacin, tigecycline, amox/clav

Pasteurella multocida[143,144]	Sepsis, abscesses, animal bite wound	Penicillin G (AIII); ampicillin (AIII); amoxicillin (AIII)	Amox/clav, pip/tazo, doxycycline, ceftriaxone, cefpodoxime, cefuroxime, TMP/SMX, levofloxacin. Cephalexin may not demonstrate adequate activity. Not usually susceptible to clindamycin or erythromycin.
Peptostreptococcus[145]	Sepsis, deep head/neck space and intra-abdominal infection	Penicillin G (AII); ampicillin (AII)	Clindamycin, vancomycin, meropenem, imipenem, metronidazole
Plesiomonas shigelloides[146,147]	Diarrhea, neonatal sepsis, meningitis	Antibiotics may not be necessary to treat diarrhea: ciprofloxacin (BIII); 2nd- and 3rd-generation cephalosporins (AIII); azithromycin (BIII). For meningitis/sepsis: ceftriaxone.	Meropenem, amox/clav Increasing resistance to TMP/SMX
Prevotella (formerly *Bacteroides*) spp,[148] *melaninogenica*	Deep head/neck space abscess; dental abscess	Metronidazole (AII); meropenem or imipenem (AII)	Pip/tazo, cefoxitin, clindamycin, tigecycline
Propionibacterium (now *Cutibacterium*) *acnes*[78,79]	In addition to acne, invasive infection: sepsis, postoperative wound/shunt infection	Penicillin G (AIII); vancomycin (AIII)	Ceftriaxone, doxycycline, clindamycin, linezolid, daptomycin Resistant to metronidazole

D. PREFERRED THERAPY FOR SPECIFIC BACTERIAL AND MYCOBACTERIAL PATHOGENS *(continued)*

Organism	Clinical Illness	Drug of Choice (evidence grade)	Alternatives
Proteus mirabilis[149]	UTI, sepsis, meningitis	Ceftriaxone (AII) for ESBL-negative strains; cefepime; ciprofloxacin; gentamicin PO therapy: amox/clav; TMP/SMX, ciprofloxacin	Carbapenem; pip/tazo; cefiderocol; increasing resistance to ampicillin, TMP/SMX, and fluoroquinolones, particularly in nosocomial isolates Rarely contain plasmid-mediated ampC beta-lactamase Colistin resistant
Proteus vulgaris, other spp (indole-positive strains)[4–6,57,58,88]	UTI, sepsis, meningitis	Cefepime; ciprofloxacin; gentamicin (BIII); meropenem for ESBL producers Potential ampC hyper-producer (and some strains with ESBLs), so at risk for resistance to 3rd-generation cephalosporins	Imipenem, ertapenem, TMP/SMX, cefiderocol, CAZ/AVI for carbapenem resistance Colistin resistant
Providencia spp[57,58,150]	Sepsis	Cefepime; ciprofloxacin, pip/tazo, gentamicin (BIII)	Meropenem or other carbapenem for ESBL producer; TMP/SMX; CAZ/AVI for carbapenem resistance Colistin and tigecycline resistant
Pseudomonas aeruginosa[151–154]	UTI	Cefepime (AII); other antipseudomonal beta-lactams; tobramycin	Amikacin, ciprofloxacin

	Nosocomial sepsis, pneumonia	Cefepime (AI), OR meropenem (AI), OR pip/tazo AND tobramycin (BI), OR ceftazidime AND tobramycin (BII)	Ciprofloxacin AND tobramycin; cefiderocol; colistin.[57] There is controversy regarding additional clinical benefit in outcomes when newer, more potent beta-lactams are used over aminoglycoside combinations, but combinations may increase the likelihood of empiric active coverage and decrease the emergence of resistance.[155,156] Prolonged infusion of beta-lactam antibiotics will allow greater therapeutic exposure to high-MIC pathogens.
	Pneumonia in cystic fibrosis[157–160] (See Cystic Fibrosis in Chapter 1, Table 1F.)	Cefepime (AII) or meropenem (AI); OR ceftazidime AND tobramycin (BII) (AI). Azithromycin provides benefit in prolonging interval between exacerbations.	Inhalational antibiotics for prevention of acute exacerbations (but insufficient evidence to recommend for treatment of exacerbation): tobramycin; aztreonam; colistin. Many organisms are MDR; consider ciprofloxacin or colistin parenterally; in vitro synergy testing may suggest effective combinations.
Pseudomonas cepacia, mallei, or *pseudomallei* (See *Burkholderia* entries earlier in this table.)			
Rhodococcus equi[161]	Necrotizing pneumonia	Vancomycin AND imipenem for immunocompromised hosts, single-drug therapy for normal hosts (AIII)	Ciprofloxacin or levofloxacin AND azithromycin or rifampin; doxycycline; linezolid

D. PREFERRED THERAPY FOR SPECIFIC BACTERIAL AND MYCOBACTERIAL PATHOGENS *(continued)*

Organism	Clinical Illness	Drug of Choice (evidence grade)	Alternatives
Rickettsia[162,163]	Rocky Mountain spotted fever, Q fever, typhus, rickettsialpox, *Ehrlichia* infection, *Anaplasma* infection	Doxycycline (all ages) (AII)	Chloramphenicol is less effective than doxycycline. A single course of doxycycline is not associated with detectable dental staining.
Salmonella, non-Typhi strains[164–166]	Gastroenteritis (may not require therapy if clinically improving and not immunocompromised). Consider treatment for those with higher risk for invasion (<1 y [or, with highest risk, those <3 mo], immunocompromised, and with focal infections or bacteremia).	Azithromycin (AII) or ceftriaxone (AII); cefixime (AII)	For susceptible strains when culture results available: ciprofloxacin; TMP/SMX; ampicillin
Salmonella Typhi[165,167,168]	Typhoid fever	Azithromycin (AII); ceftriaxone (AII); TMP/SMX (AII); ciprofloxacin (AII)	Obtain blood and stool cultures before treatment to allow for selection of most narrow spectrum antibiotic. Prefer antibiotics with high intracellular concentrations (eg, TMP/SMX, fluoroquinolones). Amoxicillin acceptable for susceptible strains.

Serratia marcescens[57,58,87–89]	Nosocomial sepsis, pneumonia	Cefepime; meropenem; pip/tazo (BII) Potential ampC hyper-producer (and some strains with ESBLs), so at risk for resistance to 3rd-generation cephalosporins	One of the enteric bacilli that have inducible chromosomal ampC beta-lactamases (active against 2nd- and 3rd-generation cephalosporins) that may be constitutively produced by organisms within a population; ertapenem, imipenem, TMP/SMX, ciprofloxacin, ceftriaxone AND gentamicin Resistant to colistin
Shewanella spp[169,170]	Wound infection, nosocomial pneumonia, peritoneal-dialysis peritonitis, ventricular shunt infection, neonatal sepsis	Ceftazidime (AIII); gentamicin (AIII)	Ampicillin, meropenem, pip/tazo, ciprofloxacin Resistant to TMP/SMX and colistin
Shigella spp[171–174]	Enteritis, UTI, prepubertal vaginitis	Ceftriaxone (AII); ciprofloxacin[174] (AII); azithromycin[174] (AII); cefixime (AII)	Substantial (30%) resistance to azithromycin now reported in the United States.[174] Use most narrow spectrum agent active against pathogen: PO ampicillin (not amoxicillin for enteritis); TMP/SMX.
Sphingomonas paucimobilis[175,176]	Bacteremia, wound infection, ocular infection, osteomyelitis	Antipseudomonal penicillins, carbapenems (BIII)	Aminoglycosides, TMP/SMX
Spirillum minus[177]	Rat-bite fever (sodoku)	Penicillin G IV (AII); for endocarditis, ADD gentamicin or streptomycin (AIII).	Ampicillin, doxycycline, ceftriaxone, vancomycin, streptomycin

D. PREFERRED THERAPY FOR SPECIFIC BACTERIAL AND MYCOBACTERIAL PATHOGENS *(continued)*

Organism	Clinical Illness	Drug of Choice (evidence grade)	Alternatives
Staphylococcus aureus (See Chapter 1 for specific infections.)[178,179]			
– Mild to moderate infections	Skin infections, mild to moderate	MSSA: a 1st-generation cephalosporin (cefazolin IV, cephalexin PO) (AI); oxacillin/nafcillin IV (AI), dicloxacillin PO (AI) MRSA: clindamycin (if susceptible) IV or PO, ceftaroline IV,[180] vancomycin IV, or TMP/SMX PO (AII)	For MSSA: amox/clav. For CA-MRSA: linezolid IV, PO; daptomycin IV has been studied and FDA approved for use in children >1 y.[181]
– Moderate to severe infections, empiric treatment of CA-MRSA	Pneumonia, sepsis, myositis, osteomyelitis, etc	MSSA: oxacillin/nafcillin IV (AI); a 1st-generation cephalosporin (cefazolin IV) (AI) ± gentamicin (AIII) MRSA: clindamycin (if susceptible) (AII) OR ceftaroline (AII) OR vancomycin if MIC is ≤2 (AII)[182] Combination therapy with gentamicin and/or rifampin not prospectively studied	For CA-MRSA: linezolid (AII); OR daptomycin[183] for non-pulmonary infection (AII) (studies published in children); ceftaroline IV (FDA approved for children) Approved for adults (primarily for treatment of MRSA): dalbavancin (once-weekly dosing), oritavancin (once-weekly dosing), tedizolid (See Chapter 12.)
Staphylococcus, coagulase negative[184,185]	Nosocomial bacteremia (neonatal bacteremia), infected intravascular catheters, CNS shunts, UTI	Empiric: vancomycin (AII) OR ceftaroline (AII)	If susceptible: nafcillin (or other antistaphylococcal beta-lactam); rifampin (in combination); clindamycin, linezolid; ceftaroline IV; daptomycin for age >1 y (but not for pneumonia)

Stenotrophomonas maltophilia[186–188]	Sepsis	TMP/SMX (AII)	Ceftazidime, levofloxacin, doxycycline, minocycline, tigecycline, and colistin, and as of 2020, cefiderocol is approved for adults.[188]
Streptobacillus moniliformis[177,189]	Rat-bite fever (Haverhill fever)	Penicillin G (AIII); ampicillin (AIII); for endocarditis, ADD gentamicin or streptomycin (AIII).	Doxycycline, ceftriaxone, carbapenems, clindamycin, vancomycin
Streptococcus, group A[190]	Pharyngitis, impetigo, adenitis, cellulitis, necrotizing fasciitis	Penicillin (AI); amoxicillin (AI)	A 1st-generation cephalosporin (cefazolin or cephalexin) (AI), clindamycin (AI), a macrolide (AI), vancomycin (AIII). For recurrent streptococcal pharyngitis, clindamycin or amox/clav, or the addition of rifampin to the last 4 days of penicillin therapy (AIII). The addition of clindamycin may decrease toxin production in overwhelming infection.
Streptococcus, group B[191]	Neonatal sepsis, pneumonia, meningitis	Penicillin (AII) or ampicillin (AII)	Gentamicin is used initially for presumed synergy for group B streptococcus until a clinical/microbiological response has been documented (AIII).

D. PREFERRED THERAPY FOR SPECIFIC BACTERIAL AND MYCOBACTERIAL PATHOGENS *(continued)*

Organism	Clinical Illness	Drug of Choice (evidence grade)	Alternatives
Streptococcus, milleri/anginosus group (*Streptococcus intermedius, anginosus,* and *constellatus;* includes some ß-hemolytic group C and group G streptococci)[192,193]	Pneumonia, sepsis, skin and soft tissue infection,[192,193] sinusitis,[194] arthritis, brain abscess, epidural abscess, subdural empyema, meningitis	Penicillin G (AIII); ampicillin (AIII); ADD gentamicin for serious infection (AIII); ceftriaxone. Many strains show decreased susceptibility to penicillin, requiring higher dosages to achieve adequate antibiotic exposure, particularly in the CNS.	Clindamycin, vancomycin Potential for PO step-down therapy for intracranial complications with fluoroquinolones[195]
Streptococcus, viridans group (α-hemolytic streptococci, most commonly *Streptococcus sanguinis, oralis* [*mitis*], *salivarius, mutans, morbillorum*)	Endocarditis[196]; oropharyngeal, deep head/neck space infections	Penicillin G ± gentamicin (AII) OR ceftriaxone ± gentamicin (AII)	Vancomycin
Streptococcus pneumoniae[197–199] With widespread use of conjugate pneumococcal vaccines, antibiotic resistance in pneumococci has decreased.[199]	Sinusitis, otitis[200]	Amoxicillin, high-dose (90 mg/kg/day div bid) (AII); standard dose (40–45 mg/kg/day div tid) is now likely to be effective in otherwise healthy children following widespread use of PCV13 vaccines.[198,199]	Amox/clav, cefdinir, cefpodoxime, cefuroxime, clindamycin, OR ceftriaxone IM
	Meningitis	Ceftriaxone (AI); vancomycin is no longer required for possible ceftriaxone resistance; ceftriaxone-resistant strains have not been reported to cause meningitis in the post-PCV13 era (AIII).	Penicillin G alone for pen-S strains; ceftriaxone alone for ceftriaxone-susceptible strains

	Pneumonia, osteomyelitis/arthritis,[197,199] sepsis	Ampicillin (AII); ceftriaxone (AI)	Penicillin G alone for pen-S strains; ceftriaxone alone for ceftriaxone-susceptible strains
Treponema pallidum[51,200]	Syphilis (See chapters 1 and 2.)	Penicillin G (AII)	Desensitize to penicillin preferred to alternative therapies. Doxycycline, ceftriaxone.
Ureaplasma urealyticum[51,201]	Genitourinary infections	Azithromycin (AII)	Erythromycin; doxycycline, ofloxacin (for adolescent genital infections)
	Neonatal pneumonia	Azithromycin (AIII) (effective clearing of *U urealyticum* in preterm neonates demonstrated, but randomized trial to treat pneumonia not yet performed[201])	
Vibrio cholerae[202,203]	Cholera	Doxycycline (AI)	A single treatment course of doxycycline is not associated with tooth staining. If susceptible, azithromycin (AII): ciprofloxacin (AII), TMP/SMX.
Vibrio vulnificus[204–206]	Sepsis, necrotizing fasciitis	Doxycycline AND ceftazidime (AII)	Ciprofloxacin AND ceftriaxone
Yersinia enterocolitica[207,208]	Diarrhea, mesenteric enteritis, reactive arthritis, sepsis	TMP/SMX for enteritis (AIII); ceftriaxone or ciprofloxacin for invasive infection (AIII)	Gentamicin, doxycycline
Yersinia pestis[209–211]	Plague	Gentamicin (AII) OR levofloxacin (AII)	Doxycycline, ciprofloxacin
Yersinia pseudotuberculosis[207]	Mesenteric adenitis; Far East scarlet-like fever[212]; reactive arthritis	Ceftriaxone, TMP/SMX, or ciprofloxacin (AIII)	Gentamicin

4. Choosing Among Antibiotics Within a Class: Beta-lactams and Beta-lactamase Inhibitors, Macrolides, Aminoglycosides, and Fluoroquinolones

Antibiotics should be compared with others regarding (1) antimicrobial spectrum; (2) degree of antibiotic exposure (a function of the pharmacokinetics of the nonprotein-bound drug at the site of infection and the pharmacodynamic properties of the drug); (3) demonstrated efficacy in adequate and well-controlled clinical trials; (4) tolerance, toxicity, and side effects; and (5) cost. When a new antibiotic is approved, it is helpful to compare the new agent with other agents, particularly those in a class of antibiotics already approved for children. If there is no substantial benefit for efficacy or safety for one antimicrobial over another for the isolated or presumed bacterial pathogen(s), one should opt for using an older, more extensively used agent (with presumably better-defined efficacy and safety) that is usually less expensive and is preferably narrower in its spectrum of activity.

Beta-lactams and Beta-lactamase Inhibitors

Beta-lactam (BL)/Beta-lactamase Inhibitor (BLI) Combinations. Increasingly studied and approved by the US Food and Drug Administration (FDA) are BL/BLI combinations that target antibiotic resistance for pathogens with resistance to current BLs based on the presence of many newly emerging beta-lactamases. The BL antibiotic may have initially demonstrated activity against a pathogen, but if a new beta-lactamase is present in that pathogen, it will hydrolyze the BL ring structure and inactivate the antibiotic. The BLI is usually a BL structure, which explains why it binds readily to certain beta-lactamases and can inhibit their activity; however, the BLI does not usually demonstrate direct antibiotic activity itself (although some BLIs with activity are currently in clinical trials). Just as different BL antibiotics bind bacterial target sites with varying affinity (creating a range of susceptibilities based on their ability to bind and inhibit function), different BLIs will bind the different bacterial beta-lactamases with varying affinity. A BLI that binds well to the *Haemophilus influenzae* beta-lactamase may not bind to and inhibit a *Staphylococcus aureus* beta-lactamase or may not bind well to one of the many *Pseudomonas* beta-lactamases. As amoxicillin and ampicillin were used extensively against *H influenzae* following their approval, resistance increased based on the presence of a beta-lactamase that hydrolyzes the BL ring of amoxicillin/ampicillin (with up to 40% of isolates still demonstrating resistance in some regions). Clavulanate, a BLI that binds to and inactivates the *H influenzae* beta-lactamase, allows amoxicillin/ampicillin to "survive" and inhibit cell wall formation, leading to the death of the organism. The first oral BL/BLI combination of amoxicillin/clavulanate, originally known as Augmentin, has been very effective. Similar combinations, primarily intravenous (IV), have now been studied, pairing penicillins, cephalosporins, and carbapenems with other BLIs such as tazobactam, sulbactam, and avibactam, as well as new investigational BLIs such as vaborbactam and relebactam.

Beta-lactam Antibiotics

Oral Cephalosporins (cephalexin, cefadroxil, cefaclor, cefprozil, cefuroxime, cefixime, cefdinir, cefpodoxime, cefditoren [tablet only], and ceftibuten). As a class, the oral cephalosporins have the advantage over oral penicillins of somewhat greater spectrum of activity. The serum half-lives of cefpodoxime, ceftibuten, and cefixime are greater than 2 hours. This pharmacokinetic feature accounts for the fact that they may be given in 1 or 2 doses per day for certain indications, particularly otitis media in which the middle ear fluid half-life is likely to be much longer than the serum half-life and urinary tract infections because of the renal elimination of most of these antibiotics. For more resistant pathogens, twice daily is preferred (see Chapter 11). The spectrum of activity for gram-negative organisms increases as one goes from the first-generation cephalosporins (cephalexin and cefadroxil), to the second generation (cefaclor, cefprozil, and cefuroxime) that demonstrates activity against *H influenzae* (including beta-lactamase–producing strains), to the third generation (cefixime, cefdinir, cefpodoxime, cefditoren, and ceftibuten) that has enhanced coverage of many enteric gram-negative bacilli (eg, *Escherichia coli, Klebsiella* spp). However, ceftibuten and cefixime, in particular, have a disadvantage of less activity against *Streptococcus pneumoniae* than the others, particularly against penicillin non-susceptible strains. No oral current cephalosporins exist with activity against the extended-spectrum beta-lactamases (ESBLs) of *E coli/Klebsiella, Pseudomonas,* or methicillin-resistant *S aureus* (MRSA).

Parenteral Cephalosporins. First-generation cephalosporins, such as cefazolin, are used mainly for treatment of gram-positive infections caused by *S aureus* (excluding MRSA) and group A streptococcus and for surgical prophylaxis; the gram-negative spectrum is limited but more extensive than ampicillin. Cefazolin is well tolerated on intramuscular or IV injection.

A second-generation cephalosporin (cefuroxime) and the cephamycins (cefoxitin and cefotetan) provide increased activity against many gram-negative organisms, particularly *H influenzae* and *E coli*. Cefoxitin has additional activity against up to 80% of strains of *Bacteroides fragilis*. In empiric therapy for mild to moderate infections at low risk of being caused by *B fragilis*, cefoxitin can be considered for use in place of the more active agents such as metronidazole or carbapenems.

Third-generation cephalosporins (ceftriaxone and ceftazidime) all have enhanced potency against many enteric gram-negative bacilli. As with all cephalosporins, though, they are less active against enterococci and *Listeria* at readily achievable serum concentrations. Only ceftazidime has significant activity against *Pseudomonas*. Ceftriaxone has been used very successfully to treat meningitis caused by pneumococcus (mostly penicillin-susceptible strains), *H influenzae* type b, meningococcus, and susceptible strains of *E coli* meningitis. The drug has the greatest usefulness for treating gram-negative bacillary infections due to their safety, compared with other classes of antibiotics (including aminoglycosides). Because ceftriaxone is excreted to a large extent via the liver, it can be used with little dosage adjustment in patients with renal failure. With a serum half-life of 4 to 7 hours, it can be given once a day for all infections, including meningitis, that are caused by susceptible organisms.

Cefepime, a fourth-generation cephalosporin approved for use in children in 1999, exhibits (1) enhanced antipseudomonal activity over ceftazidime; (2) the gram-positive activity of second-generation cephalosporins; (3) better activity than earlier generations against gram-negative enteric bacilli; and (4) stability against the inducible ampC beta-lactamases of *Enterobacter* and *Serratia* (and some strains of *Proteus* and *Citrobacter*) that can hydrolyze third-generation cephalosporins. It can be used as single-drug antibiotic therapy against these pathogens, rather than paired with an aminoglycoside, as is commonly done with third-generation cephalosporins designed to decrease the emergence of ampC-resistant strains. However, cefepime is hydrolyzed by many of the most widely circulating ESBL enzymes (and carbapenemases) and should not be used if an ESBL *E coli* or *Klebsiella* is suspected.

Ceftaroline is a fifth-generation cephalosporin, the first of the cephalosporins with activity against MRSA. Ceftaroline was approved by the FDA for adults in 2010, approved for children in 2016 for treatment of complicated skin infections (including MRSA) and community-acquired pneumonia, and approved for neonates in 2019. The pharmacokinetics of ceftaroline have been evaluated in all pediatric age-groups, including neonates, and in children with cystic fibrosis; clinical studies for pediatric community-acquired pneumonia and complicated skin infection are published.[1,2] Based on these published data and postmarketing experience for infants and children, we believe that ceftaroline should be as effective as and safer than vancomycin for treatment of MRSA infections. Just as BLs such as cefazolin are preferred over vancomycin for methicillin-susceptible *S aureus* infections, ceftaroline should be considered preferred treatment over vancomycin for MRSA infection. Neither renal function nor drug levels need to be followed with ceftaroline therapy. Limited pharmacokinetic and clinical data also support the use of ceftaroline in neonates in which coagulase-negative staphylococci are the most common pathogens causing catheter-related bloodstream infections.

Cefiderocol[3] is an advanced-spectrum cephalosporin, recently approved for adults with complicated urinary tract infections (cUTIs), and nosocomial pneumonia (including ventilator-associated pneumonia), with a unique mechanism of entry into bacterial cells. It covers some difficult multidrug-resistant gram-negative pathogens, including *Acinetobacter, Pseudomonas,* and *Stenotrophomonas,* so we are looking forward to reviewing pediatric data when available, hopefully next year. Both COVID-19 and events in Ukraine, where many antibiotics are very capably studied, have caused unavoidable delays in pediatric clinical trials.

Penicillinase-Resistant Penicillins (dicloxacillin [capsules only]; nafcillin and oxacillin [parenteral only]). "Penicillinase" refers specifically to the beta-lactamase produced by *S aureus* in this case and not those produced by gram-negative bacteria. These antibiotics are active against penicillin-resistant *S aureus* but not against MRSA. Nafcillin differs pharmacologically from the others because it is excreted primarily by the liver rather than by the kidneys, which may explain the relative lack of nephrotoxicity when this penicillin is compared with methicillin, which is no longer available in the United States. Nafcillin pharmacokinetics are erratic in persons with liver disease, and the drug often causes phlebitis with IV infusion.

Antipseudomonal and Anti-enteric Gram-negative BLs (piperacillin/tazobactam, aztreonam, ceftazidime, cefepime, meropenem, imipenem, and ertapenem). Piperacillin/tazobactam (Zosyn) and ceftazidime/avibactam (Avycaz) (both FDA approved for children), and, still under investigation in children, ceftolozane/tazobactam (Zerbaxa), imipenem/relebactam (Recarbrio), and meropenem/vaborbactam (Vabomere), represent BL/BLI combinations, as noted previously. The BLI (clavulanic acid, tazobactam, avibactam, or vaborbactam in these combinations) binds irreversibly to and neutralizes specific beta-lactamase enzymes produced by the organism. The combination adds to the spectrum of the original antibiotic only when the mechanism of resistance is a beta-lactamase enzyme and only when the BLI is capable of binding to and inhibiting that particular organism's beta-lactamase enzyme(s). The combinations extend the spectrum of activity of the primary antibiotic to include many beta-lactamase–positive bacteria, including some strains of enteric gram-negative bacilli (*E coli, Klebsiella,* and *Enterobacter*), *S aureus,* and *B fragilis.* Piperacillin/tazobactam, ceftolozane/tazobactam, ceftazidime/avibactam, and imipenem/relebactam may still be inactive against *Pseudomonas* because many other non–beta-lactamase mechanisms of resistance may also be active.

Pseudomonas has an intrinsic capacity to develop resistance following exposure to any BL, based on the activity of several inducible chromosomal beta-lactamases, upregulated efflux pumps, and changes in the permeability of the cell wall, as well as mutational changes in the antibacterial target sites. Because development of resistance during therapy is somewhat common (particularly beta-lactamase–mediated resistance against ceftazidime), an aminoglycoside such as tobramycin is often used in combination, assuming that the tobramycin may kill strains developing resistance to the BLs. Cefepime, meropenem, and imipenem are relatively stable to the beta-lactamases induced while a patient is receiving therapy and can be used as single-agent therapy for most *Pseudomonas* infections, but resistance may still develop to these agents based on other mechanisms of resistance. For *Pseudomonas* infections in compromised hosts or in life-threatening infections, these drugs, too, should be used in combination with an aminoglycoside or a second active agent. The benefits of the additional antibiotic should be weighed against the potential for additional toxicity and alteration of host flora.

Aminopenicillins (amoxicillin and amoxicillin/clavulanate [oral formulations only, in the United States], ampicillin [oral and parenteral], and ampicillin/sulbactam [parenteral only]). Amoxicillin is very well absorbed, good tasting, and associated with very few side effects. Augmentin is a combination of amoxicillin and clavulanate (as noted previously) that is available in several fixed proportions that permit amoxicillin to remain active against many beta-lactamase–producing bacteria, including *H influenzae* and *S aureus* (but not MRSA). Amoxicillin/clavulanate has undergone many changes in formulation since its introduction. The ratio of amoxicillin to clavulanate was originally 4:1, based on susceptibility data of pneumococcus and *Haemophilus* during the 1970s. With the emergence of penicillin-resistant pneumococcus, recommendations for increasing the dosage of amoxicillin were made, particularly for upper respiratory tract infections. However, if one increases the dosage of clavulanate even slightly, the incidence of diarrhea increases dramatically. By keeping the dosage of clavulanate constant while increasing the dosage of amoxicillin, one can treat the relatively resistant pneumococci while not increasing gastrointestinal side effects of the combination. The original 4:1 ratio is present in suspensions containing 125 and 250 mg of amoxicillin per 5 mL and the 125- and 250-mg chewable tablets. A higher 7:1 ratio is present in the suspensions containing 200 and 400 mg of amoxicillin per 5 mL and in the 200- and 400-mg chewable tablets. A still higher ratio of 14:1 is present in the suspension formulation Augmentin ES-600 that contains 600 mg of amoxicillin per 5 mL; this preparation is designed to deliver 90 mg/kg/day of amoxicillin, divided twice daily, for the treatment of ear (and sinus) infections. The high serum and middle ear fluid concentrations achieved with 45 mg/kg/dose, combined with the long middle ear fluid half-life (4–6 hours) of amoxicillin, allow for a therapeutic antibiotic exposure to pathogens in the middle ear with a twice-daily regimen. However, the prolonged half-life in the middle ear fluid is not necessarily found in other infection sites (eg, skin, lung tissue, joint tissue), for which dosing of amoxicillin and Augmentin should continue to be 3 times daily for most susceptible pathogens.

For older children who can swallow tablets, the amoxicillin to clavulanate ratios are as follows: 500-mg tablet (4:1); 875-mg tablet (7:1); 1,000-mg tablet (16:1).

Sulbactam, another BLI like clavulanate, is combined with ampicillin in the parenteral formulation Unasyn. The relatively narrow spectrum of activity of ampicillin against enteric bacilli limits the activity of this combination, compared with the more broad spectrum of activity of agents such as piperacillin and ceftazidime when used in BL/BLI combinations. Sulbactam inhibits only beta-lactamases that prevent ampicillin from killing these gram-negative bacilli; it does not increase the spectrum of activity beyond what ampicillin can potentially achieve.

Carbapenems. Meropenem, imipenem, and ertapenem are currently available carbapenems with a broader spectrum of activity than of any other class of BL currently available. Meropenem, imipenem, and ertapenem are approved by the FDA for use in children. At present, we recommend them for treatment of infections caused by bacteria resistant to standard therapy or for mixed infections involving aerobes and anaerobes. Imipenem has greater central nervous system (CNS) irritability than other carbapenems, leading to an increased risk for seizures in children with meningitis, but this is not clinically significant in children without underlying CNS inflammation. Meropenem was not associated with an increased rate of seizures, compared with cefotaxime in children with meningitis. Imipenem and meropenem are active against virtually all coliform bacilli, including ceftriaxone-resistant (ESBL- or ampC-producing) strains; against *Pseudomonas aeruginosa* (including most ceftazidime-resistant strains); and against anaerobes, including

B fragilis. While ertapenem lacks the excellent activity against *P aeruginosa* of the other carbapenems, it has the advantage of a prolonged serum half-life, which allows for once-daily dosing in adults and children 13 years and older and twice-daily dosing in younger children. Newly emerging strains of *Klebsiella pneumoniae* (and *E coli*) may contain *K pneumoniae* carbapenemases (KPC) that degrade and inactivate all the carbapenems. Less common in North America are the New Delhi metallo-beta-lactamase (NDM)–carrying enteric bacilli (*E coli* and *Klebsiella*) that are also resistant to carbapenems. Multidrug-resistant strains have spread to many parts of the world, reinforcing the need to keep track of your local antibiotic susceptibility patterns. Carbapenems have been paired with BLIs (eg, vaborbactam, relebactam) that inhibit KPC but do not inhibit the metallo-beta-lactamase enzymes. New BLIs that can inhibit NDM are under investigation.

Macrolides

Erythromycin is the prototype of macrolide antibiotics. Almost 30 macrolides have been produced, but only 3 are FDA approved for children in the United States: erythromycin, azithromycin (also called an "azalide"), and clarithromycin, while a fourth, telithromycin (also called a "ketolide"), is approved for adults and available only in tablet form. As a class, these drugs achieve greater concentrations intracellularly than in serum, particularly with azithromycin and clarithromycin. As a result, measuring serum concentrations is usually not clinically useful. Gastrointestinal intolerance to erythromycin is caused by the breakdown products of the macrolide. This is much less of a problem with azithromycin and clarithromycin. Azithromycin, clarithromycin, and telithromycin extend the clinically relevant activity of erythromycin to include *Haemophilus;* azithromycin and clarithromycin also have substantial activity against certain mycobacteria. Azithromycin is also active in vitro and effective against many enteric gram-negative pathogens, including *Salmonella* and *Shigella,* when given orally. For many infections, the ability of azithromycin to concentrate intracellularly with drug accumulation over multiple doses allows dosing just once daily for 3 to 5 days to create site-of-infection concentrations that are equivalent to 7 to 10 days for more traditionally eliminated antibiotics.

Aminoglycosides

Although 5 aminoglycoside antibiotics are available in the United States, only 3 are widely used for systemic therapy of aerobic gram-negative infections and for synergy in the treatment of certain gram-positive and gram-negative infections: gentamicin, tobramycin, and amikacin. Streptomycin and kanamycin have more limited utility than the other agents due to increased toxicity. Resistance in gram-negative bacilli to aminoglycosides is caused by bacterial enzymes that adenylate, acetylate, or phosphorylate the aminoglycoside, resulting in inactivity. The specific activities of each enzyme against each aminoglycoside in each pathogen are highly variable. As a result, antibiotic susceptibility tests must be done for each aminoglycoside drug separately. There are small differences in toxicities to the kidneys and eighth cranial nerve hearing/vestibular function, although it is uncertain whether these small differences are clinically significant. For all children receiving a full treatment course of a week or more, it is advisable to monitor peak and trough serum concentrations early in the course of therapy, as the degree of drug exposure correlates with toxicity and the elevated trough concentrations may predict impending drug accumulation. With amikacin, desired peak concentrations are 20 to 35 mcg/mL and trough drug concentrations are less than 10 mcg/mL; for gentamicin and tobramycin, depending on the frequency of dosing, peak concentrations should be 5 to 10 mcg/mL and trough concentrations less than 2 mcg/mL. In the past, children with cystic fibrosis have required greater dosages to achieve equivalent therapeutic serum concentrations due to enhanced clearance, although with improvements in nutrition and pulmonary function over the past decade, the differences are less prominent. Inhaled tobramycin has been very successful in children with cystic fibrosis as an adjunctive therapy for gram-negative bacillary infections. The role of inhaled aminoglycosides in other gram-negative pneumonias (eg, ventilator-associated pneumonia) has not yet been defined.

Once-Daily Dosing of Aminoglycosides. Once-daily dosing of 5 to 7.5 mg/kg of gentamicin or tobramycin has been studied in adults and in some neonates and children; peak serum concentrations are greater than those achieved with dosing 3 times daily. Aminoglycosides demonstrate concentration-dependent killing of pathogens, suggesting a potential benefit to higher serum concentrations achieved with once-daily dosing. Regimens giving the daily dosage as a single infusion (rather than as traditionally split doses every 8 hours) are effective and safe for normal adults and immunocompromised hosts with fever and neutropenia and may be less toxic than 8-hourly dosing. Experience with once-daily dosing in children is increasing, with similar encouraging results as noted for adults. A recent Cochrane review for children (and adults) with cystic fibrosis comparing once-daily with 3-times–daily administration showed equal efficacy with decreased toxicity in children.[2] Once-daily dosing should be considered as effective as multiple, smaller doses per day and is likely to be safer for children; therefore, it should be the preferred regimen for treatment.

Fluoroquinolones

Fluoroquinolone (FQ) toxicity to cartilage in weight-bearing joints of experimental juvenile animals was first documented to be dose and duration-of-therapy dependent more than 40 years ago. Pediatric studies were therefore not initially undertaken with ciprofloxacin or other FQs. However, with increasing antibiotic resistance in pediatric pathogens and an accumulating database in pediatrics suggesting that joint toxicity may be uncommon, the FDA allowed prospective studies to proceed in 1998. As of July 2021, no cases of FQ-attributable joint toxicity have been documented to occur in children with FQs that are approved for use in the United States. Limited published data are available from prospective, blinded studies to accurately assess this risk, although some retrospective published data are reassuring.[4] A prospective, randomized, double-blind study of moxifloxacin for intra-abdominal infection, with 1-year follow-up specifically designed to assess tendon/joint toxicity, demonstrated no concern for toxicity.[5] Unblinded studies with levofloxacin for respiratory tract infections and unpublished randomized studies comparing ciprofloxacin with other agents for cUTI suggest the possibility of an uncommon, reversible FQ-attributable arthralgia, but these data should be interpreted with caution. The use of FQs in situations of antibiotic resistance where no other active agent is available is reasonable, while weighing the benefits of treatment against the low risk for toxicity from this class of antibiotics. The use of an oral FQ when the only alternative is parenteral therapy is also justified.[6] For clinicians reading this book, a well-documented case of FQ joint toxicity in a child is publishable (and reportable to the FDA), and the editors would be very happy to support such a report. Please feel free to contact us if you have a case.

Ciprofloxacin usually has very good gram-negative activity (with great regional variation in susceptibility) against enteric bacilli (*E coli, Klebsiella, Enterobacter, Salmonella,* and *Shigella*) and against *P aeruginosa.* However, it lacks substantial gram-positive coverage and should not be used to treat streptococcal, staphylococcal, or pneumococcal infections. Newer-generation FQs are more active against these pathogens; levofloxacin has documented efficacy and safety in pediatric clinical trials for respiratory tract infections, acute otitis media, and community-acquired pneumonia. Children with any question of joint/tendon/bone toxicity in the levofloxacin studies were followed up to 5 years after treatment, with no difference in joint/tendon outcomes in these randomized studies, compared to the outcomes of standard FDA-approved antibiotics used in these studies.[7] None of the newer-generation FQs are significantly more active against gram-negative pathogens than ciprofloxacin. Quinolone antibiotics are bitter tasting. Ciprofloxacin and levofloxacin are currently available in a suspension form; ciprofloxacin is FDA approved in pediatrics for cUTIs and inhalation anthrax, while levofloxacin is approved for plague and inhalation anthrax. Regarding levofloxacin, Johnson & Johnson chose not to apply to the FDA for approval for pediatric respiratory tract infection indications, despite successful clinical trials in children. For reasons of safety and to prevent the emergence of widespread resistance, FQs should still not be used for primary therapy for pediatric infections and should be limited to situations in which safe and effective alternative oral therapy does not exist.

5. Preferred Therapy for Specific Fungal Pathogens

NOTES

- See Chapter 6 for discussion of the differences between polyenes, azoles, and echinocandins.
- **Abbreviations:** ABLC, amphotericin B lipid complex (Abelcet); AmB, amphotericin B; AmB-D, amphotericin B deoxycholate, the conventional standard amphotericin B (original trade name Fungizone); bid, twice daily; CNS, central nervous system; CSF, cerebrospinal fluid; CT, computed tomography; div, divided; ECMO, extracorporeal membrane oxygenation; HAART, highly active antiretroviral therapy; IV, intravenous; L-AmB, liposomal amphotericin B (AmBisome); max, maximum; PO, orally; q, every; qd, once daily; qid, 4 times daily; spp, species; TMP/SMX, trimethoprim/sulfamethoxazole.

A. OVERVIEW OF MORE COMMON FUNGAL PATHOGENS AND THEIR USUAL PATTERN OF ANTIFUNGAL SUSCEPTIBILITIES

Fungal Species	Amphotericin B Formulations	Fluconazole	Itraconazole	Voriconazole	Posaconazole	Isavuconazole	Flucytosine	Caspofungin, Micafungin, or Anidulafungin
Aspergillus calidoustus	++	–	–	–	–	–	–	++
Aspergillus fumigatus	+	–	±	++	+	++	–	+
Aspergillus terreus	–	–	+	++	+	++	–	+
Blastomyces dermatitidis	++	+	++	+	+	+	–	–
Candida albicans	+	++	+	+	+	+	+	++
Candida auris	±	–	±	±	+	+	±	++
Candida glabrata	+	–	±	±	±	±	+	±
Candida guilliermondii	+	±	+	+	+	+	+	±
Candida krusei	+	–	–	+	+	+	+	++
Candida lusitaniae	–	++	+	+	+	+	+	+
Candida parapsilosis	++	++	+	+	+	+	+	+
Candida tropicalis	+	+	+	+	+	+	+	++

Coccidioides immitis	++	++	+	+	++	+	–	–
Cryptococcus spp	++	+	+	+	+	+	++	–
Fusarium spp	±	–	–	++	+	+	–	–
Histoplasma capsulatum	++	+	++	+	+	+	–	–
Lomentospora (formerly *Scedosporium*) *prolificans*	–	–	±	±	±	±	–	±
Mucor spp	++	–	±	–	+	++	–	–
Paracoccidioides spp	+	+	++	+	+	+	–	–
Penicillium spp	±	–	++	+	+	+	–	–
Rhizopus spp	++	–	–	–	+	+	–	–
Scedosporium apiospermum	–	–	±	+	+	+	–	±
Sporothrix spp	+	+	++	+	+	+	–	–
Trichosporon spp	–	+	+	++	+	+	–	–

NOTE: ++ = preferred; **+** = acceptable; **±** = possibly effective (see text for further discussion); **–** = unlikely to be effective.

B. SYSTEMIC INFECTIONS

Infection

When treating invasive fungal disease with azoles, it is important to document therapeutic serum concentrations, particularly when using oral therapy. The editors use laboratories that provide high-performance liquid chromatography/mass spectrometry techniques with rapid results compared with the older microbiological techniques. One laboratory that provides this service is the University of Texas Health Science Center at San Antonio Fungus Testing Laboratory (https://lsom.uthscsa.edu/pathology/reference-labs/fungus-testing-laboratory/antifungal-drug-levels; 210/567-4029).

	Therapy (evidence grade)	Comments
Prophylaxis		
Prophylaxis of invasive fungal infection in patients with hematologic malignancies[1–11]	Caspofungin was superior to fluconazole in a randomized controlled trial of neutropenic children with acute myeloid leukemia (AI),[12] yet compared to triazoles, caspofungin did not significantly reduce incidence of invasive fungal disease in pediatric recipients of allogeneic hematopoietic cell transplants.[13] Micafungin is safe and effective as prophylaxis in pediatric autologous hematopoietic stem cell transplant (AII).[14] Fluconazole 6 mg/kg/day for prevention of infection (AII). Posaconazole for prevention of infection has been well studied in adults (AI) and offers anti-mold coverage.[4]	Fluconazole is not effective against molds and some strains of *Candida*. Posaconazole PO, voriconazole PO, and micafungin IV are effective in adults in preventing yeast and mold infections but are not well studied in children for this indication.[15]
Prophylaxis of invasive fungal infection in patients with solid-organ transplants[16–20]	Fluconazole 6 mg/kg/day for prevention of infection (AII)	AmB, caspofungin, micafungin, voriconazole, or posaconazole may be effective in preventing infection.

Treatment		
Aspergillosis[1,21–32]	Voriconazole (AI) 18 mg/kg/day IV div q12h as a loading dose on the first day, then 16 mg/kg/day IV div q12h as a maintenance dose for children 2–12 y or 12–14 y and weighing <50 kg. In children ≥15 y or 12–14 y and weighing >50 kg, use adult dosing (load 12 mg/kg/day IV div q12h on the first day, then 8 mg/kg/day div q12h as a maintenance dose) (AII). When stable, may switch from voriconazole IV to voriconazole PO at a dose of 18 mg/kg/day div bid for children 2–12 y and at least 400 mg/day div bid for children >12 y (AII). Dosing in children <2 y is less clear, but doses are generally higher due to more rapid clearance (AIII). These are only initial dosing recommendations; it is critical to understand that continued dosing in all ages is guided by close monitoring of trough serum voriconazole concentrations in individual patients (AII). Unlike in adults, voriconazole oral bioavailability in children is about only 50%–60%, so trough levels are crucial when using PO.[33] Alternatives for primary therapy when voriconazole cannot be administered: isavuconazole (AI), posaconazole (AI), or L-AmB 5 mg/kg/day (AII). Dosing of isavuconazole in children <13 y is 10 mg/kg (q8h on days 1 and 2 and qd thereafter).[34] ABLC is another alternative. Echinocandin primary monotherapy should not be used for treating invasive aspergillosis (CII). AmB-D should be used only in resource-limited settings in which no alternative agent is available (AII).	Voriconazole is the current guideline-recommended primary antifungal therapy for all clinical forms of aspergillosis. A recent randomized controlled trial showed that posaconazole is non-inferior to voriconazole for invasive aspergillosis (AI).[35] An earlier randomized controlled trial showed that isavuconazole was non-inferior to voriconazole for invasive aspergillosis (AI).[30] Early initiation of therapy in patients with strongly suspected disease is important while a diagnostic evaluation is conducted. Optimal voriconazole trough serum concentrations (generally thought to be 2–5 mcg/mL) are essential. Check trough level 2–5 days after initiation of therapy, and repeat the following week to verify and 4 days after a change of dose.[32] It is critical to monitor trough concentrations to guide therapy due to high inter-patient variability.[36] Low voriconazole concentrations are a consistent leading cause of clinical failure. Younger children (especially <3 y) often have lower trough voriconazole levels and need much higher dosing. Dosing for younger children should begin as listed but will invariably need to be increased. Total treatment course is for a minimum of 6 wk, largely dependent on the degree and duration of immunosuppression and evidence of disease improvement. A recent expert panel agreed that primary therapy, with confirmed appropriate therapeutic drug levels, should be given for at least 8 days to show an effect.[37]

(*Continued on next page*)

B. SYSTEMIC INFECTIONS *(continued)*

	Therapy (evidence grade)	Comments
Aspergillosis[1,20–31] *(continued)*		Current guidelines recommend that salvage antifungal therapy options after failed primary therapy include a change of antifungal class (by using L-AmB or an echinocandin), a switch to isavuconazole, a switch to posaconazole (serum trough concentrations ≥1 mcg/mL), or use of combination antifungal therapy. Most experts would recommend a switch to L-AmB. Azole monotherapy is not usually recommended after azole prophylaxis has failed. Combination antifungal therapy with voriconazole plus an echinocandin may be considered in select patients. The addition of anidulafungin to voriconazole as combination therapy showed some statistical benefit to the combination over voriconazole monotherapy in only certain patients.[38] In vitro data suggest some synergy with 2 (but not 3) drug combinations: an azole plus an echinocandin is the most well studied. If combination therapy is used, this is likely best done initially, when voriconazole trough concentrations may not yet be appropriate. Routine antifungal susceptibility testing is not recommended but is suggested for patients who are suspected of having an azole-resistant isolate or who are unresponsive to therapy. Azole-resistant *Aspergillus fumigatus* is increasing. If local epidemiology suggests >10% azole resistance, initial empiric therapy should be voriconazole + echinocandin OR + L-AmB, and subsequent therapy guided based on antifungal susceptibilities.[39] Micafungin likely has equal efficacy to caspofungin against aspergillosis.[40]

		Return of immune function is paramount to treatment success; for children receiving corticosteroids, decreasing the corticosteroid dosage or changing to steroid-sparing protocols is important.
Bipolaris, Cladophialophora, Curvularia, Exophiala, Alternaria, and other agents of **phaeohyphomycosis** (dematiaceous, pigmented molds)[41–48]	Voriconazole (AI) 18 mg/kg/day IV div q12h as a loading dose on the first day, then 16 mg/kg/day IV div q12h as a maintenance dose for children 2–12 y or 12–14 y and weighing <50 kg. In children ≥15 y or 12–14 y and weighing >50 kg, use adult dosing (load 12 mg/kg/day IV div q12h on the first day, then 8 mg/kg/day div q12h as a maintenance dose) (AII). When stable, may switch from voriconazole IV to voriconazole PO at a dose of 18 mg/kg/day div bid for children 2–12 y and at least 400 mg/day div bid for children >12 y (AII). Dosing in children <2 y is less clear, but doses are generally higher due to more rapid clearance (AIII). These are only initial dosing recommendations; continued dosing in all ages is guided by close monitoring of trough serum voriconazole concentrations in individual patients (AII). Unlike in adults, voriconazole oral bioavailability in children is about only 50%–60%, so trough levels are crucial.[33] Alternatives could include posaconazole (trough concentrations >1 mcg/mL) or combination therapy with an echinocandin + azole or an echinocandin + L-AmB (BIII).	Aggressive surgical debulking/excision is essential for CNS lesions. These can be highly resistant infections, so strongly recommend antifungal susceptibility testing to guide therapy and consultation with a pediatric infectious diseases expert. Antifungal susceptibilities are often variable, but empiric therapy with voriconazole is the best start. Optimal voriconazole trough serum concentrations (generally thought to be 2–5 mcg/mL) are important for success. Check trough level 2–5 days after initiation of therapy and repeat the following week to verify and 4 days after a change of dose. It is critical to monitor trough concentrations to guide therapy due to high inter-patient variability.[36] Low voriconazole concentrations are a leading cause of clinical failure. Younger children (especially <3 y) often have lower voriconazole levels and need much higher dosing. Some experts will recommend higher trough levels for difficult CNS lesions.

B. SYSTEMIC INFECTIONS *(continued)*

	Therapy (evidence grade)	Comments
Blastomycosis (North American)[49–55]	For moderate to severe pulmonary disease: L-AmB 5 mg/kg IV daily for 1–2 wk or until improvement noted, followed by step-down therapy with itraconazole oral solution 10 mg/kg/day div bid (max 400 mg/day) for a total of 6–12 mo (AIII). ABLC is an alternative formulation if L-AmB is not available. Itraconazole loading dose (double dose for first 2 days) is recommended in adults but has not been studied in children (but is likely helpful). For mild to moderate pulmonary disease: itraconazole oral solution 10 mg/kg/day div bid (max 400 mg/day) for a total of 6–12 mo (AIII). Itraconazole loading dose (double dose for first 2 days) is recommended in adults but has not been studied in children (but is likely helpful). For CNS blastomycosis: L-AmB or ABLC (preferred over AmB-D) for 4–6 wk, followed by an azole (fluconazole is preferred, at 12 mg/kg/day after a loading dose of 25 mg/kg; alternatives for CNS disease are voriconazole or itraconazole), for a total of at least 12 mo and until resolution of CSF abnormalities (AII). Some experts suggest combination therapy with L-AmB/ABLC plus high-dose fluconazole as induction therapy in CNS blastomycosis until clinical improvement (BIII).	New international guidelines exist.[56] All forms of blastomycosis should be treated. Itraconazole oral solution provides greater and more reliable absorption than capsules, and only the oral solution should be used (on an empty stomach); serum concentrations of itraconazole should be determined 5 days after start of therapy to ensure adequate drug exposure. For blastomycosis, maintain trough itraconazole concentrations 1–2 mcg/mL (values for both itraconazole and hydroxyl-itraconazole are added together). If only itraconazole capsules are available, use 20 mg/kg/day div q12h taken with cola drink to increase gastric acidity and bioavailability. Alternative to itraconazole: 12 mg/kg/day fluconazole (BIII) after a loading dose of 25 mg/kg/day. A case series has shown that outcomes of voriconazole are like those of itraconazole, and there is little experience with posaconazole or isavuconazole. Patients with extrapulmonary blastomycosis should receive at least 12 mo of total therapy; long courses are recommended for CNS or bone involvement. If induction with L-AmB alone is failing, add itraconazole or high-dose fluconazole until clinical improvement. Lifelong itraconazole if immunosuppression cannot be reversed.
Candidiasis[57–61] (See Chapter 6.)		
– Cutaneous	Topical therapy (alphabetic order): ciclopirox, clotrimazole, econazole, haloprogin, ketoconazole, miconazole, oxiconazole, sertaconazole, sulconazole	Fluconazole 6 mg/kg/day PO qd for 5–7 days Relapse common in cases of chronic mucocutaneous disease, and antifungal susceptibilities critical to drive appropriate therapy

– Disseminated infection, acute (including catheter fungemia)	An echinocandin is recommended as initial therapy. Caspofungin 70 mg/m^2 IV loading dose on day 1 (max dose 70 mg), followed by 50 mg/m^2 IV (max dose 70 mg) on subsequent days (AII); OR micafungin 2 mg/kg/day q24h (children weighing <40 kg), with max dose 100 mg/day (AII).[62] ABLC or L-AmB 5 mg/kg/day IV q24h (BII) is an effective but less attractive alternative due to potential toxicity (AII). Fluconazole (12 mg/kg/day q24h, after a loading dose of 25 mg/kg/day) is an alternative for patients who are not critically ill and have had no prior azole exposure (CIII). A fluconazole loading dose is standard of care in adult patients but has been studied only in infants (not yet in children)[63]; however, it is very likely that the beneficial effect of a loading dose extends to children. Fluconazole can be used as step-down therapy in stable neutropenic patients with susceptible isolates and documented bloodstream clearance (CIII). For children of all ages receiving ECMO, fluconazole is dosed as a 35 mg/kg loading dose on day 1, followed by 12 mg/kg/day (BII).[64] Transition from an echinocandin to fluconazole (usually within 5–7 days) is recommended for non-neutropenic patients who are clinically stable, have isolates that are susceptible to fluconazole (eg, *Candida albicans*), and have negative repeated blood cultures following initiation of antifungal therapy (AII).	Prompt removal of infected IV catheter or any infected devices is absolutely critical to success (AII). For infections with *Candida krusei* or *Candida glabrata*, an echinocandin is preferred; however, there are increasing reports of some *C glabrata* resistance to echinocandins (treatment would, therefore, be lipid formulation L-AmB or ABLC) (BIII). There are increasing reports of some *Candida tropicalis* resistance to fluconazole. Lipid formulation AmB (5 mg/kg daily) is a reasonable alternative if there is intolerance, limited availability, or resistance to other antifungal agents (AI). Transition from a lipid AmB to fluconazole is recommended after 5–7 days among patients who have isolates that are susceptible to fluconazole, who are clinically stable, and in whom repeated cultures on antifungal therapy are negative (AI). Voriconazole (18 mg/kg/day div q12h loading dose, followed by 16 mg/kg/day div q12h) is effective for candidemia but offers little advantage over fluconazole as initial therapy. Voriconazole is recommended as step-down oral therapy for select cases of candidemia due to *C krusei* or if mold coverage is needed. Follow-up blood cultures should be performed qd or every other day to establish the time point at which candidemia has been cleared (AIII). Duration of therapy is for 2 wk AFTER negative cultures in pediatric patients without obvious metastatic complications and after symptom resolution (AII). In neutropenic patients, ophthalmologic findings of choroidal and vitreous infection are minimal until recovery from neutropenia; therefore, dilated funduscopic examinations should be performed within the first week after recovery from neutropenia (AIII).

(*Continued on next page*)

B. SYSTEMIC INFECTIONS *(continued)*

	Therapy (evidence grade)	Comments
– Disseminated infection, acute (including catheter fungemia) (*continued*)	For CNS infections: L-AmB/ABLC (5 mg/kg/day), and AmB-D (1 mg/kg/day) as an alternative, combined with or without flucytosine 100 mg/kg/day PO div q6h (AII) until initial clinical response, followed by step-down therapy with fluconazole (12 mg/kg/day q24h, after a loading dose of 25 mg/kg/day); echinocandins do not achieve therapeutic concentrations in CSF.	All non-neutropenic patients with candidemia should ideally have a dilated ophthalmologic examination, preferably performed by an ophthalmologist, within the first week after diagnosis (AIII).
– Disseminated infection, chronic (hepatosplenic)	Initial therapy with lipid formulation AmB (L-AmB or ABLC, 5 mg/kg daily) OR an echinocandin (caspofungin 70 mg/m^2 IV loading dose on day 1 [max dose 70 mg], followed by 50 mg/m^2 IV [max dose 70 mg] on subsequent days OR micafungin 2 mg/kg/day q24h in children weighing <40 kg [max dose 100 mg]) for several weeks, followed by oral fluconazole in patients unlikely to have a fluconazole-resistant isolate (12 mg/kg/day q24h, after a loading dose of 25 mg/kg/day) (AIII). Therapy should continue until lesions resolve on repeated imaging; they usually resolve after several months. Premature discontinuation of antifungal therapy can lead to relapse (AIII).	If chemotherapy or hematopoietic cell transplant is required, it should not be delayed because of the presence of chronic disseminated candidiasis, and antifungal therapy should be continued throughout the period of high risk to prevent relapse (AIII).
– Neonatal[60] (See Chapter 2.)	AmB-D (1 mg/kg/day) is recommended therapy (AII).[65] Fluconazole (12 mg/kg/day q24h, after a loading dose of 25 mg/kg/day) is an alternative if patient has not been receiving fluconazole prophylaxis (AII).[66] For treatment of neonates and young infants (<120 days) receiving ECMO, fluconazole is loaded with 35 mg/kg on day 1, followed by 12 mg/kg/day q24h (BII).	In nurseries with high rates of candidiasis (>10%), IV or oral fluconazole prophylaxis (AI) (3–6 mg/kg twice weekly for 6 wk) in high-risk neonates (birth weight <1,000 g) is recommended. Oral nystatin, 100,000 U 3 times daily for 6 wk, is an alternative to fluconazole in neonates with birth weights <1,500 g when availability or resistance precludes the use of fluconazole (CII).

	Lipid formulation AmB is an alternative but carries a theoretical risk of penetrating the urinary tract less than AmB-D (CIII) would. Duration of therapy for candidemia without obvious metastatic complications is for 2 wk AFTER documented clearance and resolution of symptoms (therefore, generally 3 wk total). Echinocandins should be used with caution and generally limited to salvage therapy or to situations in which resistance or toxicity precludes the use of AmB-D or fluconazole (CIII). A recent randomized trial of caspofungin vs AmB-D showed similar fungal-free survival.[67] Role of flucytosine in neonates with meningitis is questionable and not routinely recommended due to toxicity concerns. The addition of flucytosine (100 mg/kg/day div q6h) may be considered as salvage therapy in patients who have not had a clinical response to initial AmB therapy, but adverse effects are frequent (CIII).	Lumbar puncture and dilated retinal examination recommended for neonates with cultures positive for *Candida* spp from blood and/or urine (AIII). Same recommended for all neonates with birth weight <1,500 g with candiduria with or without candidemia (AIII). CT or ultrasound imaging of genitourinary tract, liver, and spleen should be performed if blood cultures are persistently positive (AIII). Meningoencephalitis in the neonate occurs at a higher rate than in older children/adults. Central venous catheter removal is strongly recommended. Infected CNS devices, including ventriculostomy drains and shunts, should be removed if possible.
– Oropharyngeal, esophageal[57]	Mild oropharyngeal disease: clotrimazole 10-mg troches PO 5 times daily OR nystatin 100,000 U/mL, 4–6 mL qid for 7–14 days. Alternatives also include miconazole mucoadhesive buccal 50-mg tablet to the mucosal surface over the canine fossa qd for 7–14 days OR 1–2 nystatin pastilles (200,000 U each) qid for 7–14 days (AII). Moderate to severe oropharyngeal disease: fluconazole 6 mg/kg PO qd for 7–14 days (AII). Esophageal candidiasis: oral fluconazole (6–12 mg/kg/day, after a loading dose of 25 mg/kg/day) for 14–21 days (AI). If cannot tolerate oral therapy, use fluconazole IV OR ABLC/L-AmB/AmB-D OR an echinocandin (AI).	A meta-analysis showed that clotrimazole is less effective than fluconazole but as effective as other topical therapies.[68] For fluconazole-refractory oropharyngeal or esophageal disease: itraconazole oral solution OR posaconazole OR AmB IV OR an echinocandin for up to 28 days (AII). Esophageal disease always requires systemic antifungal therapy. A diagnostic trial of antifungal therapy for esophageal candidiasis is appropriate before performing an endoscopic examination (AI). Chronic suppressive therapy (3 times weekly) with fluconazole is recommended for recurrent infections (AI).

B. SYSTEMIC INFECTIONS *(continued)*

	Therapy (evidence grade)	Comments
– Urinary tract infection	Cystitis: fluconazole 6 mg/kg qd IV or PO for 2 wk (AII). For fluconazole-resistant *C glabrata* or *C krusei,* AmB-D for 1–7 days (AIII). Pyelonephritis: fluconazole 12 mg/kg qd IV or PO for 2 wk (AIII) after a loading dose of 25 mg/kg/day. For fluconazole-resistant *C glabrata* or *C krusei,* AmB-D with or without flucytosine for 1–7 days (AIII).	Treatment is NOT recommended in asymptomatic candiduria unless high risk for dissemination; neutropenic low birth weight neonate (<1,500 g); or patient to undergo urologic manipulation (AIII). Neutropenic patients and low birth weight neonates should be treated as recommended for candidemia (AIII). Removing Foley catheter, if present, may lead to a spontaneous cure in the normal host; check for additional upper urinary tract disease. AmB-D bladder irrigation is not generally recommended due to high relapse rate (an exception may be in fluconazole-resistant *Candida*) (CIII). For renal collecting-system fungus balls, surgical debridement may be required in non-neonates (BIII). Echinocandins have poor urinary concentrations. AmB-D has greater urinary penetration than L-AmB/ABLC.
– Vulvovaginal[66]	Topical vaginal cream/tablets/suppositories (alphabetic order): butoconazole, clotrimazole, econazole, fenticonazole, miconazole, sertaconazole, terconazole, or tioconazole for 3–7 days (AI) OR fluconazole 10 mg/kg (max 150 mg) as a single dose (AII)	For uncomplicated vulvovaginal candidiasis, no topical agent is clearly superior. Avoid azoles during pregnancy. For severe disease, fluconazole 150 mg given q72h for 2–3 doses (AI). For recurring disease, consider 10–14 days of induction with topical agent or fluconazole, followed by fluconazole once weekly for 6 mo (AI). In a phase 2 study, ibrexafungerp was effective and well tolerated (AII).[69]

Chromoblastomycosis (subcutaneous infection by dematiaceous fungi)[70–74]	Itraconazole oral solution 10 mg/kg/day div bid for 12–18 mo, in combination with surgical excision or repeated cryotherapy (AII). Itraconazole oral solution provides greater and more reliable absorption than capsules, and only the oral solution should be used (on an empty stomach); serum concentrations of itraconazole should be determined 5 days after start of therapy to ensure adequate drug exposure. Maintain trough itraconazole concentrations 1–2 mcg/mL (values for both itraconazole and hydroxyl-itraconazole are added together).	Alternative: terbinafine plus surgery; heat and potassium iodide; posaconazole. Lesions are recalcitrant and difficult to treat.

B. SYSTEMIC INFECTIONS *(continued)*

	Therapy (evidence grade)	Comments
Coccidioidomycosis[75–83]	For moderate infections: fluconazole 12 mg/kg IV/PO q24h (AII) after loading dose of 25 mg/kg/day. For severe pulmonary disease: AmB-D 1 mg/kg/day IV q24h OR ABLC/L-AmB 5 mg/kg/day IV q24h (AIII) as initial therapy for several weeks until clear improvement, followed by an oral azole for total therapy of at least 12 mo, depending on genetic or immunocompromised risk factors. For meningitis: fluconazole 12 mg/kg/day IV q24h (AII) after loading dose of 25 mg/kg/day (AII). Itraconazole has also been effective (BIII). If no response to azole, use intrathecal AmB-D (0.1–1.5 mg/dose) with or without fluconazole (AIII). Lifelong azole suppressive therapy required due to high relapse rate. Adjunctive corticosteroids in meningitis have resulted in less secondary cerebrovascular events.[84] For extrapulmonary (non-meningeal), particularly for osteomyelitis, an oral azole such as fluconazole or itraconazole solution 10 mg/kg/day div bid for at least 12 mo (AIII), and L-AmB/ABLC as an alternative (less toxic than AmB-D) for severe disease or if worsening. Itraconazole oral solution provides greater and more reliable absorption than capsules, and only the oral solution should be used (on an empty stomach); serum concentrations of itraconazole should be determined 5 days after start of therapy to ensure adequate drug exposure. Maintain trough itraconazole concentrations 1–2 mcg/mL (values for both itraconazole and hydroxyl-itraconazole are added together).	New international guidelines exist.[56] Mild pulmonary disease does not require routine therapy in the normal host and only requires periodic reassessment. Treatment with fluconazole or itraconazole should be given to all patients with underlying immunosuppression, prolonged infection, underlying cardiopulmonary comorbidities, or complement fixation titers of ≥1:32. There is experience with posaconazole for disease in adults but little experience in children. Isavuconazole experience in adults is increasing. Treat until titers of serum cocci complement fixation drop to 1:8 or 1:4, at about 3–6 mo. Disease in immunocompromised hosts may need to be treated longer, including potentially lifelong azole secondary prophylaxis. Watch for relapse up to 1–2 y after therapy.

Cryptococcosis[85–89]	For mild to moderate pulmonary disease: fluconazole 12 mg/kg/day (max 400 mg) IV/PO q24h after loading dose of 25 mg/kg/day for 6–12 mo (AII). Itraconazole is alternative if cannot tolerate fluconazole. For meningitis or severe pulmonary disease: induction therapy with AmB-D 1 mg/kg/day IV q24h OR ABLC/L-AmB 5 mg/kg/day q24h; AND flucytosine 100 mg/kg/day PO div q6h for a minimum of 2 wk and a repeated CSF culture is negative, followed by consolidation therapy with fluconazole (12 mg/kg/day with max dose 400 mg after a loading dose of 25 mg/kg/day) for a minimum of 8 more wk (AI). Then use maintenance therapy with fluconazole (6 mg/kg/day) for 6–12 mo (AI). Alternative induction therapies for meningitis or severe pulmonary disease (order of preference): AmB product for 4–6 wk (AII); AmB product plus fluconazole for 2 wk, followed by fluconazole for 8 wk (BII); fluconazole plus flucytosine for 6 wk (BII).	Serum flucytosine concentrations should be obtained after 3–5 days to achieve a 2-h post-dose peak <100 mcg/mL (ideally 30–80 mcg/mL) to prevent neutropenia. For HIV-positive patients, continue maintenance therapy with fluconazole (6 mg/kg/day) indefinitely. Initiate HAART 2–10 wk after commencement of antifungal therapy to avoid immune reconstitution inflammatory syndrome. In organ transplant recipients, continue maintenance fluconazole (6 mg/kg/day) for 6–12 mo after consolidation therapy with higher-dose fluconazole. For cryptococcal relapse, restart induction therapy (this time for 4–10 wk), repeat CSF analysis q2wk until sterile, and determine antifungal susceptibility of relapse isolate. Successful use of voriconazole, posaconazole, and isavuconazole for cryptococcosis has been reported in adult patients. In resource-limited settings, a recent clinical trial of a single 10 mg/kg dose of L-AmB plus 14 days of flucytosine + fluconazole was non-inferior to standard therapy.[90]

B. SYSTEMIC INFECTIONS *(continued)*

	Therapy (evidence grade)	Comments
Fusarium, Lomentospora (formerly ***Scedosporium***) ***prolificans, Pseudallescheria boydii*** (and its asexual form, ***Scedosporium apiospermum***),[41,91–95] and other agents of hyalohyphomycosis	Voriconazole (AII) 18 mg/kg/day IV div q12h as a loading dose on the first day, then 16 mg/kg/day IV div q12h as a maintenance dose for children 2–12 y or 12–14 y and weighing <50 kg. In children ≥15 y or 12–14 y and weighing >50 kg, use adult dosing (load 12 mg/kg/day IV div q12h on the first day, then 8 mg/kg/day div q12h as a maintenance dose) (AII). When stable, may switch from voriconazole IV to voriconazole PO at a dose of 18 mg/kg/day div bid for children 2–12 y and at least 400 mg/day div bid for children >12 y (AII). Dosing in children <2 y is less clear, but doses are generally higher due to more rapid clearance (AIII). These are only initial dosing recommendations; continued dosing in all ages is guided by close monitoring of trough serum voriconazole concentrations in individual patients (AII). Unlike in adults, voriconazole oral bioavailability in children is about only 50%–60%, so trough levels are crucial at this stage.[33]	These can be highly resistant infections, so strongly recommend antifungal susceptibility testing against a wide range of agents to guide specific therapy and consultation with a pediatric infectious diseases expert. Optimal voriconazole trough serum concentrations (generally thought to be 2–5 mcg/mL) are important for success. Check trough level 2–5 days after initiation of therapy and repeat the following week to verify and 4 days after a change of dose. It is critical to monitor trough concentrations to guide therapy due to high inter-patient variability.[36] Low voriconazole concentrations are a leading cause of clinical failure. Younger children (especially <3 y) often have lower voriconazole levels and need much higher dosing. Often resistant to AmB in vitro. Alternatives: posaconazole (trough concentrations >1 mcg/mL) can be active; echinocandins have been reportedly successful as salvage therapy in combination with azoles; while there are reports of promising in vitro combinations with terbinafine, terbinafine does not obtain therapeutic tissue concentrations required for these disseminated infections; miltefosine (for leishmaniasis) use has been reported. Olorofim is an investigational agent with excellent activity against these recalcitrant pathogens.

Histoplasmosis[96–98]	For severe acute pulmonary disease: ABLC/L-AmB 5 mg/kg/day q24h for 1–2 wk, followed by itraconazole 10 mg/kg/day div bid (max 400 mg daily) to complete a total of 12 wk (AIII). Add methylprednisolone (0.5–1.0 mg/kg/day) for first 1–2 wk in patients with hypoxia or significant respiratory distress. For mild to moderate acute pulmonary disease: if symptoms persist for >1 mo, itraconazole oral solution 10 mg/kg/day div bid for 6–12 wk (AIII). For progressive disseminated histoplasmosis: ABLC/L-AmB 5 mg/kg/day q24h for 4–6 wk; alternative treatment is lipid AmB for 1–2 wk followed by itraconazole 10 mg/kg/day div bid (max 400 mg daily) to complete a total of at least 12 mo (AIII).	New international guidelines exist.[56] Mild pulmonary disease may not require therapy and, in most cases, resolves in 1 mo. CNS histoplasmosis requires initial L-AmB/ABLC (less toxic than AmB-D) therapy for 4–6 wk, followed by itraconazole for at least 12 mo and until CSF antigen resolution. Itraconazole oral solution provides greater and more reliable absorption than capsules, and only the oral solution should be used (on an empty stomach); serum concentrations of itraconazole should be determined 5 days after start of therapy to ensure adequate drug exposure. Maintain trough itraconazole concentrations at >1–2 mcg/mL (values for both itraconazole and hydroxyl-itraconazole are added together). If only itraconazole capsules are available, use 20 mg/kg/day div q12h taken with cola drink to increase gastric acidity and bioavailability. Potential lifelong suppressive itraconazole if cannot reverse immunosuppression. Corticosteroids recommended for 2 wk for pericarditis with hemodynamic compromise. Voriconazole and posaconazole use has been reported. Fluconazole is inferior to itraconazole.

B. SYSTEMIC INFECTIONS *(continued)*

	Therapy (evidence grade)	Comments
Mucormycosis (previously known as zygomycosis)[31,99–105]	Aggressive surgical debridement combined with induction antifungal therapy: L-AmB at 5–10 mg/kg/day q24h (AII) for 3 wk. Lipid formulations of AmB are preferred to AmB-D due to increased penetration and decreased toxicity. Some experts advocate induction or salvage combination therapy with combination of L-AmB plus posaconazole[106] or L-AmB plus an echinocandin (although data are largely in diabetic patients with rhinocerebral disease) (CIII).[107] For salvage therapy, isavuconazole (AII)[108] or posaconazole (AIII). Following successful induction antifungal therapy (for at least 3 wk), can continue consolidation therapy with posaconazole (or use intermittent L-AmB) (BII).	Latest international mucormycosis guidelines recommend L-AmB as primary therapy.[109] Following clinical response with AmB, long-term oral step-down therapy with posaconazole (trough concentrations ideally for mucormycosis at >2 mcg/mL) can be attempted for 2–6 mo. Dosing of isavuconazole in children <13 y is 10 mg/kg (q8h on days 1 and 2 and qd thereafter).[34] Voriconazole has NO activity against mucormycosis or other zygomycetes. Return of immune function is paramount to treatment success; for children receiving corticosteroids, decreasing the corticosteroid dosage or changing to steroid-sparing protocols is also important. Antifungal susceptibility is key if can be obtained. CNS disease likely benefits from higher doses such as L-AmB at 10 mg/kg/day q24h. Likely no benefit at >10 mg/kg/day and only increased toxicity.
Paracoccidioidomycosis[110–113]	Itraconazole oral solution 10 mg/kg/day (max 400 mg daily) div bid for 6 mo (AIII) OR voriconazole (for dosing, see Aspergillosis earlier in this table under Treatment) (BI). Itraconazole is superior to TMP/SMX.	New international guidelines exist.[56] Alternatives: fluconazole; isavuconazole; sulfadiazine or TMP/SMX for 3–5 y. Voriconazole is similarly efficacious and useful in cases with CNS involvement. AmB is recommended for immunocompromised patients.

Pneumocystis jiroveci (formerly ***carinii***) pneumonia[114–116]	Severe disease: preferred regimen is TMP/SMX 15–20 mg TMP component/kg/day IV div q8h (AI) OR, for TMP/SMX intolerance or TMP/SMX treatment failure, pentamidine isethionate 4-mg base/kg/day IV qd (BII), for 3 wk. Mild to moderate disease: start with IV therapy, then, after acute pneumonitis is resolved, TMP/SMX 20 mg TMP component/kg/day PO div qid for 3-wk total treatment course (AII).	Alternatives: TMP AND dapsone; OR primaquine AND clindamycin; OR atovaquone. Prophylaxis: preferred regimen is TMP/SMX (5 mg TMP component/kg/day) PO div bid 3 times/wk on consecutive days; OR same dose, given qd; OR atovaquone: 30 mg/kg/day for infants 1–3 mo; 45 mg/kg/day for infants/children 4–24 mo; and 30 mg/kg/day for children >24 mo; OR dapsone 2 mg/kg (max 100 mg) PO qd, OR dapsone 4 mg/kg (max 200 mg) PO once weekly. Use steroid therapy for more severe disease.
Sporotrichosis[117,118]	For cutaneous/lymphocutaneous: itraconazole oral solution 10 mg/kg/day div bid for 2–4 wk after all lesions gone (generally total of 3–6 mo) (AII) For serious pulmonary or disseminated infection or disseminated sporotrichosis: ABLC/L-AmB at 5 mg/kg/day q24h until favorable response, then step-down therapy with itraconazole PO for at least a total of 12 mo (AIII) For less severe disease, itraconazole for 12 mo	New international guidelines exist.[56] If no response for cutaneous disease, treat with higher itraconazole dose, terbinafine, or saturated solution of potassium iodide. Fluconazole is less effective. Obtain serum concentrations of itraconazole after 2 wk of therapy; want serum trough concentration >1 mcg/mL. For meningeal disease, initial L-AmB/ABLC (less toxic than AmB-D) should be 4–6 wk before change to itraconazole for at least 12 mo of therapy. Surgery may be necessary in osteoarticular or pulmonary disease.

C. LOCALIZED MUCOCUTANEOUS INFECTIONS

Infection	Therapy (evidence grade)	Comments
Dermatophytoses		
– Scalp (tinea capitis, including kerion)[119–124]	Griseofulvin ultramicrosize 10–15 mg/kg/day or microsize 20–25 mg/kg/day PO qd for 6–12 wk (AII) (taken with milk or fatty foods to augment absorption) generally for 8 wk. For kerion, treat concurrently with prednisone (1–2 mg/kg/day for 1–2 wk) (AIII). Terbinafine can be used for only 2–4 wk. Terbinafine dosing is 62.5 mg/day (<20 kg), 125 mg/day (20–40 kg), or 250 mg/day (>40 kg) (AII).	Griseofulvin is superior for *Microsporum* infections, but terbinafine is superior for *Trichophyton* infections.[125] *Trichophyton tonsurans* predominates in United States. No need to routinely follow liver function tests in normal, healthy children taking griseofulvin. Alternatives: itraconazole oral solution 5 mg/kg qd or fluconazole. 2.5% selenium sulfide shampoo, or 2% ketoconazole shampoo, 2–3 times weekly should be used concurrently to prevent recurrences.
– Tinea corporis (infection of the trunk/limbs/face) – Tinea cruris (infection of the groin) – Tinea pedis (infection of the toes/feet)	Topical agents (alphabetic order): butenafine, ciclopirox, clotrimazole, econazole, haloprogin, ketoconazole, miconazole, naftifine, oxiconazole, sertaconazole, sulconazole, terbinafine, and tolnaftate (AII); apply daily for 4 wk.	For unresponsive tinea lesions, use griseofulvin PO in dosages provided for scalp (tinea capitis, including kerion); fluconazole PO; itraconazole PO; OR terbinafine PO. For tinea pedis: terbinafine PO or itraconazole PO is preferred over other oral agents. Keep skin as clean and dry as possible, particularly for tinea cruris and tinea pedis.
– Tinea unguium (onychomycosis)[121,126,127]	Terbinafine 62.5 mg/day (<20 kg), 125 mg/day (20–40 kg), or 250 mg/day (>40 kg). Use for at least 6 wk (fingernails) or 12–16 wk (toenails) (AII).	Recurrence or partial response common. Pulse terbinafine (1 wk per mo or 1 wk q3mo) or itraconazole has similar efficacy to that of continuous treatment.[128,129] Alternative: itraconazole pulse therapy with 10 mg/kg/day div q12h for 1 wk per mo. Two pulses for fingernails and 3 pulses for toenails. Alternatives: fluconazole, griseofulvin.

– Tinea versicolor (also called "pityriasis versicolor")[121,130,131]	Apply topically: selenium sulfide 2.5% lotion or 1% shampoo daily, leave on 30 min, then rinse; for 7 days, then monthly for 6 mo (AIII); OR ciclopirox 1% cream for 4 wk (BII); OR terbinafine 1% solution (BII); OR ketoconazole 2% shampoo daily for 5 days (BII). For small lesions, topical clotrimazole, econazole, haloprogin, ketoconazole, miconazole, or naftifine.	For lesions that fail to clear with topical therapy or for extensive lesions: fluconazole PO or itraconazole PO is equally effective. Recurrence common.

6. Choosing Among Antifungal Agents: Polyenes, Azoles, and Echinocandins

Separating antifungal agents by class, much like navigating the myriad of antibacterial agents, allows one to best understand the underlying mechanisms of action and then appropriately choose which agent would be optimal for empiric therapy or a directed approach. There are certain helpful generalizations that should be considered; for example, echinocandins are fungicidal against yeasts and fungistatic against molds, while azoles are the opposite. Coupled with these concepts is the need for continued surveillance for fungal epidemiology and resistance patterns. While some fungal species (spp) are inherently or very often resistant to specific agents or even classes, there are an increasing number of fungal isolates that are developing resistance due to environmental pressure or chronic use in individual patients. Additionally, new (often resistant) fungal spp emerge that deserve special attention, such as *Candida auris,* which can be multidrug resistant. In 2023, there are 15 individual antifungal agents approved by the US Food and Drug Administration (FDA) for systemic use, and several more in development, including entirely new classes. Many of these new antifungals currently in development will likely be approved and available soon (fosmanogepix, rezafungin, olorofim, oteseconazole, and others). This chapter focuses on only the most commonly used systemic agents and does not highlight the many anticipated new agents until they are approved for use in patients. For each agent, there are sometimes several formulations, each with unique pharmacokinetics that one must understand to optimize the agent, particularly in patients who are critically ill. Therefore, it is more important than ever to establish a firm conceptual foundation in understanding both how these antifungal agents work to optimize pharmacokinetics and where they work best to target fungal pathogens most appropriately.

Polyenes

Amphotericin B (AmB) is a polyene antifungal antibiotic that has been available since 1958. A *Streptomyces* species, isolated from the soil in Venezuela, produced 2 antifungals whose names originated from the drug's amphoteric property of reacting as an acid as well as a base. Amphotericin A was not as active as AmB, so only AmB is used clinically. Nystatin is another polyene antifungal, but, due to systemic toxicity, it is used only in topical preparations. Nystatin was named after the New York State Department of Health, where the discoverers were working at the time. AmB remains the most broad-spectrum antifungal available for clinical use. This lipophilic drug binds to ergosterol, the major sterol in the fungal cell membrane, and for years it was thought to create transmembrane pores that compromise the integrity of the cell membrane and create a rapid fungicidal effect through osmotic lysis. However, new biochemical studies suggest a mechanism of action more related to inhibiting ergosterol synthesis. Toxicity is likely due to cross-reactivity with the human cholesterol bi-lipid membrane, which resembles fungal ergosterol. The toxicity of the conventional formulation, AmB deoxycholate (AmB-D)—the parent molecule coupled with an ionic detergent for clinical use—can be substantial from the standpoints of systemic reactions (eg, fever, rigors) and acute and chronic renal toxicity. Premedication with acetaminophen, diphenhydramine, and meperidine has historically been used to prevent systemic reactions during infusion. Renal dysfunction develops primarily as decreased glomerular filtration with a rising serum creatinine concentration, but substantial tubular nephropathy is associated with potassium and magnesium wasting, requiring supplemental potassium for many neonates and children, regardless of clinical symptoms associated with infusion. Fluid loading with saline pre– and post–AmB-D infusion seems to somewhat mitigate renal toxicity.

Three lipid preparations approved in the mid-1990s decrease toxicity with no apparent decrease in clinical efficacy. Decisions on which lipid AmB preparation to use should, therefore, largely focus on side effects and costs. Two clinically useful lipid formulations exist: one in which ribbonlike lipid complexes of AmB are created (AmB lipid complex [ABLC]), Abelcet, and one in which AmB is incorporated into true liposomes (liposomal AmB [L-AmB]), AmBisome. The classic clinical dosage used of these preparations is 5 mg/kg/day, in contrast to the 1 mg/kg/day of AmB-D. In most studies, the side effects of L-AmB were somewhat less than those of ABLC, but both have significantly fewer side effects than AmB-D. The advantage of the lipid preparations is the ability to safely deliver a greater overall dose of the parent AmB drug. The cost of conventional AmB-D is substantially less than that of either lipid formulation. A colloidal dispersion of AmB in cholesteryl sulfate, Amphotec, which is no longer available in the United States, with decreased nephrotoxicity but infusion-related side effects, is closer to AmB-D than to the lipid formulations and precludes recommendation for its use. The decreased nephrotoxicity of the 3 lipid preparations is thought to be due to the preferential binding of its AmB to high-density lipoproteins, compared to AmB-D binding to low-density lipoproteins. Despite in vitro concentration-dependent killing, a clinical trial comparing L-AmB at doses of 3 mg/kg/day with 10 mg/kg/day showed no efficacy benefit for the higher dose and only greater toxicity.[1] Recent pharmacokinetic analyses of L-AmB showed that while children receiving L-AmB at lower doses exhibit linear pharmacokinetics, a significant proportion of children receiving L-AmB at daily doses greater than 5 mg/kg/day exhibit nonlinear pharmacokinetics with significantly higher peak concentrations and some toxicity.[2,3] Therefore, it is generally not recommended to use any lipid AmB preparations at very high dosages (>5 mg/kg/day), as it will likely incur only greater toxicity with no real therapeutic advantage. There are reports of using higher dosing in very difficult infections where a lipid AmB formulation is the first-line therapy (eg, mucormycosis), and while experts remain divided on this practice, it is clear that at least 5 mg/kg/day of a lipid AmB formulation should be used in such a setting. AmB has a long terminal half-life, and, coupled with the concentration-dependent killing, the agent is best used as single daily doses. These pharmacokinetics explain the use in some studies of once-weekly, or even once-every-2-weeks,[4] AmB for antifungal prophylaxis or preemptive therapy, albeit with mixed clinical results. If the overall AmB exposure needs to be decreased due to toxicity, it is best to increase the dosing interval (eg, 3 times weekly) but retain the full milligram per kilogram dose for optimal pharmacokinetics. There are ongoing efforts to develop novel delivery mechanisms for AmB, such as nanoparticles with encochleated AmB as an oral formulation, which are not ready for clinical use yet.

AmB-D has been used for nonsystemic purposes, such as bladder washes, intraventricular instillation, intrapleural instillation, and other modalities, but there are no firm data supporting those clinical indications, and it is likely that the local toxicities outweigh the theoretic benefits. One exception is aerosolized AmB for antifungal prophylaxis (not treatment) in lung transplant recipients due to the different pathophysiology of invasive aspergillosis (often originating at the bronchial anastomotic site, more so than parenchymal disease) in that specific patient population. This aerosolized prophylaxis approach, while indicated for lung transplant recipients, has not been shown to be effective in other patient populations. Due to the lipid chemistry, the L-AmB does not interact well with renal tubules and L-AmB is recovered from the urine at lower levels than AmB-D, so there is a theoretic concern with using a lipid formulation, as opposed to AmB-D, when treating isolated urinary fungal disease. This theoretic concern is likely outweighed by the real concern of toxicity with AmB-D. Most experts believe AmB-D should be reserved for use in resource-limited settings in which no alternative agents (eg, lipid formulations) are available. An exception is in neonates, where limited retrospective data suggest that the AmB-D formulation has better efficacy for invasive candidiasis.[5] Importantly, there are several pathogens that are inherently or functionally resistant to AmB, including *Candida lusitaniae, Trichosporon* spp, *Aspergillus terreus, Fusarium* spp, and *Pseudallescheria boydii* (*Scedosporium apiospermum*) or *Lomentospora prolificans.*

Azoles

This class of systemic agents was first approved in 1981 and is divided into imidazoles (ketoconazole), triazoles (fluconazole and itraconazole), and second-generation triazoles (voriconazole, posaconazole, and isavuconazole) based on the number of nitrogen atoms in the azole ring. All the azoles work by inhibition of ergosterol synthesis (fungal cytochrome P450 [CYP] sterol 14-demethylation) that is required for fungal cell membrane integrity. While the polyenes are rapidly fungicidal, the azoles are fungistatic against yeasts and fungicidal against molds. However, it is important to note that ketoconazole and fluconazole have no mold activity. The only systemic imidazole is ketoconazole, which is primarily active against *Candida* spp and is available in an oral formulation. Three azoles (itraconazole, voriconazole, and posaconazole) need therapeutic drug monitoring with trough levels within the first 4 to 7 days (when the patient is at a pharmacokinetic steady state); at present it is unclear if isavuconazole will require drug-level monitoring. It is less clear if therapeutic drug monitoring is required during primary azole prophylaxis, although low levels have been associated with a higher probability of breakthrough infection.

Fluconazole is active against a broader range of fungi than ketoconazole and includes clinically relevant activity against *Cryptococcus, Coccidioides,* and *Histoplasma.* The pediatric treatment dose is 12 mg/kg/day, which targets exposures that are observed in critically ill adults who receive 800 mg of fluconazole per day. Like most other azoles, fluconazole requires a loading dose on the first day, and this approach is routinely used in adult patients. A loading dose of 25 mg/kg on the first day has been nicely studied in infants[6,7] but has not been definitively studied in all children; yet it is likely also beneficial and the patient will reach steady-state concentrations more quickly based on adult and neonatal studies. The exception where it has been formally studied is children of all ages receiving extracorporeal membrane oxygenation, for whom, because of the higher volume of distribution, a higher loading dose (35 mg/kg) is required to achieve comparable exposure.[8,9] Compared with AmB, fluconazole achieves relatively high concentrations in urine and cerebrospinal fluid (CSF) due to its low lipophilicity, with urinary concentrations often so high that treatment against even "resistant" pathogens that are isolated only in the urine is possible. Fluconazole remains one of the most active and, so far, one of the safest systemic antifungal agents for the treatment of most *Candida* infections. *Candida albicans* remains generally sensitive to fluconazole, although resistance is increasingly present in many non-*albicans Candida* spp as well as in *C albicans* in children repeatedly exposed to fluconazole. For instance, *Candida krusei* is considered inherently resistant to fluconazole, *Candida glabrata* demonstrates dose-dependent resistance to fluconazole (and, usually, voriconazole), *Candida tropicalis* is developing more resistant strains, and the newly identified *C auris* is generally fluconazole resistant. Fluconazole is available in parenteral and oral (with >90% bioavailability) formulations, and toxicity is unusual and primarily hepatic.

Itraconazole is active against an even broader range of fungi and, unlike fluconazole, includes molds such as *Aspergillus*. It is currently available as a capsule or an oral solution (the intravenous [IV] form was discontinued); the oral solution provides about 30% higher and more consistent serum concentrations than capsules and should be used preferentially. Absorption using itraconazole oral solution is improved on an empty stomach and not influenced by gastric pH (unlike with the capsule form, which is best administered under fed conditions or with a more acidic cola beverage to increase absorption), and monitoring itraconazole serum concentrations, as with most azole antifungals, is a key principal in management. Generally, itraconazole serum trough levels should be 1 to 2 mcg/mL, greater than 1 mcg/mL for treatment, and greater than 0.5 mcg/mL for prophylaxis; trough levels greater than 5 mcg/mL may be associated with increased toxicity. Concentrations should be checked after 5 days of therapy to ensure adequate drug exposure. When measured by high-pressure liquid chromatography, itraconazole and its bioactive hydroxy-itraconazole metabolite are reported, the sum of which should be considered in assessing drug levels. In adult patients, itraconazole is recommended to be loaded at 200 mg twice daily for 2 days, followed by 200 mg daily starting on the third day. Loading dose studies have not been performed in children. Itraconazole in children requires twice-daily dosing throughout treatment, compared with once-daily maintenance dosing in adults, and the key to treatment success is following drug levels. Limited pharmacokinetic data are available in children; itraconazole has not been approved by the FDA for pediatric indications. Itraconazole is indicated in adults for therapy for mild to moderate disease with blastomycosis, histoplasmosis, and others. Although it possesses antifungal activity, itraconazole is not indicated as primary therapy against invasive aspergillosis, as voriconazole is a far superior option. Itraconazole is not active against mucormycosis. Toxicity in adults is primarily hepatic.

Voriconazole was approved in 2002 and is FDA approved for children 2 years and older.[10] Voriconazole is a fluconazole derivative, so think of it as having the greater tissue and CSF penetration of fluconazole but the added antifungal spectrum of itraconazole to include molds. While the bioavailability of voriconazole in adults is about 96%, multiple studies have shown that it is about only 50% to 60% in children, requiring clinicians to carefully monitor voriconazole trough concentrations in patients taking the oral formulation, further complicated by great inter-patient variability in clearance. Voriconazole serum concentrations are tricky to interpret, but monitoring these concentrations is essential to using this drug, as with all azole antifungals, and is especially important in circumstances of suspected treatment failure or possible toxicity. Most experts suggest voriconazole trough concentrations of 2 mcg/mL (at a minimum, 1 mcg/mL) or greater, which would generally exceed the pathogen's minimum inhibitory concentration. Generally, toxicity will not be seen until concentrations of about 6 mcg/mL or greater. Trough levels should be monitored 2 to 5 days after initiation of therapy and monitored again the following week to confirm that the patient remains in the therapeutic range or again 4 days after a change of dose. One important point is the acquisition of an accurate trough concentration, one obtained just before the next dose is due (not hours before solely for phlebotomy convenience) and not obtained through a catheter infusing the drug. These simple trough parameters will make interpretation possible. The fundamental voriconazole pharmacokinetics are different in adults versus children; in adults, voriconazole is metabolized in a nonlinear fashion, whereas in children, the drug is metabolized in a linear fashion. This explains the increased pediatric loading dosing for voriconazole at 9 mg/kg/dose versus loading with 6 mg/kg/dose in adult patients. Younger children, especially those younger than 3 years, require even higher dosages of voriconazole and have a larger therapeutic window for dosing. However, many studies have shown an inconsistent relationship, on a population level, between dosing and levels, highlighting the need for close monitoring after the initial dosing scheme and then dose adjustment as needed in the individual patient. For children younger than 2 years, some studies have even proposed 3-times–daily dosing to achieve sufficient serum levels.[11] Given the poor clinical and microbiological response of *Aspergillus* infections to AmB, voriconazole is clearly the treatment of choice for invasive aspergillosis and many other invasive mold infections (eg, pseudallescheriasis, fusariosis). Importantly, infections with mucormycosis are resistant to voriconazole. Voriconazole retains activity against most *Candida* spp, including some that are fluconazole resistant, but it is unlikely to replace fluconazole for treatment of fluconazole-susceptible *Candida* infections. Importantly, there are increasing reports of *C glabrata* resistance to voriconazole. Voriconazole produces some unique transient visual field abnormalities in about 10% of adults and children. There are an increasing number of reports, seen in as high as 20% of patients, of a photosensitive sunburn-like erythema that is not aided by sunscreen (only sun avoidance). In some rare long-term (mean of 3 years of therapy) cases, this voriconazole phototoxicity has developed into cutaneous squamous cell carcinoma. Discontinuing voriconazole is recommended in patients experiencing chronic phototoxicity. The rash is the most common indication for switching from voriconazole to posaconazole/isavuconazole if a triazole antifungal is required. Other voriconazole chronic toxicities reported include fluorosis and periostitis. Hepatotoxicity is uncommon, occurring in only 2% to 5% of patients. Voriconazole is CYP metabolized (CYP2C19), and allelic polymorphisms in the population could lead to personalized dosing.[12] Results have shown that some patients of certain ethnicities will face higher toxic serum concentrations than other patients, again reiterating the need for close trough level monitoring. Voriconazole also interacts with many similarly P450-metabolized drugs to produce some profound changes in serum concentrations of many concurrently administered drugs.

Posaconazole, an itraconazole derivative, was FDA approved in 2006 as an oral suspension for adolescents 13 years and older. A delayed-release tablet formulation was approved in November 2013, also for adolescents 13 years and older, and an IV formulation was approved in March 2014 for patients 18 years and older. Effective absorption of the oral suspension strongly requires taking the medication with food, ideally a high-fat meal; taking posaconazole on an empty stomach will result in about one-fourth of the absorption as in the fed state. The tablet formulation has significantly better absorption due to its delayed release in the small intestine, but absorption will still be slightly increased with food. If the patient can take the (relatively large) tablets, the delayed-release tablet is the much-preferred form due to the ability to easily obtain higher and more consistent drug levels. Due to the low pH (<5) of IV posaconazole, a central venous catheter is required for administration. The IV formulation contains only slightly lower amounts of the cyclodextrin vehicle than voriconazole, so similar theoretic renal accumulation concerns exist. The pediatric oral suspension dose recommended by some experts for treating invasive disease is estimated to be at least 18 mg/kg/day divided 3 times daily, but even that dose has not achieved target levels.[13] A study with a new pediatric formulation for suspension, essentially the tablet form that is able to be suspended, has recently been completed and showed good tolerability. In that study, a dose of 6 mg/kg (given twice a day as a loading dose on the first day and then once daily) as an IV or formulation for oral suspension achieved target exposures that were necessary for antifungal prophylaxis, with a safety profile like that for adult patients.[14] In that study, the IV formulation led to greater levels than the formulation for suspension, but both achieved target levels. A subsequent study suggests that posaconazole dosing for the delayed-release tablets and IV formulation requires likely greater daily doses for children younger than 13 years.[15] However, the exact pediatric dosing for posaconazole requires consultation with a pediatric infectious disease expert. Importantly, the delayed-release tablet cannot be broken for use due to its chemical coating. Pediatric dosing with the current IV or extended-release tablet dosing is not yet fully defined, but adolescents can likely follow the adult dosing schemes. In adult patients, IV posaconazole is loaded at 300 mg twice daily on the first day and then 300 mg once daily starting on the second day. Similarly, in adult patients, the extended-release tablet is dosed as 300 mg twice daily on the first day and then 300 mg once daily starting on the second day. In adult patients, the maximum amount of posaconazole oral suspension given is 800 mg/day due to its excretion, and that has been given as 400 mg twice daily or 200 mg 4 times a day in severely ill patients due to saturable absorption and findings of a marginal increase in exposure with more frequent dosing. Greater than 800 mg/day is not indicated in any patient. As with voriconazole and itraconazole, trough levels should be monitored, and most experts feel that posaconazole levels for treatment should be greater than or equal to 1 mcg/mL (and >0.7 mcg/mL for prophylaxis). Monitor posaconazole trough levels on day 5 of therapy or soon after. The in vitro activity of posaconazole against *Candida* spp is better than that of fluconazole and like that of voriconazole. Overall in vitro antifungal activity against *Aspergillus* is also equivalent to voriconazole, but, notably, it is the first triazole with substantial activity against some mucormycosis pathogens, including *Rhizopus* spp and *Mucor* spp, as well as activity against *Coccidioides, Histoplasma,* and *Blastomyces* and the pathogens of phaeohyphomycosis. Posaconazole treatment of invasive aspergillosis in patients with chronic granulomatous disease appears to be superior to voriconazole in this specific patient population for an unknown reason. Posaconazole is eliminated by hepatic glucuronidation but does demonstrate inhibition of the CYP3A4 enzyme system, leading to many drug interactions with other P450-metabolized drugs. It is currently approved for prophylaxis of *Candida* and *Aspergillus* infections in high-risk adults and for treatment of *Candida* oropharyngeal disease or esophagitis in adults. Posaconazole, like itraconazole, has generally poor CSF penetration.

Isavuconazole is a new triazole that was FDA approved in March 2015 for treatment of invasive aspergillosis and invasive mucormycosis with oral (capsules only) and IV formulations. Isavuconazole has not only a similar antifungal spectrum as voriconazole but also, very importantly, activity against mucormycosis. A phase 3 clinical trial in adult patients demonstrated non-inferiority versus voriconazole against invasive aspergillosis and other mold infections,[16] and an open-label study showed activity against mucormycosis.[17] New international mucormycosis guidelines recommend isavuconazole in the setting of preexisting renal compromise (when L-AmB, the recommended primary therapy, is, therefore, not recommended).[18] Isavuconazole is actually dispensed as the prodrug isavuconazonium sulfate. Dosing in adult patients is loading with isavuconazole at 200 mg (equivalent to 372-mg isavuconazonium sulfate) every 8 hours for 2 days (6 doses), followed by 200 mg once daily for maintenance dosing. A recently completed pediatric pharmacokinetic study reports that a dose of 10 mg/kg (every 8 hours on days 1 and 2 and once daily thereafter) resulted in similar exposures and safety as seen in adults.[19] The half-life is long (>5 days), there is 98% bioavailability in adults, and there is no reported food effect with oral isavuconazole. The manufacturer suggests no need for therapeutic drug monitoring, but some experts suggest trough levels may be needed in difficult-to-treat infections, and, absent well-defined therapeutic targets, the mean concentrations from phase II/III studies suggest that a range of 2 to 3 mcg/mL after day 5 is adequate exposure. Another study suggests a range of 2 to 5 mcg/mL.[20] To date, it seems that isavuconazole requires less dose modifications than voriconazole. Unlike voriconazole, the IV formulation does not contain the vehicle cyclodextrin, a difference that could make it more attractive in patients with renal failure. Early experience suggests a much lower rate of photosensitivity and skin disorders as well as visual disturbances, compared with voriconazole. Pediatric studies for treatment of invasive aspergillosis and mucormycosis are currently ongoing.

Echinocandins

This class of systemic antifungal agents was first approved in 2001. The echinocandins inhibit cell wall formation (in contrast to acting on the cell membrane by the polyenes and azoles) by noncompetitively inhibiting beta-1,3-glucan synthase, an enzyme present in fungi but absent in mammalian cells. These agents are generally very safe, as there is no beta-1,3-glucan in humans. The echinocandins are not metabolized through the CYP system, so fewer drug interactions are problematic, compared with the azoles. There is no need to adjust dose in renal failure, but one needs a lower dosage in the setting of very severe hepatic dysfunction. As a class, these antifungals generally have poor CSF penetration, although animal studies have shown adequate brain parenchyma levels, and do not penetrate the urine well. While the 3 clinically available echinocandins each individually have some unique and important dosing and pharmacokinetic parameters, especially in children, efficacy is generally equivalent. Opposite the azole class, the echinocandins are fungicidal against yeasts but fungistatic against molds. The fungicidal activity against yeasts has elevated the echinocandins to the preferred therapy against invasive candidiasis. Echinocandins are thought to be best used against invasive aspergillosis only as salvage therapy if a triazole fails or in a patient with suspected triazole resistance, never as primary monotherapy against invasive aspergillosis or any other invasive mold infection. Improved efficacy with combination therapy with the echinocandins and triazoles against *Aspergillus* infections is unclear, with disparate results in multiple smaller studies and a definitive clinical trial demonstrating minimal benefit over voriconazole monotherapy in only certain patient populations. Some experts have used combination therapy in invasive aspergillosis with a triazole plus echinocandin only during the initial phase of waiting for triazole drug levels to be appropriately high. There are reports of echinocandin resistance in *Candida* spp, as high as 12% in *C glabrata* in some studies, and the echinocandins as a class have previously been shown to be somewhat less active against *Candida parapsilosis* isolates (about 10%–15% respond poorly, but most are still susceptible, and guidelines still recommend echinocandin empiric therapy for invasive candidiasis). There is no therapeutic drug monitoring required for the echinocandins.

Caspofungin received FDA approval for children and teens aged 3 months to 17 years in 2008 for empiric therapy for presumed fungal infections in febrile, neutropenic patients; treatment of candidemia as well as *Candida* esophagitis, peritonitis, and empyema; and salvage therapy for invasive aspergillosis. A study in children with acute myeloid leukemia demonstrated that caspofungin prophylaxis resulted in significantly lower incidence of invasive fungal disease, compared with fluconazole prophylaxis.[21] A study comparing caspofungin with triazole prophylaxis in pediatric allogeneic hematopoietic cell transplant recipients showed no difference in the agents.[22] Due to its earlier approval, there are generally more reports with caspofungin than with the other echinocandins. Caspofungin dosing in children is calculated according to body surface area, with a loading dose on the first day of 70 mg/m^2, followed by daily maintenance dosing of 50 mg/m^2, and not to exceed 70 mg regardless of the calculated dose. Dose adjustment is unnecessary in children with mild liver dysfunction.[23] Significantly higher doses of caspofungin have been studied in adult patients without any clear added benefit in efficacy, but if the 50 mg/m^2 dose is tolerated and does not provide adequate clinical response, the daily dose can be increased to 70 mg/m^2. Dosing for caspofungin in neonates is 25 mg/m^2/day.

Micafungin was approved in 2005 for adults for treatment of candidemia, *Candida* esophagitis and peritonitis, and prophylaxis of *Candida* infections in stem cell transplant recipients and in 2013 for pediatric patients 4 months and older. Micafungin has the most pediatric and neonatal data available of all 3 echinocandins, including more extensive pharmacokinetic studies surrounding dosing and several efficacy studies.[24–26] Micafungin dosing in children is age dependent, as clearance increases dramatically in the younger age-groups (especially neonates), necessitating higher doses for younger children. Doses in children are generally thought to be 2 mg/kg/day, with higher doses likely needed for neonates, infants,[27] and younger patients and 10 mg/kg/day given to preterm neonates. Adult micafungin dosing (100 or 150 mg once daily) is to be used in patients who weigh more than 40 kg. Unlike with the other echinocandins, a loading dose is not required for micafungin. A recent prospective pediatric study showed that micafungin prophylaxis was safe and effective in children with autologous hematopoietic stem cell transplant.[28]

Anidulafungin was approved for adults for candidemia and *Candida* esophagitis in 2006 and is not officially approved for pediatric patients. Like the other echinocandins, anidulafungin is not P450 metabolized and has not demonstrated significant drug interactions. Limited pediatric pharmacokinetic data suggest weight-based dosing (3 mg/kg/day loading dose, followed by 1.5 mg/kg/day maintenance dosing).[29] This dosing achieves similar exposure levels in neonates and infants.[29] The adult dose for invasive candidiasis is a loading dose of 200 mg on the first day, followed by 100 mg daily. An open-label study of pediatric invasive candidiasis in children showed similar efficacy and minimal toxicity, comparable to those of the other echinocandins.[30] An additional study showed similar and acceptable pharmacokinetics in patients 1 month to 2 years of age.[31]

Triterpenoid

Ibrexafungerp was approved in June 2021 for adults with vulvovaginal candidiasis following 2 phase III studies (VANISH 203 and VANISH 306). This is the first new class of antifungals (also called "fungerps") approved since 2001. Enfumafungin, structurally distinct from the echinocandins, was discovered through screening of natural products and modified to develop this semisynthetic derivative for clinical use. Like the echinocandins, ibrexafungerp not only noncompetitively inhibits beta-1,3-glucan synthase but also destroys the fungi *Candida* and inhibits the fungi *Aspergillus*. The binding site on the glucan-synthase enzyme is not the same as on the echinocandins. Resistance or reduced susceptibility to the echinocandins is largely through 2 hot spot alterations in the *FKS1* gene, while many resistance alterations to ibrexafungerp are due to the *FKS2* gene, and ibrexafungerp has activity against some echinocandin-resistant isolates. Ibrexafungerp is the first orally available glucan-synthase inhibitor and has a long half-life, suggesting once-daily dosing for clinical use. As with the echinocandins, initial studies show limited to no distribution to the central nervous system and variable distribution to the eye. In a phase II study, ibrexafungerp as step-down therapy following initial echinocandin therapy for invasive candidiasis was well tolerated and achieved a favorable global response, like the standard of care.[32] There is an ongoing coadministration study with voriconazole in pulmonary invasive aspergillosis (SCYNERGIA), as well as an ongoing recurrent vulvovaginal candidiasis study (CANDLE), yet no completed pediatric studies.

7. Preferred Therapy for Specific Viral Pathogens

NOTE

- **Abbreviations:** AASLD, American Association for the Study of Liver Diseases; ART, antiretroviral therapy; ARV, antiretroviral; bid, twice daily; BSA, body surface area; CDC, Centers for Disease Control and Prevention; CLD, chronic lung disease; CMV, cytomegalovirus; CrCl, creatinine clearance; DAA, direct-acting antiviral; div, divided; EBV, Epstein-Barr virus; ECMO, extracorporeal membrane oxygenation; EUA, Emergency Use Authorization; FDA, US Food and Drug Administration; G-CSF, granulocyte colony-stimulating factor; HAART, highly active antiretroviral therapy; HBeAg, hepatitis B e antigen; HBV, hepatitis B virus; HCV, hepatitis C virus; HHS, US Department of Health and Human Services; HSV, herpes simplex virus; IFN, interferon; IG, immune globulin; IM, intramuscular; IV, intravenous; max, maximum; NRTI, nucleoside reverse transcriptase inhibitor; PEP, postexposure prophylaxis; PMA, postmenstrual age (weeks of gestation since most recent menstrual period PLUS weeks of chronologic age since birth); PO, orally; PrEP, preexposure prophylaxis; PTLD, posttransplant lymphoproliferative disorder; q, every; qd, once daily; qid, 4 times daily; RAE, retinol activity equivalent; RSV, respiratory syncytial virus; SQ, subcutaneous; tab, tablet; TAF, tenofovir alafenamide; tid, 3 times daily; WHO, World Health Organization.

A. OVERVIEW OF NON-HIV, NON–HEPATITIS B OR C VIRAL PATHOGENS AND USUAL PATTERN OF SUSCEPTIBILITY TO ANTIVIRALS

Virus	Acyclovir	Baloxavir	Cidofovir	Famciclovir	Foscarnet	Ganciclovir
Cytomegalovirus			+		+	+
Herpes simplex virus	++			+	+	+
Influenza A and B viruses		+				
Varicella-zoster virus	++			+	+	+

Virus	Letermovir	Oseltamivir	Peramivir	Valacyclovir	Valganciclovir	Zanamivir
Cytomegalovirus	+				++	
Herpes simplex virus				++	+	
Influenza A and B viruses		++	+			+
Varicella-zoster virus				++		

NOTE: ++ = preferred; + = acceptable; [blank cell] = untested.

B. OVERVIEW OF HEPATITIS B OR C VIRAL PATHOGENS AND USUAL PATTERN OF SUSCEPTIBILITY TO ANTIVIRALS

Virus	Daclatasvir Plus Sofosbuvir	Elbasvir/ Grazoprevir (Zepatier)	Entecavir	Glecaprevir/ Pibrentasvir (Mavyret)	Interferon alfa-2b
Hepatitis B virus			++		+
Hepatitis C virus[a]	+[c]	+[b,d]		++[e,f]	

Virus	Lamivudine	Ombitasvir/ Paritaprevir/ Ritonavir Co-packaged With Dasabuvir (Viekira Pak)	Pegylated Interferon Alfa-2a	Sofosbuvir/ Ledipasvir (Harvoni)	Sofosbuvir Plus Ribavirin
Hepatitis B virus	+		+		
Hepatitis C virus[a]		+[g]		++[e,h]	++[e,i]

Virus	Sofosbuvir/ Velpatasvir (Epclusa)	Sofosbuvir/ Velpatasvir/ Voxilaprevir (Vosevi)	Telbivudine	Tenofovir
Hepatitis B virus			+	++
Hepatitis C virus[a]	++[e,f]	+[j]		

NOTE: ++ = preferred; **+** = acceptable; [blank cell] = untested.

[a] HCV treatment guidelines from the Infectious Diseases Society of America and the AASLD available at www.hcvguidelines.org (accessed September 29, 2022).

[b] Approved ≥12 y of age.

[c] Treats genotypes 1 and 3. Not approved for children.

[d] Treats genotypes 1 and 4.

[e] Approved ≥3 y of age.

[f] Treats genotypes 1 through 6.

[g] Treats genotype 1. Not approved for children.

[h] Treats genotypes 1, 4, 5, and 6.

[i] In children, treats genotypes 2 and 3; in adults, 1 through 4.

[j] Not approved for children.

C. PREFERRED THERAPY FOR SPECIFIC VIRAL PATHOGENS

Infection	Therapy (evidence grade)	Comments
Adenovirus (pneumonia or disseminated infection in immunocompromised hosts)[1]	Cidofovir and ribavirin are active in vitro, but no prospective clinical data exist and both have significant toxicity. Two cidofovir dosing schedules have been used in clinical settings: (1) 5 mg/kg/dose IV once weekly or (2) 1–1.5 mg/kg/dose IV 3 times/wk. If parenteral cidofovir is used, IV hydration and oral probenecid should be used to reduce renal toxicity.	Brincidofovir, the PO bioavailable lipophilic derivative of cidofovir also known as CMX001, has been evaluated for the treatment of adenovirus in immunocompromised hosts. It is not yet commercially available.
Coronavirus (SARS-CoV-2) See www.aap.org/Nelsons for coronavirus updates.	Remdesivir is approved for use in patients aged ≥28 d and weighing at least 3 kg with positive results of direct SARS-CoV-2 viral testing, who are hospitalized or who are not hospitalized and have mild to moderate COVID-19 and risk factors for progression to severe COVID-19: Adults and pediatric patients weighing ≥40 kg: Single IV loading dose of 200 mg on day 1, followed by maintenance IV doses of 100 mg qd on and after day 2 Pediatric patients aged ≥28 d and weighing 3–<40 kg: Single IV loading dose of 5.0 mg/kg on day 1, followed by maintenance IV doses of 2.5 mg/kg qd on and after day 2 Nirmatrelvir/ritonavir (Paxlovid) has EUA from the FDA for the treatment of mild to moderate COVID-19 in persons aged ≥12 y and weighing ≥40 kg: 300 mg nirmatrelvir with 100 mg ritonavir PO bid for 5 days	Treatment duration for remdesivir is 10 days for hospitalized patients requiring invasive mechanical ventilation and/or ECMO. Treatment duration for remdesivir is 5 days for hospitalized patients not requiring invasive mechanical ventilation and/or ECMO (can be extended for up to 5 additional days based on initial clinical response). Treatment duration for remdesivir is 3 days for nonhospitalized patients diagnosed with mild to moderate COVID-19 and having risk factors for progression to severe COVID-19. Nirmatrelvir/ritonavir (Paxlovid) has numerous drug-drug interactions. Consult the listing on the FDA or Pfizer website before prescribing. Molnupiravir has EUA from the FDA for the treatment of mild to moderate COVID-19 in adults aged ≥18 y.

Cytomegalovirus		
– Neonatal[2]	See Chapter 2.	
– Immunocompromised (HIV, chemotherapy, transplant-related)[3–15]	For induction: ganciclovir 10 mg/kg/day IV div q12h for 14–21 days (AII) (may be increased to 15 mg/kg/day IV div q12h). For maintenance: 5 mg/kg IV q24h for 5–7 days per week. Duration dependent on degree of immunosuppression (AII). CMV hyperimmune globulin may decrease morbidity in bone marrow transplant patients with CMV pneumonia (AII).	Use foscarnet or cidofovir for ganciclovir-resistant strains; for HIV-positive children on HAART, CMV may resolve without anti-CMV therapy. Also used for prevention of CMV disease posttransplant for 100–120 days. Data on valganciclovir dosing in young children for treatment of retinitis are unavailable, but consideration can be given to transitioning from IV ganciclovir to oral valganciclovir after improvement of retinitis is noted. Limited data on oral valganciclovir in infants[16,17] (32 mg/kg/day PO div bid) and children (dosing by BSA [dose (milligrams) = 7 × BSA × CrCl]).[5] Maribavir (400 mg PO bid) is approved for the treatment of adult and pediatric patients (aged ≥12 y and weighing at least 35 kg) with posttransplant CMV infection/disease that is refractory to treatment (with or without genotypic resistance) with ganciclovir, valganciclovir, cidofovir, or foscarnet.

C. PREFERRED THERAPY FOR SPECIFIC VIRAL PATHOGENS *(continued)*

Infection	Therapy (evidence grade)	Comments
– Prophylaxis of infection in immunocompromised hosts[4,18]	Ganciclovir 5 mg/kg IV daily (or 3 times/wk) (started at engraftment for stem cell transplant patients) (BII) Valganciclovir at total dose in milligrams = 7 × BSA × CrCl (use max CrCl 150 mL/min/1.73 m^2) PO qd with food for children and teens 4 mo–16 y (max dose 900 mg/day) for primary prophylaxis in HIV patients[19] who are CMV antibody positive and have severe immunosuppression (CD4 count <50/mm^3 in children ≥6 y; CD4 percentage <5% in children <6 y) (CIII) Letermovir (adults ≥18 y, CMV-seropositive recipients [R+] of an allogeneic hematopoietic stem cell transplant) 480 mg administered PO qd or as IV infusion over 1 h through 100 days posttransplant (BI)[20]	Neutropenia is a complication with ganciclovir and valganciclovir prophylaxis and may be addressed with G-CSF. Prophylaxis and preemptive treatment strategies are effective, but preemptive treatment in high-risk adult liver transplant recipients is superior to prophylaxis.[9] Letermovir being studied in children, but no dosing information available at this time.
Ebola	Atoltivimab/maftivimab/odesivimab-ebgn (brand name: Inmazeb) Ansuvimab-zykl (brand name: Ebanga)	For treatment of *Zaire ebolavirus* infections
Enterovirus	Supportive therapy; no antivirals currently FDA approved	Pocapavir PO is currently under investigation for enterovirus (poliovirus). Pleconaril PO is currently under consideration for submission to FDA for approval for treatment of neonatal enteroviral sepsis syndrome.[21] As of June 2022, it is not available for compassionate use.

Epstein-Barr virus		
– Mononucleosis, encephalitis[22–24]	Limited data suggest small clinical benefit of valacyclovir in adolescents for mononucleosis (3 g/day div tid for 14 days) (CIII). For EBV encephalitis: ganciclovir IV OR acyclovir IV (AIII).	No prospective data on benefits of acyclovir IV or ganciclovir IV in EBV clinical infections of normal hosts. Patients suspected to have infectious mononucleosis should not be given ampicillin or amoxicillin, which causes nonallergic morbilliform rashes in a high proportion of patients with active EBV infection (AII). Therapy with short-course corticosteroids (prednisone 1 mg/kg/day PO [max 20 mg/day] for 7 days with subsequent tapering) may have a beneficial effect on acute symptoms in patients with marked tonsillar inflammation with impending airway obstruction, massive splenomegaly, myocarditis, hemolytic anemia, or hemophagocytic lymphohistiocytosis (BIII).
– Posttransplant lymphoproliferative disorder[25,26]	Ganciclovir (AIII)	Decrease immunosuppression if possible, as this approach has the most effect on control of EBV; rituximab, methotrexate have been used but without controlled data. Preemptive treatment with ganciclovir may decrease PTLD in solid-organ transplants.

C. PREFERRED THERAPY FOR SPECIFIC VIRAL PATHOGENS *(continued)*

Infection	Therapy (evidence grade)	Comments
Hepatitis B virus (chronic)[27–45]	AASLD-preferred treatments of children and adolescents[46]: IFN alfa-2b for children 1–18 y: 3 million U/m^2 BSA SQ 3 times/wk for 1 wk, followed by dose escalation to 6 million U/m^2 BSA (max 10 million U/dose); OR entecavir for children ≥2 y (optimum duration of therapy unknown [BII]) Entecavir dosing IF no prior nucleoside therapy: ≥16 y: 0.5 mg qd 2–15 y: 10–11 kg: 0.15 mg oral solution qd >11–14 kg: 0.2 mg oral solution qd >14–17 kg: 0.25 mg oral solution qd >17–20 kg: 0.3 mg oral solution qd >20–23 kg: 0.35 mg oral solution qd >23–26 kg: 0.4 mg oral solution qd >26–30 kg: 0.45 mg oral solution qd >30 kg: 0.5 mg oral solution or tab qd If prior nucleoside therapy: Double the dosage in each weight bracket for entecavir listed previously; OR tenofovir dipivoxil fumarate for adolescents ≥12 y and adults 300 mg qd. **NOTE:** TAF is also a preferred treatment of adults (25 mg daily) but has not been studied in children.	AASLD-nonpreferred treatments of children and adults: Lamivudine 3 mg/kg/day (max 100 mg) PO q24h for 52 wk for children ≥2 y (children coinfected with HIV and HBV should use the approved dose for HIV) (AII). Lamivudine approved for children ≥2 y, but antiviral resistance develops on therapy in 30%; OR adefovir for children ≥12 y (10 mg PO q24h for a minimum of 12 mo; optimum duration of therapy unknown) (BII); OR telbivudine (adult dose 600 mg qd). There are not sufficient clinical data to identify the appropriate dose for use in children. Indications for treatment of chronic HBV infection, with or without HIV coinfection, are (1) evidence of ongoing HBV viral replication, as indicated by serum HBV DNA (>20,000 without HBeAg positivity or >2,000 IU/mL with HBeAg positivity) for >6 mo and persistent elevation of serum transaminase levels for >6 mo, or (2) evidence of chronic hepatitis on liver biopsy (BII). Antiviral therapy is not warranted in children without necroinflammatory liver disease (BIII). Treatment is not recommended for children with immunotolerant chronic HBV infection (ie, normal serum transaminase levels despite detectable HBV DNA) (BII). All patients with HBV and HIV coinfection should initiate ART, regardless of CD4 count. This should include 2 drugs that have HBV activity as well, specifically tenofovir (dipivoxil fumarate or alafenamide) plus lamivudine or emtricitabine.[46] Patients who are already receiving effective ART that does not include a drug with HBV activity should have treatment changed to include tenofovir (dipivoxil fumarate or alafenamide) plus lamivudine or emtricitabine; alternatively, entecavir is reasonable if patients are receiving a fully suppressive ART regimen.

Hepatitis C virus (chronic)[47–54]	Genotypes 1–6: daily fixed-dose combination of sofosbuvir/velpatasvir (Epclusa) (<17 kg: 37.5 mg velpatasvir with 150 mg sofosbuvir qd; 17–<30 kg: 50 mg velpatasvir with 200 mg sofosbuvir; ≥30 kg: 100 mg velpatasvir with 400 mg sofosbuvir) for patients ≥3 y with genotype 1–6 who are treatment-naive or IFN-experienced without cirrhosis or with compensated cirrhosis OR Daily fixed-dose combination of glecaprevir/pibrentasvir (Mavyret) for patients ≥3 y with genotype 1–6 who are treatment-naive or treatment-experienced without cirrhosis or with compensated cirrhosis: ≥12 y or ≥45 kg: glecaprevir 300 mg with pibrentasvir 120 mg qd 3–11 y: <20 kg: glecaprevir 150 mg with pibrentasvir 60 mg qd 20–<30 kg: glecaprevir 200 mg with pibrentasvir 80 mg qd 30–<45 kg: glecaprevir 250 mg with pibrentasvir 100 mg qd Genotype 1: daily fixed-dose combination of ledipasvir (90 mg)/sofosbuvir (400 mg) (Harvoni) for patients with genotype 1 who are treatment-naive without cirrhosis or with compensated cirrhosis, or treatment-experienced with or without cirrhosis OR for patients ≥12 y elbasvir (50 mg)/grazoprevir (100 mg) (Zepatier) qd	Treatment of HCV infections in adults has been revolutionized in recent years with the licensure of numerous highly effective DAAs for use in adults, adolescents, and children as young as 3 y. Given the efficacy of these new treatment regimens in adults (AI),[55–70] treatment of children should consist only of IFN-free regimens, and an age-appropriate antiviral should be given to all HCV-infected children ≥3 y. The following treatment is recommended, based on viral genotype[71]: Sofosbuvir (Sovaldi) and sofosbuvir in a fixed-dose combination tab with ledipasvir (Harvoni) are now approved for patients ≥3 y; sofosbuvir/velpatasvir (Epclusa) is now approved for patients ≥3 y; and glecaprevir/pibrentasvir (Mavyret) is now approved for patients ≥3 y. (See www.hcvguidelines.org/unique-populations/children [accessed September 29, 2022] for additional information [BI].)

(*Continued on next page*)

C. PREFERRED THERAPY FOR SPECIFIC VIRAL PATHOGENS *(continued)*

Infection	Therapy (evidence grade)	Comments
Hepatitis C virus (chronic)[47–54] *(continued)*	Genotype 2: daily sofosbuvir (400 mg) plus weight-based ribavirin (see below) for patients with genotype 2 who are treatment-naive or treatment-experienced without cirrhosis or with compensated cirrhosis Genotype 3: daily sofosbuvir (400 mg) plus weight-based ribavirin (see below) for patients with genotype 3 who are treatment-naive or treatment-experienced without cirrhosis or with compensated cirrhosis Genotype 4 in patients ≥12 y: elbasvir (50 mg)/grazoprevir (100 mg) (Zepatier) qd Genotype 4, 5, or 6: daily fixed-dose combination of ledipasvir (90 mg)/sofosbuvir (400 mg) (Harvoni) for patients with genotype 4, 5, or 6 who are treatment-naive or treatment-experienced without cirrhosis or with compensated cirrhosis Dosing for ribavirin in combination therapy with sofosbuvir for adolescents ≥12 y or ≥35 kg: <47 kg: 15 mg/kg/day in 2 div doses 47–59 kg: 800 mg/day in 2 div doses 60–73 kg: 400 mg in morning and 600 mg in evening >73 kg: 1,200 mg/day in 2 div doses	

Herpes simplex virus		
– Third trimester maternal suppressive therapy[72–74]	Acyclovir or valacyclovir maternal suppressive therapy in pregnant women reduces HSV recurrences and viral shedding at the time of delivery but does not fully prevent neonatal HSV[73] (BIII).	
– Neonatal	See Chapter 2.	
– Mucocutaneous (normal host)	Acyclovir 80 mg/kg/day PO div qid (max dose 800 mg) for 5–7 days, or 15 mg/kg/day IV as 1- to 2-h infusion div q8h (AII). Valacyclovir 20 mg/kg/dose (max dose 1 g) PO bid[75] for 5–7 days (BII). Suppressive therapy for frequent recurrence (no pediatric data): acyclovir 20 mg/kg/dose bid or tid (max dose 400 mg) for 6–12 mo, then reevaluate need (AIII).	Foscarnet for acyclovir-resistant strains. Immunocompromised hosts may require 10–14 days of therapy. Topical acyclovir not efficacious and, therefore, not recommended.
– Genital	Adult doses: acyclovir 400 mg PO tid for 7–10 days; OR valacyclovir 1 g PO bid for 10 days; OR famciclovir 250 mg PO tid for 7–10 days (AI)	All 3 drugs have been used as prophylaxis to prevent recurrence. Topical acyclovir not efficacious and, therefore, not recommended.
– Encephalitis	Acyclovir 60 mg/kg/day IV as 1- to 2-h infusion div q8h; for 21 days for infants ≤4 mo. For older infants and children, 45 mg/kg/day IV as 1- to 2-h infusion div q8h (AIII).	Safety of high-dose acyclovir (60 mg/kg/day) not well-defined beyond the neonatal period; can be used but monitor for neurotoxicity and nephrotoxicity.
– Keratoconjunctivitis	1% trifluridine OR 0.15% ganciclovir ophthalmic gel (AII)	Consultation with ophthalmologist required for assessment and management (eg, concomitant use of topical steroids in certain situations)

C. PREFERRED THERAPY FOR SPECIFIC VIRAL PATHOGENS *(continued)*

Infection	Therapy (evidence grade)	Comments
HIV		
Current information on HIV treatment and opportunistic infections of children[77] is posted at https://clinicalinfo.hiv.gov/en/guidelines (accessed September 29, 2022); other information on HIV programs is available at www.cdc.gov/hiv/policies/index.html (accessed September 29, 2022). Consult with an HIV expert, if possible, for current recommendations, as treatment options are complicated and constantly evolving.		
– Therapy for HIV infection		
State-of-the-art therapy is rapidly evolving with introduction of new agents and combinations; currently there are many individual and fixed-dose combination ARV agents approved for use by the FDA that have pediatric indications and that continue to be actively used; guidelines for children and adolescents are continually updated on the ClinicalInfo.HIV.gov and CDC websites given previously.	Effective therapy (HAART) consists of ≥3 agents, including 2 NRTIs, plus a protease inhibitor, a non-NRTI, or an integrase inhibitor; many different combination regimens give similar treatment outcomes; choice of agents depends on the age of the child, viral load, consideration of potential viral resistance, and extent of immune depletion, in addition to judging the child's ability to adhere to the regimen. "Rapid initiation" of ART is recommended for all children, meaning initiation within days of HIV diagnosis.	Assess drug toxicity (based on the agents used) and virologic/immunologic response to therapy (quantitative plasma HIV and CD4 count) initially monthly and then q3–6mo during the maintenance phase.
– Children of any age	Any child with AIDS or significant HIV-related symptoms (clinical category C and most B conditions) should be treated (AI). Guidance from the WHO and HHS guidelines committees now recommends treatment of **all children** regardless of age, CD4 count, or clinical status, with situation-specific levels of urgency.	Adherence counseling and appropriate ARV formulations are critical for successful implementation. Recently, the combination of an integrase inhibitor with 2 NRTIs has become the preferred treatment regimen for children (as well as adults). Alternative regimens may use either an NRTI or a protease inhibitor.

– First 4 wk after birth	HAART with ≥3 drugs is recommended for **all infants and children** regardless of clinical status or laboratory values (AI).	Preferred therapy in the first 2 wk after birth is zidovudine and lamivudine PLUS either nevirapine or raltegravir. Preferred therapy from 2–4 wk: zidovudine and lamivudine PLUS either lopinavir/ritonavir (toxicity concerns preclude its use until a PMA of 42 wk and a postnatal age of at least 14 days is reached) or raltegravir.
– HIV-infected children 1 mo–12 y	**Treat all** with any CD4 count (AI).	Preferred regimens: 4 wk–6 y: 2 NRTIs PLUS dolutegravir (alternatives to dolutegravir include raltegravir or elvitegravir [>25 kg]). 6–12 y: 2 NRTIs PLUS dolutegravir OR bictegravir (alternatives to dolutegravir or bictegravir include raltegravir OR elvitegravir OR atazanavir/ritonavir OR darunavir/ritonavir).
– HIV-infected youth ≥12 y	**Treat all** regardless of CD4 count (AI).	Preferred regimens comprise TAF or tenofovir (adolescents/Tanner stage 4 or 5) plus emtricitabine OR abacavir plus lamivudine PLUS dolutegravir, raltegravir, or bictegravir. **NOTE:** A recent report suggests the possibility of neural tube defects developing in offspring of women who become pregnant while taking dolutegravir and/or use it during the first trimester. Subsequent studies have supported safety, and the guidelines panel now recommends dolutegravir as preferred therapy for women who are planning a pregnancy (AIII) or who are pregnant (AII). **NOTE:** Cabenuva (injectable, long-acting cabotegravir plus rilpivirine) has recently been approved for treatment of HIV infection for 12- to 18-year-olds. It requires an oral lead-in dosing period followed by injections q2mo (one each for cabotegravir and rilpivirine). For this treatment regimen, initiation by a pediatric/adult HIV specialist team is strongly recommended.

C. PREFERRED THERAPY FOR SPECIFIC VIRAL PATHOGENS (continued)

Infection	Therapy (evidence grade)	Comments
– Antiretroviral-experienced child	Consult with HIV specialist.	Consider treatment history and drug resistance testing and assess adherence.
– HIV exposures, nonoccupational	Therapy recommendations for exposures available on the CDC website at www.cdc.gov/hiv/guidelines/preventing.html (accessed September 29, 2022)	PEP remains unproven, but substantial evidence supports its use; consider individually regarding risk, time from exposure, and likelihood of adherence; prophylactic regimens administered for 4 wk.
– Negligible exposure risk (urine, nasal secretions, saliva, sweat, or tears—no visible blood in secretions) OR >72 h since exposure	Prophylaxis not recommended (BIII)	
– Significant exposure risk (blood, semen, vaginal, or rectal secretions from a known HIV-infected individual) AND <72 h since exposure	Prophylaxis recommended (BIII) Preferred regimens: 4 wk–<2 y: zidovudine PLUS lamivudine PLUS either raltegravir or lopinavir/ritonavir 2–12 y: tenofovir PLUS emtricitabine PLUS raltegravir ≥13 y: tenofovir PLUS emtricitabine PLUS either raltegravir or dolutegravir	Consultation with a pediatric HIV specialist is advised.
– Significant exposure risk **PrEP**	Truvada (tenofovir [300 mg]/emtricitabine [200 mg]): 1 tab daily	Daily PrEP has proven efficacy for prevention of HIV infection in individuals at high risk. It is FDA approved for adolescents/youth (13–24 y; ≥35 kg). Strategies for use include both episodic and continuous administration. Baseline HIV and renal function testing is indicated, and it is recommended to evaluate HIV infection status and renal function about q3mo while receiving PrEP.

– HIV exposure, occupational[78]	See guidelines on the CDC website at www.cdc.gov/hiv/guidelines/preventing.html (accessed September 29, 2022).	
Human herpesvirus 6		
– Immunocompromised children[76]	No prospective comparative data; ganciclovir 10 mg/kg/day IV div q12h used in case report (AIII)	May require high dose to control infection; safety and efficacy not defined at high doses
Influenza virus		
Recommendations for the treatment of influenza can vary from season to season; access the American Academy of Pediatrics website (www.aap.org) and the CDC website (www.cdc.gov/flu/professionals/antivirals/summary-clinicians.htm; accessed September 29, 2022) for the most current, accurate information.		

C. PREFERRED THERAPY FOR SPECIFIC VIRAL PATHOGENS *(continued)*

Infection	Therapy (evidence grade)	Comments
Influenza A and B		
– Treatment[79–81]	Oseltamivir Preterm, <38 wk of PMA: 1 mg/kg/dose PO bid[79] Preterm, 38–40 wk of PMA: 1.5 mg/kg/dose PO bid[79] Preterm, >40 wk of PMA: 3 mg/kg/dose PO bid Full-term, birth–8 mo: 3 mg/kg/dose PO bid 9–11 mo: 3.5 mg/kg/dose PO bid[80] 12–23 mo: 30 mg/dose PO bid 2–12 y: ≤15 kg: 30 mg bid 16–23 kg: 45 mg bid 24–40 kg: 60 mg bid >40 kg: 75 mg bid ≥13 y: 75 mg bid OR Zanamivir ≥7 y: 10 mg by inhalation bid for 5 days OR Peramivir (BII) 6 mo–<13 y: single IV dose 12 mg/kg, up to 600 mg ≥13 y: single IV dose 600 mg OR Baloxavir (BII) ≥5 y: <20 kg: single dose 2 mg/kg PO 20–79 kg: single dose 40 mg PO ≥80 kg: single dose 80 mg PO	Oseltamivir is currently drug of choice for treatment of influenza. For patients 12–23 mo, the original FDA-approved unit dose of 30 mg/dose may provide inadequate drug exposure; 3.5 mg/kg/dose PO bid has been studied,[80] but study population sizes were small. Studies of parenteral zanamivir have been completed in children.[82] However, this formulation of the drug is not approved in the United States and is not available for compassionate use. The adamantanes, amantadine and rimantadine, are currently not effective for treatment due to near-universal resistance of influenza A virus. Resistance to baloxavir is being monitored carefully across the world. Problems with resistance have limited use of baloxavir in Japan.

– Chemoprophylaxis	Oseltamivir 3 mo–12 y: the milligram dose given for prophylaxis is the same as for the treatment dose for all ages, but it is given qd for prophylaxis instead of bid for treatment. Zanamivir ≥5 y: 10 mg by inhalation qd for as long as 28 days (community outbreaks) or 10 days (household setting) Baloxavir ≥5 y: <20 kg: single dose 2 mg/kg PO 20–79 kg: single dose 40 mg PO ≥80 kg: single dose 80 mg PO	Oseltamivir is currently drug of choice for chemoprophylaxis of influenza. Unless the situation is judged critical, oseltamivir chemoprophylaxis is not routinely recommended for patients <3 mo because of limited safety and efficacy data in this age-group. The adamantanes, amantadine and rimantadine, are currently not effective for chemoprophylaxis due to near-universal resistance of influenza A virus.
Measles[83]	No prospective data on antiviral therapy. Ribavirin is active against measles virus in vitro. Vitamin A is beneficial in children with measles and is recommended by WHO for all children with measles regardless of their country of residence (qd dosing for 2 days): for children ≥1 y: 200,000 IU (60,000 mcg RAE); for infants 6–12 mo: 100,000 IU (30,000 mcg RAE); for infants <6 mo: 50,000 IU (15,000 mcg RAE) (BII). An additional (ie, a third) age-specific dose of vitamin A should be given 2–6 wk later to children with clinical signs and symptoms of vitamin A deficiency. Even in countries where measles is not usually severe, vitamin A should be given to all children with severe measles (eg, requiring hospitalization). Parenteral and oral formulations are available in the United States.	IG prophylaxis for exposed, unimmunized children: 0.5 mL/kg (max 15 mL) IM

C. PREFERRED THERAPY FOR SPECIFIC VIRAL PATHOGENS (*continued*)

Infection	Therapy (evidence grade)	Comments
Monkeypox	Following consultation with the CDC, treatment may be considered in patients experiencing severe disease that prompts hospitalization or in patients likely to experience severe disease (ie, immunocompromised patients, children <8 y, pregnant/breastfeeding women): CDC-held Emergency Access Investigational New Drug protocol allows use of tecovirimat for non–variola *Orthopoxvirus* infection (eg, monkeypox). CDC-held Emergency Access Investigational New Drug Protocol allows use of vaccinia immune globulin intravenous for non–variola *Orthopoxvirus* infection (eg, monkeypox).	PrEP vaccination may be available for health care professionals, and PEP vaccination (within 4 days from date of exposure) may be available with the 2 attenuated virus vaccines that are FDA approved, through the CDC (800/CDC-INFO [800/232-4636]). Cidofovir and brincidofovir may be effective, but no data exist on either drug for treatment of monkeypox in humans (www.cdc.gov/poxvirus/monkeypox/clinicians/treatment.html, reviewed September 15, 2022; accessed September 29, 2022).
Respiratory syncytial virus[84,85]		
– Therapy (severe disease in compromised host)	Ribavirin (6-g vial to make 20-mg/mL solution in sterile water), aerosolized over 18–20 h daily for 3–5 days (BII)	Aerosol ribavirin provides only a small benefit and should be considered only for use for life-threatening infection with RSV. Airway reactivity with inhalation precludes routine use.
– Prophylaxis (palivizumab, Synagis for high-risk infants) (BI)[84,85]	Prophylaxis: palivizumab (a monoclonal antibody) 15 mg/kg IM monthly (max 5 doses) for the following high-risk infants (AI): In first year after birth, palivizumab prophylaxis is recommended for infants born before 29 wk 0 days' gestation.	Palivizumab does not provide benefit in the treatment of an active RSV infection. Palivizumab prophylaxis may be considered for children <24 mo who will be profoundly immunocompromised during the RSV season.

Palivizumab prophylaxis is not recommended for otherwise healthy infants born at ≥29 wk 0 days' gestation.

In first year after birth, palivizumab prophylaxis is recommended for preterm infants with CLD of prematurity, defined as birth at <32 wk 0 days' gestation and a requirement for >21% oxygen for at least 28 days after birth.

Clinicians may administer palivizumab prophylaxis in the first year after birth to certain infants with hemodynamically significant heart disease.

Palivizumab prophylaxis is not recommended in the second year after birth except for children who required at least 28 days of supplemental oxygen after birth and who continue to require medical support (supplemental oxygen, chronic corticosteroid therapy, or diuretic therapy) during the 6-mo period before the start of the second RSV season.

Monthly prophylaxis should be discontinued in any child who experiences a breakthrough RSV hospitalization.

Children with pulmonary abnormality or neuromuscular disease that impairs the ability to clear secretions from the upper airways may be considered for prophylaxis in the first year after birth.

Insufficient data are available to recommend palivizumab prophylaxis for children with cystic fibrosis or Down syndrome.

The burden of RSV disease and costs associated with transport from remote locations may result in a broader use of palivizumab for RSV prevention in Alaska Native populations and possibly in select other American Indian populations.

Palivizumab prophylaxis is not recommended for prevention of health care–associated RSV disease.

C. PREFERRED THERAPY FOR SPECIFIC VIRAL PATHOGENS

Infection	Therapy (evidence grade)	Comments
Varicella-zoster virus[86]	For prophylaxis/preemptive therapy following exposure in an asymptomatic child, see Chapter 15.	
– Infection in a normal host	Acyclovir 80 mg/kg/day (max single dose 800 mg) PO div qid for 5 days (AI)	The sooner antiviral therapy can be started, the greater the clinical benefit.
– Severe primary chickenpox, disseminated infection (cutaneous, pneumonia, encephalitis, hepatitis); immunocompromised host with primary chickenpox or disseminated zoster	Acyclovir 30 mg/kg/day IV as 1- to 2-h infusion div q8h for 10 days (acyclovir doses of 45–60 mg/kg/day in 3 div doses IV should be used for disseminated or central nervous system infection). Dosing can also be provided as 1,500 mg/m^2/day IV div q8h. Duration in immunocompromised children: 7–14 days, based on clinical response (AI).	Oral valacyclovir, famciclovir, foscarnet also active

8. Choosing Among Antiviral Agents

As a general rule, antiviral agents are specific to certain families of viruses. That is, the anti-herpesvirus drugs do not work against influenza, the anti-hepatitis C drugs do not work against hepatitis B, and so on. While some antiviral agents (eg, ribavirin, remdesivir) may have cross-family coverage, an antiviral drug that is broad enough in spectrum to cover multiple types of viruses and, thus, be used empirically in many situations simply does not exist at this point. It, therefore, is imperative that clinicians think through what viruses need to be covered when they are selecting which specific antiviral agent to use. For this reason, this chapter is structured by virus family.

Anti-herpesvirus Drugs

Broadly speaking, anti-herpesvirus drugs should be considered by subfamily within the broader Herpesviridae family. Herpes simplex virus (HSV) and varicella-zoster virus (VZV) are in the alpha subfamily, cytomegalovirus is in the beta subfamily, and Epstein-Barr virus (EBV) is in the gamma subfamily.

The antiviral drug of choice for the alpha herpesviruses (ie, HSV, gingivostomatitis/fever blisters, genital infection, neonatal infection; VZV, chickenpox, shingles) is acyclovir, a nucleoside analogue that is available intravenously or orally. Orally administered acyclovir (given in divided doses 4 or 5 times each day as tablets, capsules, or suspension) is poorly absorbed. However, the valine ester prodrug of acyclovir, valacyclovir, has enhanced bioavailability and twice-daily dosing that makes it an attractive option if the patient is old enough to be able to take it. Valacyclovir does not come in a liquid formulation, but there is a recipe for creation of a suspension in the package insert that allows for the compounding of a product that has a 28-day shelf life. There are data for dosing of valacyclovir in pediatric patients, although not in very young infants. Famciclovir (the prodrug of penciclovir), also a nucleoside analogue like acyclovir, is approved in adults for genital HSV and shingles, but there are far less pediatric data on efficacy. Although pediatric dosing recommendations are provided in the package label for infants and children, no suspension formulation has been approved; we prefer acyclovir to famciclovir based on much more extensive published pediatric data. Resistance to this class of antiviral may occur with repeated treatment courses. Alternatives include cidofovir and foscarnet, but each of these has significant toxicity issues that limit their use more widely.

For the beta herpesviruses, ganciclovir (another nucleoside analogue) is the antiviral agent of choice, also available either intravenously or orally. When oral dosing is an option, the valine ester prodrug of ganciclovir, valganciclovir, is used. Valganciclovir has improved bioavailability relative to oral ganciclovir. Cidofovir and foscarnet also have activity against the beta herpesviruses but, as mentioned previously, have toxicity issues that limit the use. The newest antiviral drug with activity against human cytomegalovirus that is approved for use in adults is letermovir, a DNA terminase complex inhibitor. Studies of letermovir in the pediatric population are underway.

There are no antiviral agents with excellent activity against the gamma herpesviruses. In general, ganciclovir or its prodrug, valganciclovir, is used when activity is desired against EBV. The degree of benefit that either of these drugs provides, though, is unproven.

Anti-influenza Drugs

The drug of choice for influenza treatment in children is oseltamivir, a neuraminidase inhibitor, which is available only as an oral formulation. Zanamivir, also a neuraminidase inhibitor, is an active antiviral agent against most current strains of influenza but is available only in the United States as an inhalation formulation. Zanamivir is about as effective as oseltamivir, but its inhaled delivery mechanism has limited its use. Peramivir is another neuraminidase inhibitor given only intravenously as a single dose for uncomplicated outpatient influenza for patients down to 6 months of age; starting an intravenous line and infusing peramivir over 15 to 30 minutes may be difficult in many clinic settings. All the neuraminidase inhibitors should be given as early as possible in the influenza illness, preferably within 48 hours of onset of illness. Influenza may mutate to develop resistance to the neuraminidase inhibitors at any time, but the Centers for Disease Control and Prevention keeps track of global resistance patterns and shares current information on its website.

Baloxavir is the first approved endonuclease inhibitor drug in this class for influenza; it prevents replication of virus at a very early stage in cell infection. It requires only a single dose for treatment of uncomplicated outpatient influenza infection in adults, with published data in children down to 1 year of age documenting similar efficacy. Studies for complicated influenza in hospitalized adults (multiple daily doses) have not yet been published, and trials in children for complicated influenza have not begun. Experience with this drug is limited in the United States at this time, but we are concerned about the relative rapid development of resistance, which has been a major problem with baloxavir use globally.

In addition to treating active infection, oseltamivir, zanamivir, and baloxavir are also approved for prophylaxis following influenza exposure.

Anti-hepatitis Drugs

The development of drugs that are active against hepatitis C virus (HCV) has been one of the most remarkable aspects of antiviral drug development over the past 10 years. There are currently 4 antiviral drugs with activity against HCV that are approved for use in children 3 years and older: sofosbuvir/ledipasvir (Harvoni), sofosbuvir plus ribavirin, sofosbuvir/velpatasvir (Epclusa), and glecaprevir/pibrentasvir (Mavyret). Mavyret and Epclusa demonstrate transgenotype activity and, therefore, can be used with any genotype of HCV. There is also 1 HCV antiviral drug approved for use in children 12 years and older: elbasvir/grazoprevir (Zepatier). Given the pace of development, it is reasonable to anticipate that additional antiviral drugs with HCV activity are likely to be approved in children over the upcoming months and years. The American Academy of Pediatrics recommends that all HCV-infected children 3 years and older be treated with an age-approved antiviral regimen.

Anti-coronavirus Drugs

As of June 2022, remdesivir is the only antiviral drug with activity against coronaviruses. It is approved for use in persons 6 months and older for use against SARS-CoV-2. In addition, nirmatrelvir/ritonavir (Paxlovid) has received Emergency Use Authorization from the US Food and Drug Administration for the treatment of mild to moderate COVID-19 disease in persons aged 12 years and older and weighing 40 kg or more. Molnupiravir has received Emergency Use Authorization for treatment of mild to moderate COVID-19 disease in persons 18 years and older.

9. Preferred Therapy for Specific Parasitic Pathogens

NOTES

- Many of the parasitic infections listed in this chapter are not common, and current advice from your local infectious disease/tropical medicine/global health specialist may be invaluable. For some parasitic diseases, therapy may be available only from the Centers for Disease Control and Prevention (CDC), as noted. The CDC also provides up-to-date information about parasitic diseases and current treatment recommendations at www.cdc.gov/parasites (accessed September 30, 2022). Consultation is available from the CDC for parasitic disease diagnostic services (www.cdc.gov/dpdx; accessed September 30, 2022); for parasitic disease testing and experimental therapy, 404/639-3670; and for malaria, 770/488-7788 or 855/856-4713 toll-free, Monday through Friday, 9:00 am to 5:00 pm (ET), and the emergency number is 770/488-7100 for after hours, weekends, and holidays (correct as of September 30, 2022). Antiparasitic drugs available from the CDC Drug Service can be reviewed and requested at www.cdc.gov/laboratory/drugservice/index.html (accessed September 30, 2022).
- Additional information about many of the organisms and diseases mentioned here, along with treatment recommendations, can be found in the appropriate sections in the American Academy of Pediatrics *Red Book*.
- **Abbreviations:** AmB, amphotericin B; A-P, atovaquone/proguanil; ASTMH, American Society of Tropical Medicine and Hygiene; bid, twice daily; CDC, Centers for Disease Control and Prevention; CNS, central nervous system; CrCl, creatinine clearance; CSF, cerebrospinal fluid; CT, computed tomography; DEC, diethylcarbamazine; div, divided; DS, double-strength; FDA, US Food and Drug Administration; G6PD, glucose-6-phosphate dehydrogenase; GI, gastrointestinal; IDSA, Infectious Diseases Society of America; IM, intramuscular; IND, investigational new drug; IV, intravenous; LP, lumbar puncture; max, maximum; MF, microfilariae; MRI, magnetic resonance imaging; NECT, nifurtimox-eflornithine combination therapy; PAIR, puncture, aspiration, injection, re-aspiration; PHMB, polyhexamethylene biguanide; PO, orally; q, every; qd, once daily; qid, 4 times daily; qod, every other day; spp, species; SQ, subcutaneous; tab, tablet; TB, tuberculosis; TD, travelers diarrhea; tid, 3 times daily; TMP/SMX, trimethoprim/sulfamethoxazole.

A. SELECT COMMON PATHOGENIC PARASITES AND SUGGESTED AGENTS FOR TREATMENT

	Albendazole/ Mebendazole	Triclabendazole	Metronidazole/ Tinidazole	Praziquantel	Ivermectin	Nitazoxanide	DEC	Pyrantel Pamoate	Paromomycin	TMP/SMX
Ascariasis	++				+	+		+		
Blastocystis spp			+			+			+	+
Cryptosporidiosis						+			+	
Cutaneous larva migrans	++				++					
Cyclosporiasis			–			+				++
Cystoisospora spp						+				++
Dientamoebiasis	–		++			+			+	
Liver fluke *Clonorchis* and *Opisthorchis*	+			++						
Fasciola hepatica and *Fasciola gigantica*		++				+				
Lung fluke	–			++						
Giardia spp	+		++			++			+	
Hookworm	++				–			+		
Loiasis	+						++			
Mansonella ozzardi	–				+		–			
Mansonella perstans	±			–	–		±			

Onchocerciasis				++			
Pinworm	++						++
Schistosomiasis			++				
Strongyloides spp	+			++			
Tapeworm			++		+		
Toxocariasis	++					+	
Trichinellosis	++						
Trichomoniasis		++					
Trichuriasis	++						
Wuchereria bancrofti	+					++	

NOTE: ++ = preferred; **+** = acceptable; **±** = possibly effective (see text for further discussion); **—** = unlikely to be effective; [blank cell] = untested.

B. PREFERRED THERAPY FOR SPECIFIC PARASITIC PATHOGENS

Disease/Organism	Treatment (evidence grade)	Comments
Acanthamoeba	See Amebic meningoencephalitis later in this table.	
Amebiasis[1–5]		
Entamoeba histolytica		
– Asymptomatic intestinal colonization	Paromomycin 25–35 mg/kg/day PO div tid for 7 days; OR iodoquinol 30–40 mg/kg/day (max 650 mg/dose) PO div tid for 20 days; OR diloxanide furoate (not commercially available in United States) 20 mg/kg/day PO div tid (max 500 mg/dose) for 10 days (CII)	Follow-up stool examination to ensure eradication of carriage; screen/treat positive close contacts. *Entamoeba dispar, Entamoeba moshkovskii*, and *Entamoeba polecki* do not require treatment.
– Mild to moderate intestinal disease	Metronidazole 35–50 mg/kg/day (max 500–750 mg/dose) PO div tid for 7–10 days; OR tinidazole (age >3 y) 50 mg/kg/day PO (max 2 g) qd for 3 days; OR nitazoxanide (age ≥12 y, 500 mg bid for 3 days; ages 4–11 y, 200 mg bid for 3 days; ages 1–3 y, 100 mg bid for 3 days) FOLLOWED BY paromomycin or iodoquinol, as above, to eliminate cysts (BII)	Treatment options for severe and extraintestinal disease are like those for mild to moderate disease except that the need for broad-spectrum antibiotics should be considered in the event of superimposed bacterial infection and the need for site-specific treatment in extraintestinal infection such as liver abscess. Use of paromomycin for clearance of intestinal infection should be delayed if there is concern for intestinal perforation. Avoid antimotility drugs, steroids. Tinidazole (evaluated by the FDA for children ≥3 y), when available, may be more effective with fewer adverse events than metronidazole. Take tinidazole with food to decrease GI side effects; pharmacists can crush tabs and mix with syrup for those unable to take tabs. Avoid alcohol ingestion with metronidazole and tinidazole. Preliminary data support use of nitazoxanide to treat clinical infection, but it may not prevent parasitological failure.

– Liver abscess, extraintestinal disease	Metronidazole 35–50 mg/kg/day IV q8h, switch to PO when tolerated, for 7–10 days; OR tinidazole (age >3 y) 50 mg/kg/day PO (max 2 g) qd for 5 days; OR nitazoxanide (age ≥12 y, 500 mg bid for 3 days; ages 4–11 y, 200 mg bid for 3 days; ages 1–3 y, 100 mg bid for 3 days) FOLLOWED BY paromomycin or iodoquinol, as above, to eliminate cysts (BII).	Serologic assays >95% positive in extraintestinal amebiasis. Percutaneous or surgical drainage may be indicated for large liver abscesses or inadequate response to medical therapy. Avoid alcohol ingestion with metronidazole and tinidazole. Take tinidazole with food to decrease GI side effects; pharmacists can crush tabs and mix with syrup for those unable to take tabs.
Amebic meningoencephalitis[6–10]		
Naegleria fowleri	AmB 1.5 mg/kg/day IV div q12h for 3 days, then 1 mg/kg/day qd for 11 days; PLUS AmB intrathecally 1.5 mg qd for 2 days, then 1 mg/day qod for 8 days; PLUS azithromycin 10 mg/kg/day IV or PO (max 500 mg/day) for 28 days; PLUS fluconazole 10 mg/kg/day IV or PO qd (max 600 mg/day) for 28 days; PLUS rifampin 10 mg/kg/day qd IV or PO (max 600 mg/day) for 28 days; PLUS miltefosine <45 kg 50 mg PO bid; ≥45 kg 50 mg PO tid (max 2.5 mg/kg/day) for 28 days PLUS dexamethasone 0.6 mg/kg/day div qid for 4 days	Treatment recommendations based on regimens used for 5 known survivors; available at www.cdc.gov/parasites/naegleria/treatment-hcp.html (accessed September 30, 2022). Conventional amphotericin preferred; liposomal AmB is less effective in animal models. Treatment outcomes usually unsuccessful; early therapy (even before diagnostic confirmation if indicated) may improve survival. Miltefosine is available commercially (contact www.impavido.com for help in obtaining the drug); CDC provides expertise in treatment of patients with *N fowleri* infection (770/488-7100).

B. PREFERRED THERAPY FOR SPECIFIC PARASITIC PATHOGENS (continued)

Disease/Organism	Treatment (evidence grade)	Comments
Acanthamoeba	Combination regimens including miltefosine, fluconazole, and pentamidine favored by some experts; TMP/SMX, metronidazole, and a macrolide may be added. Other drugs that have been used alone or in combination include rifampin, other azoles, sulfadiazine, flucytosine, and caspofungin. Keratitis: topical therapies include PHMB (0.02%) or biguanide chlorhexidine, combined with propamidine isethionate (0.1%) or hexamidine (0.1%) (topical therapies not approved in United States but available at compounding pharmacies).	Optimal treatment regimens uncertain; combination therapy favored. Miltefosine is available commercially (contact www.impavido.com for help in obtaining the drug). CDC is available for consultation about management of these infections (770/488-7100). Keratitis should be evaluated by an ophthalmologist. Prolonged treatment often needed.
Balamuthia mandrillaris	Combination regimens preferred. Drugs that have been used alone or in combination include pentamidine, 5-flucytosine, fluconazole, macrolides, sulfadiazine, miltefosine, thioridazine, AmB, itraconazole, and albendazole.	Optimal treatment regimen uncertain; regimens based on case reports; prolonged treatment often needed. Surgical resection of CNS lesions may be beneficial. CDC is available for consultation about management of these infections (770/488-7100).
Ancylostoma braziliense	See Cutaneous larva migrans later in this table.	
Ancylostoma caninum	See Cutaneous larva migrans later in this table.	
Ancylostoma duodenale	See Hookworm later in this table.	

Angiostrongyliasis[11–14]		
Angiostrongylus cantonensis (cerebral disease)	Supportive care	Most patients recover without antiparasitic therapy; anthelmintic treatment may provoke worsening of neurologic symptoms. Corticosteroids, analgesics, and repeated LP may be of benefit. Prednisolone (1–2 mg/kg/day, up to 60 mg qd, in 2 div doses, for 2 wk) may shorten duration of headache and reduce need for repeated LP. Ocular disease may require surgery or laser treatment.
Angiostrongylus costaricensis (eosinophilic enterocolitis)	Supportive care	Surgery may be pursued to exclude another diagnosis, such as appendicitis, or to remove inflamed intestine.
Ascariasis (*Ascaris lumbricoides*)[15]	First line: albendazole 400 mg PO once OR mebendazole 500 mg once or 100 mg bid for 3 days (BII) Pregnant women: pyrantel pamoate 11 mg/kg, max 1 g once Alternatives: ivermectin 150–200 mcg/kg PO once (CII); nitazoxanide Ages 1–3 y: 100 mg PO bid for 3 days Ages 4–11 y: 200 mg PO bid for 3 days Age ≥12 y: 500 mg PO bid for 3 days	Follow-up stool ova and parasite examination after therapy not essential. Take albendazole with food (bioavailability increases with food, especially fatty meals). Albendazole has theoretical risk of causing seizures in patients coinfected with cysticercosis.

B. PREFERRED THERAPY FOR SPECIFIC PARASITIC PATHOGENS *(continued)*

Disease/Organism	Treatment (evidence grade)	Comments
Babesiosis (*Babesia* spp)[16–20]	Mild to moderate disease: azithromycin 10 mg/kg/day (max 500 mg/dose) PO on day 1; 5 mg/kg/day from day 2 on (max 250 mg/dose) for 7–10 days PLUS atovaquone 40 mg/kg/day (max 750 mg/dose) PO div bid (this regimen preferred due to fewer adverse events) OR clindamycin 20–40 mg/kg/day IV div tid or qid (max 600 mg/dose), PLUS quinine 24 mg/kg/day PO (max 650 mg/dose) div tid for 7–10 days Severe disease: azithromycin 5–10 mg/kg/day (max 500 mg/dose) IV for 7–10 days PLUS atovaquone 40 mg/kg/day (max 750 mg/dose) PO div bid; OR clindamycin 20–40 mg/kg/day IV div tid or qid (max 600 mg/dose), PLUS quinine 25 mg/kg/day PO (max 650 mg/dose) div tid for 7–10 days Can transition from IV to oral therapy when symptoms improve and parasitemia declines	Most asymptomatic infections with *Babesia microti* in immunocompetent individuals do not require treatment. Daily monitoring of hematocrit and percentage of parasitized red blood cells (until <5%) is helpful in guiding management. Exchange blood transfusion may be of benefit for severe disease and *Babesia divergens* infection. Higher doses of medications and prolonged therapy may be needed for asplenic or immunocompromised individuals. Clindamycin and quinine remain the regimen of choice for *B divergens*.
Balantidium coli[21]	Tetracycline (patients >7 y) 40 mg/kg/day PO div qid for 10 days (max 2 g/day) (CII); OR metronidazole 35–50 mg/kg/day PO div tid for 5 days (max 750 mg/dose); OR iodoquinol 30–40 mg/kg/day PO (max 650 mg/dose) div tid for 20 days	Optimal treatment regimen uncertain. Prompt stool examination may increase detection of rapidly degenerating trophozoites. None of these medications have been evaluated by the FDA for this indication. Nitazoxanide may also be effective.
Baylisascaris procyonis (raccoon roundworm)[22,23]	Albendazole 25–50 mg/kg/day PO for 10–20 days given as soon as possible (<3 days) after exposure (eg, proactive therapy following ingestion of raccoon feces or contaminated soil) might prevent clinical disease (CIII).	Therapy generally unsuccessful to prevent fatal outcome or severe neurologic sequelae once CNS disease present. Steroids may be of value in decreasing inflammation in CNS or ocular infection. Albendazole bioavailability increased with food, especially fatty meals.

Blastocystis spp[24,25]	Specific treatment rarely indicated. Metronidazole 35–50 mg/kg/day (max 750 mg/dose) PO div tid for 5–10 days (BII); OR tinidazole 50 mg/kg (max 2 g) once (age >3 y) (BII).	Pathogenesis debated. Asymptomatic individuals do not need treatment; diligent search for other pathogenic parasites recommended for symptomatic individuals with *Blastocystis* spp. Paromomycin, nitazoxanide (500 mg PO bid for age ≥12 y; 200 mg PO bid for 3 days for ages 4–11 y; 100 mg PO bid for 3 days for ages 1–3 y), and TMP/SMX may also be effective. Metronidazole resistance may occur. Take tinidazole with food; tabs may be crushed and mixed with flavored syrup.
Brugia malayi, Brugia timori	See Filariasis later in this table.	
Chagas disease (*Trypanosoma cruzi*)[26–28]	See Trypanosomiasis later in this table.	
Clonorchis sinensis	See Flukes later in this table.	
Cryptosporidiosis (*Cryptosporidium parvum*)[29–32]	Nitazoxanide Ages 1–3 y: 100 mg PO bid for 3 days. Ages 4–11 y: 200 mg PO bid for 3 days. Age ≥12 y: 500 mg PO bid for 3 days (BII). Paromomycin 25–35 mg/kg/day div bid–qid (CII); OR azithromycin 10 mg/kg/day for 5 days (CII); OR paromomycin AND azithromycin given as combination therapy may yield initial response but may not result in sustained cure in immunocompromised individuals.	Recovery depends largely on the immune status of the host; treatment not required in all immunocompetent individuals. Medical therapy may have limited efficacy in HIV-infected patients not receiving effective antiretroviral therapy. Longer courses (>2 wk) may be needed in solid-organ transplant patients. Nitazoxanide has been evaluated by the FDA for cryptosporidiosis and is approved for this infection.

B. PREFERRED THERAPY FOR SPECIFIC PARASITIC PATHOGENS *(continued)*

Disease/Organism	Treatment (evidence grade)	Comments
Cutaneous larva migrans or creeping eruption[33,34] (dog and cat hookworm) (*Ancylostoma caninum, Ancylostoma braziliense, Uncinaria stenocephala*)	Ivermectin 200 mcg/kg PO for 1 day (weight >15 kg) (CII); OR albendazole (age >2 y) 15 mg/kg/day (max 400 mg) PO qd for 3 days (CII)	Albendazole bioavailability increased with food, especially fatty meals. The FDA has not reviewed data on the safety and efficacy of ivermectin in children weighing <15 kg, and data on albendazole in children aged <2 y are limited. For individual children, the benefits of treatment are likely to outweigh risks.
Cyclospora spp[35–37] (cyanobacterium-like agent)	TMP/SMX 8–10 mg TMP/kg/day (max 1 DS tab bid) PO div bid for 7–10 days (BIII)	HIV-infected patients may require higher doses/longer therapy. Nitazoxanide may be an alternative for TMP/SMX-allergic patients.
Cysticercosis[38–41] (*Cysticercus cellulosae;* larva of *Taenia solium*)	Neurocysticercosis Patients with 1–2 viable parenchymal cysticerci: albendazole 15 mg/kg/day PO div bid (max 1,200 mg/day) for 10–14 days PLUS steroids (prednisone 1 mg/kg/day or dexamethasone 0.1 mg/kg/day) begun at least 1 day before antiparasitic therapy, continued during antiparasitic treatment followed by rapid taper (to reduce inflammation associated with dying organisms) Patients with >2 viable parenchymal cysticerci: albendazole 15 mg/kg/day PO div bid (max 1,200 mg/day) for 10–14 days PLUS praziquantel 50 mg/kg/day PO div tid (CII) for 10–14 days plus steroids (prednisone 1 mg/kg/day or dexamethasone 0.1 mg/kg/day) begun at least 1 day before antiparasitic therapy, continued during antiparasitic treatment followed by rapid taper (to reduce inflammation associated with dying organisms)	Collaboration with a specialist with experience treating this condition is recommended. See IDSA-ASTMH guidelines.[41] For infection caused by only 1–2 cysts, some do not use steroid therapy routinely with active treatment. Management of seizures, cerebral edema, intracranial hypertension, or hydrocephalus, when present, is the focus of initial therapy and may require antiepileptic drugs, neuroendoscopy, or surgical approaches before considering antiparasitic therapy. Imaging with both CT and MRI is recommended for classifying disease in patients newly diagnosed with neurocysticercosis. Optimal dose and duration of steroid therapy are uncertain. Screening for TB infection and *Strongyloides* is recommended for patients likely to require prolonged steroid therapy. Take albendazole with food (bioavailability increases with food, especially fatty meals).

Cystoisospora (formerly *Isospora*) *belli*[42]	Age >2 mo: TMP/SMX 8–10 mg TMP/kg/day PO (or IV) div bid for 7–10 days (max 160 mg TMP/800 mg SMX bid)	Infection often self-limited in immunocompetent hosts; consider treatment if symptoms do not resolve by 5–7 days or are severe. Pyrimethamine plus leucovorin, ciprofloxacin, and nitazoxanide are alternatives. Immunocompromised patients should be treated; longer courses or suppressive therapy may be needed for severely immunocompromised patients.
Dientamoebiasis[43,44] (*Dientamoeba fragilis*)	Metronidazole 35–50 mg/kg/day PO div tid for 10 days (max 750 mg/dose); OR paromomycin 25–35 mg/kg/day PO div tid for 7 days; OR iodoquinol 30–40 mg/kg/day (max 650 mg/dose) PO div tid for 20 days (BII)	Routine treatment of asymptomatic individuals not indicated. Treatment indicated when no other cause except *Dientamoeba* found for abdominal pain or diarrhea lasting >1 wk. Take paromomycin with meals and iodoquinol after meals. Tinidazole, nitazoxanide, tetracycline, and doxycycline may also be effective. Albendazole and mebendazole have no activity against *Dientamoeba*.
Diphyllobothrium latum	See Tapeworms later in this table.	
Dipylidium caninum	See Tapeworms later in this table.	
Echinococcosis[45,46]		
Echinococcus granulosus	Albendazole 10–15 mg/kg/day PO div bid (max 800 mg/day) for 1–6 mo alone (CIII) or as adjunctive therapy with surgery or percutaneous treatment; initiate 4–30 days before and continue for at least 1 mo after surgery.	Involvement with specialist with experience treating this condition strongly recommended. Surgery is the treatment of choice for management of complicated cysts. PAIR technique effective for appropriate cysts. Mebendazole is an alternative if albendazole is unavailable; if used, continue for 3 mo after PAIR. Take albendazole with food (bioavailability increases with food, especially fatty meals).

B. PREFERRED THERAPY FOR SPECIFIC PARASITIC PATHOGENS *(continued)*

Disease/Organism	Treatment (evidence grade)	Comments
Echinococcus multilocularis	Surgical treatment generally the treatment of choice; postoperative albendazole 10–15 mg/kg/day PO div bid (max 800 mg/day) should be administered to reduce relapse; duration uncertain (at least 2 y with long-term monitoring for relapse). Benefit of preoperative albendazole unknown.	Involvement with specialist with experience treating this condition recommended. Take albendazole with food (bioavailability increases with food, especially fatty meals).
Entamoeba histolytica	See Amebiasis earlier in this table.	
Enterobius vermicularis	See Pinworms later in this table.	
Fasciola hepatica	See Flukes later in this table.	
Fasciolopsis buski	See Flukes later in this table.	
Eosinophilic meningitis	See Angiostrongyliasis earlier in this table.	
Filariasis[47–50]		
– River blindness (*Onchocerca volvulus*)	Ivermectin 150 mcg/kg PO once (AII); repeat q3–6mo until asymptomatic and no ongoing exposure; OR if no ongoing exposure, doxycycline 4 mg/kg/day PO (max 200 mg/day div bid) for 6 wk followed by a single dose of ivermectin; may provide 1 dose of ivermectin for symptomatic relief 1 wk before beginning doxycycline.	Doxycycline targets *Wolbachia,* the endosymbiotic bacteria associated with *O volvulus.* Assess for *Loa loa* coinfection before using ivermectin if exposure occurred in settings where both *Onchocerca* and *L loa* are endemic. Optimal treatment of onchocerciasis in the setting of *L loa* infection is uncertain; consultation with a specialist familiar with these diseases is recommended. Moxidectin (8 mg PO once) was FDA approved in 2018 for adults and children ≥12 y, for treatment of onchocerciasis (to kill MF); not yet available commercially in United States. Screening for loiasis recommended before use. Safety and efficacy of repeated doses have not been studied. The FDA has not reviewed information on safety and efficacy in children <12 y.

– Tropical pulmonary eosinophilia[51]	DEC (from CDC) 6 mg/kg/day PO div tid for 14–21 days; corticosteroids to reduce inflammation; bronchodilators for bronchospasm (CII)	DEC is available from CDC Drug Service at 404/639-3670.
Loa loa	Symptomatic loiasis with MF of *L loa*/mL <8,000: DEC (from CDC) 8–10 mg/kg/day PO div tid for 21 days Symptomatic loiasis, with MF/mL ≥8,000: apheresis followed by DEC Albendazole (symptomatic loiasis, with MF/mL <8,000 and failed 2 rounds of DEC, OR symptomatic loiasis, with MF/mL ≥8,000 to reduce level to <8,000 before treatment with DEC) 200 mg PO bid for 21 days	Involvement with specialist with experience treating this condition recommended. Quantification of microfilarial levels is essential before treatment. Do not use DEC if onchocerciasis is present. Apheresis or albendazole may be used to reduce microfilarial levels before treatment with DEC.
Mansonella ozzardi	Ivermectin 200 mcg/kg PO once	DEC and albendazole not effective
Mansonella perstans	Combination therapy with DEC and mebendazole may be effective.	Relatively resistant to DEC, ivermectin, albendazole, and mebendazole; doxycycline 4 mg/kg/day PO (max 200 mg/day div bid) for 6 wk beneficial for clearing microfilaria in Mali and Ghana
Wuchereria bancrofti, Brugia malayi, Brugia timori, Mansonella streptocerca	DEC (from CDC) 6 mg/kg/day div tid for 12 days OR 6 mg/kg/day PO as a single dose (AII)	Avoid DEC with *Onchocerca* and *L loa* coinfection. Doxycycline (4 mg/kg/day PO, max 200 mg/day div bid, for 4–6 wk) may be considered; effectiveness of doxycycline in *M streptocerca* unknown. Albendazole has activity against adult worms. DEC is available from CDC (404/639-3670).
Flukes		
– Intestinal fluke (*Fasciolopsis buski*)	Praziquantel 75 mg/kg PO div tid for 1 day (BII)	
– Liver flukes[52] (*Clonorchis sinensis, Opisthorchis* spp)	Praziquantel 75 mg/kg PO div tid for 1–2 days (BII); OR albendazole 10 mg/kg/day PO for 7 days (CIII). Single 40 mg/kg dose praziquantel may be effective in light infection with *Opisthorchis viverrini*.[53]	Take praziquantel with liquids and food. Take albendazole with food (bioavailability increases with food, especially fatty meals).

B. PREFERRED THERAPY FOR SPECIFIC PARASITIC PATHOGENS *(continued)*

Disease/Organism	Treatment (evidence grade)	Comments
– Lung fluke[54,55] (*Paragonimus westermani* and other *Paragonimus* lung flukes)	Praziquantel 75 mg/kg/day PO div tid for 2 days (BII) Triclabendazole 10 mg/kg/dose PO bid for 1 day (approved for children ≥6 y for fascioliasis)	Triclabendazole should be taken with food to facilitate absorption. A short course of corticosteroids may reduce inflammatory response around dying flukes in cerebral disease.
– Sheep liver fluke[56] (*Fasciola hepatica, Fasciola gigantica*)	Triclabendazole 10 mg/kg/dose PO bid for 1 day (FDA evaluated for age ≥6 y) (BII) OR nitazoxanide PO (take with food), ages 12–47 mo, 100 mg/dose bid for 7 days; ages 4–11 y, 200 mg/dose bid for 7 days; age ≥12 y, 1 tab (500 mg)/dose bid for 7 days (CII).	Responds poorly to praziquantel; albendazole and mebendazole ineffective. Triclabendazole should be taken with food to facilitate absorption.
Giardiasis (*Giardia intestinalis* or *Giardia duodenalis* [formerly *lamblia*])[57–59]	Tinidazole 50 mg/kg/day (max 2 g) PO for 1 day (approved for age >3 y) (BII); OR nitazoxanide PO (take with food), ages 1–3 y, 100 mg/dose bid for 3 days; ages 4–11 y, 200 mg/dose bid for 3 days; age ≥12 y, 500 mg/dose bid for 3 days (BII).	Alternatives: metronidazole 15 mg/kg/day (max 250 mg/dose) PO div tid for 5–7 days (BII); albendazole 10–15 mg/kg/day (max 400 mg/dose) PO for 5 days (CII) OR mebendazole 200 mg PO tid for 5 days; OR paromomycin 30 mg/kg/day div tid for 5–10 days; furazolidone 8 mg/kg/day (max 100 mg/dose) in 4 doses for 7–10 days (not available in United States); quinacrine (refractory cases) 6 mg/kg/day PO div tid (max 100 mg/dose) for 5 days. If therapy ineffective, may try a higher dose or longer course of the same agent, or an agent in a different class; combination therapy may be considered for refractory cases. Prolonged courses may be needed for immunocompromised patients (eg, hypogammaglobulinemia). Treatment of asymptomatic carriers not usually indicated.

Hookworm[60–62] *Necator americanus, Ancylostoma duodenale*	Albendazole 400 mg once (repeated dose may be necessary) (BII); OR mebendazole 100 mg PO for 3 days OR 500 mg PO once; OR pyrantel pamoate 11 mg/kg (max 1 g/day) (BII) PO qd for 3 days.	
Hymenolepis nana	See Tapeworms later in this table.	
Isospora belli	See *Cystoisospora belli* earlier in this table under Cysticercosis.	
Leishmaniasis[63–70] (including kala-azar) *Leishmania* spp	Visceral: liposomal AmB 3 mg/kg/day on days 1–5, day 14, and day 21 (AI); OR miltefosine 2.5 mg/kg/day PO (max 150 mg/day) for 28 days (BII) (FDA-approved regimen: 50 mg PO bid for 28 days for weight 30–44 kg; 50 mg PO tid for 28 days for weight ≥45 kg); other AmB products available but not evaluated by the FDA for this indication. Cutaneous and mucosal disease: there is no generally accepted treatment of choice; treatment decisions should be individualized. Uncomplicated cutaneous: combination of debridement of eschars, cryotherapy, thermotherapy, intralesional pentavalent antimony, and topical paromomycin (not available in United States). Complicated cutaneous: oral or parenteral systemic therapy with miltefosine 2.5 mg/kg/day PO (max 150 mg/day) for 28 days (FDA-approved regimen: 50 mg PO bid for 28 days for weight 30–44 kg; 50 mg PO tid for 28 days for weight ≥45 kg) (BII); OR pentamidine isethionate 2–4 mg/kg/day IV or IM qod for 4–7 doses; OR amphotericin (various regimens); OR azoles (fluconazole 200 mg PO qd for 6 wk; or ketoconazole or itraconazole); also intralesional and topical alternatives.	Consultation with a specialist familiar with management of leishmaniasis is strongly advised, especially when treating patients with HIV coinfection. See IDSA-ASTMH guidelines for *Leishmania*.[63] Region where infection acquired, spp of *Leishmania*, skill of practitioner with some local therapies, and drugs available in United States affect therapeutic choices. For immunocompromised patients with visceral disease, FDA-approved dosing of liposomal amphotericin is 4 mg/kg on days 1–5, 10, 17, 24, 31, and 38, with further therapy on an individual basis. See guidelines for use of pentavalent antimonial drugs for visceral, mucosal, or complicated cutaneous leishmaniasis.

(Continued on next page)

B. PREFERRED THERAPY FOR SPECIFIC PARASITIC PATHOGENS *(continued)*

Disease/Organism	Treatment (evidence grade)	Comments
Leishmaniasis[63–70] (including kala-azar) *Leishmania* spp (*continued*)	Mucosal: AmB (Fungizone) 0.5–1 mg/kg/day IV qd or qod for cumulative total of about 20–45 mg/kg; OR liposomal AmB about 3 mg/kg/day IV qd for cumulative total of about 20–60 mg/kg; OR miltefosine 2.5 mg/kg/day PO (max 150 mg/day) for 28 days (FDA-evaluated regimen: 50 mg PO bid for 28 days for weight 30–44 kg; 50 mg PO tid for 28 days for weight ≥45 kg); OR pentamidine isethionate 2–4 mg/kg/day IV or IM qod or 3 times/wk for ≥15 doses (considered a lesser alternative).	
Lice *Pediculosis capitis* or *Pediculosis humanus, Phthirus pubis*[71,72]	Follow manufacturer's instructions for topical use: permethrin 1% (≥2 mo) OR pyrethrin (children ≥2 y) (BII); OR 0.5% ivermectin lotion (≥6 mo) (BII); OR spinosad 0.9% topical suspension (≥6 mo) (BII); OR malathion 0.5% (children ≥2 y) (BIII); OR oral ivermectin 200 mcg/kg PO once; repeat 7–10 days later (children >15 kg); OR abametapir lotion (children ≥6 mo; contains benzyl alcohol).	Launder bedding and clothing; for eyelash infestation, use petrolatum; for head lice, remove nits with comb designed for that purpose. Benzyl alcohol can be irritating to skin; systemic absorption may lead to toxicity; parasite resistance unlikely to develop. Consult specialist before re-treatment with ivermectin lotion; re-treatment with spinosad topical suspension not usually needed unless live lice seen 1 wk after treatment.
Malaria[73,74]		
Plasmodium falciparum, Plasmodium vivax, Plasmodium ovale, Plasmodium malariae	CDC Malaria Hotline 770/488-7788 or 855/856-4713 toll-free (Monday–Friday, 9:00 am–5:00 pm [ET]) or emergency consultation after hours 770/488-7100; online information at www.cdc.gov/parasites/malaria/index.html; accessed September 30, 2022	Consultation with a specialist familiar with management of malaria is advised, especially for severe malaria. No antimalarial drug provides absolute protection against malaria; fever after return from an endemic area should prompt an immediate evaluation. Emphasize personal protective measures (insecticides, bed nets, clothing, and avoidance of dusk–dawn mosquito exposures).

Prophylaxis		See www.cdc.gov/malaria/travelers/index.html (accessed September 30, 2022) for current information on travel and prophylaxis. Other drugs not available in United States are used globally for prevention and treatment of malaria.[73]
For areas with chloroquine-resistant *P falciparum* or *P vivax*	A-P: 5–8 kg, ½ pediatric tab/day; ≥9–10 kg, ¾ pediatric tab/day; ≥11–20 kg, 1 pediatric tab (62.5 mg atovaquone/25 mg proguanil); ≥21–30 kg, 2 pediatric tabs; ≥31–40 kg, 3 pediatric tabs; ≥40 kg, 1 adult tab (250 mg atovaquone/100 mg proguanil) PO qd starting 1–2 days before travel and continuing 7 days after last exposure; for children <5 kg, data on A-P limited (BII); OR mefloquine: for children <5 kg, 5 mg/kg; ≥5–9 kg, ⅛ tab; ≥10–19 kg, ¼ tab; ≥20–30 kg, ½ tab; ≥31–45 kg, ¾ tab; ≥45 kg (adult dose), 1 tab PO once weekly starting the wk before arrival in area and continuing for 4 wk after leaving area (BII); OR doxycycline (patients >7 y): 2 mg/kg (max 100 mg) PO qd starting 1–2 days before arrival in area and continuing for 4 wk after leaving area (BIII); OR primaquine (check for G6PD deficiency before administering): 0.5 mg/kg base qd starting 1 day before travel and continuing for 5 days after last exposure (BII)	Avoid mefloquine for persons with a history of seizures or psychosis, active depression, or cardiac conduction abnormalities; see black box warning. Avoid A-P in severe renal impairment (CrCl <30). *P falciparum* resistance to mefloquine exists along the borders between Thailand and Myanmar and Thailand and Cambodia, Myanmar and China, and Myanmar and Laos; isolated resistance has been reported in southern Vietnam. Take doxycycline with adequate fluids to avoid esophageal irritation and food to avoid GI side effects; use sunscreen and avoid excessive sun exposure. Tafenoquine FDA approved August 2018 for use in those ≥18 y; must test for G6PD deficiency before use; pregnancy testing recommended before use. Not evaluated by the FDA for those <18 y. Loading dose 200 mg daily for 3 days before travel; 200 mg weekly during travel; after return, 200 mg once 7 days after last maintenance dose; tabs must be swallowed whole. May also be used to prevent malaria in areas with chloroquine-resistant malaria.

B. PREFERRED THERAPY FOR SPECIFIC PARASITIC PATHOGENS *(continued)*

Disease/Organism	Treatment (evidence grade)	Comments
For areas without chloroquine-resistant *P falciparum* or *P vivax*	Chloroquine phosphate 5-mg base/kg (max 300-mg base) PO once weekly, beginning the wk before arrival in area and continuing for 4 wk after leaving area (available in suspension outside United States and Canada and at compounding pharmacies) (AII). After return from heavy or prolonged (months) exposure to infected mosquitoes: consider treatment with primaquine (check for G6PD deficiency before administering) 0.5-mg base/kg PO qd with final 2 wk of chloroquine for prevention of relapse with *P ovale* or *P vivax*.	
Treatment of disease		See www.cdc.gov/malaria/resources/pdf/Malaria_Treatment_Table.pdf for treatment of malaria in the United States (accessed September 30, 2022). Other drugs not available in United States are used globally for prevention and treatment of malaria.[73]
– Chloroquine-resistant *P falciparum* or *P vivax*	Oral therapy: artemether/lumefantrine 6 doses over 3 days at 0, 8, 24, 36, 48, and 60 h; <15 kg, 1 tab/dose; ≥15–25 kg, 2 tabs/dose; ≥25–35 kg, 3 tabs/dose; >35 kg, 4 tabs/dose (BII); A-P: for children <5 kg, data limited; ≥5–8 kg, 2 pediatric tabs (62.5 mg atovaquone/25 mg proguanil) PO qd for 3 days; ≥9–10 kg, 3 pediatric tabs qd for 3 days; ≥11–20 kg, 1 adult tab (250 mg atovaquone/100 mg proguanil) qd for 3 days; >20–30 kg, 2 adult tabs qd for 3 days; >30–40 kg, 3 adult tabs qd for 3 days; >40 kg, 4 adult tabs qd for 3 days (BII); OR quinine 30 mg/kg/day (max 2 g/day) PO div tid for 3–7 days AND doxycycline 4 mg/kg/day div bid for 7 days OR clindamycin 30 mg/kg/day div tid (max 900 mg tid) for 7 days.	Mild disease may be treated with oral antimalarial drugs; severe disease (impaired level of consciousness, convulsion, hypotension, or parasitemia >5%) should be treated parenterally. Avoid mefloquine for treatment of malaria, if possible, given higher dose and increased incidence of adverse events. Take clindamycin and doxycycline with plenty of liquids. Do not use primaquine or tafenoquine during pregnancy. Avoid artemether/lumefantrine and mefloquine in patients with cardiac arrhythmias, and avoid concomitant use of drugs that prolong QT interval.

	Parenteral therapy: artesunate (commercially available, but if not in stock or not available within 24 h, contact CDC Malaria Hotline). Children >20 kg: 2.4 mg/kg/dose IV at 0, 12, 24, and 48 h. Children <20 kg: 3 mg/kg/dose IV at 0, 12, 24, and 48 h (from CDC) (BI) AND follow artesunate by one of the following: artemether/lumefantrine, A-P, doxycycline (clindamycin in pregnant women), or, if no other options, mefloquine, all dosed as above. If needed, give interim treatment until artesunate arrives. See CDC website for details: www.cdc.gov/malaria/resources/pdf/Malaria_Treatment_Table.pdf (accessed September 30, 2022). For prevention of relapse with *P vivax, P ovale:* primaquine (check for G6PD deficiency before administering) 0.5-mg base/kg/day PO for 14 days.	Take A-P and artemether/lumefantrine with food or milk. Artesunate is now available commercially, but if not in stock or not available within 24 hours, contact CDC Malaria Hotline at 770/488-7788 or 855/856-4713 toll-free, Monday–Friday, 9:00 am to 5:00 pm (ET), and the emergency number is 770/488-7100 for after hours, weekends, and holidays (correct as of September 30, 2022). For relapses of primaquine-resistant *P vivax* or *P ovale,* consider re-treating with primaquine 30 mg (base) for 28 days.
– Chloroquine-susceptible *P falciparum,* chloroquine-susceptible *P vivax, P ovale, P malariae*	Oral therapy: chloroquine 10 mg/kg base (max 600-mg base) PO, then 5 mg/kg 6, 24, and 48 h after initial dose. Parenteral therapy: artesunate, as above. After return from heavy or prolonged (months) exposure to infected mosquitoes: consider treatment with primaquine (check for G6PD deficiency before administering) 0.5-mg base/kg PO qd with final 2 wk of chloroquine for prevention of relapse with *P ovale* or *P vivax.*	Alternative if chloroquine not available: hydroxychloroquine 10-mg base/kg PO immediately, followed by 5-mg base/kg PO at 6, 24, and 48 h. For relapses of primaquine-resistant *P vivax* or *P ovale,* consider re-treating with primaquine 30 mg (base) for 28 days. Tafenoquine approved July 2018 for prevention of relapse with *P vivax* malaria in those aged ≥16 y. 300 mg on the first or second day of chloroquine or hydroxychloroquine for acute malaria. Must test for G6PD deficiency before use; pregnancy testing recommended before use; tabs must be swallowed whole.
Mansonella ozzardi, Mansonella perstans, Mansonella streptocerca	See Filariasis earlier in this table.	

B. PREFERRED THERAPY FOR SPECIFIC PARASITIC PATHOGENS *(continued)*

Disease/Organism	Treatment (evidence grade)	Comments
Naegleria	See Amebic meningoencephalitis earlier in this table.	
Necator americanus	See Hookworm earlier in this table.	
Onchocerca volvulus	See Filariasis earlier in this table.	
Opisthorchis spp	See Flukes earlier in this table.	
Paragonimus westermani	See Flukes earlier in this table.	
Pinworms (*Enterobius vermicularis*)	Mebendazole 100 mg once, repeat in 2 wk; OR albendazole 400 mg PO on an empty stomach once; OR pyrantel pamoate 11 mg/kg (max 1 g) PO once (BII); repeat in 2 wk.	Treat entire household for recurrent infection (and if this fails, consider treating close child care/school contacts); re-treatment of contacts after 2 wk may be needed to prevent reinfection. Children as young as 1 y may be treated; some pediatric infectious diseases practitioners may choose to defer treatment of an exposed but uninfected infant aged <1 y. Launder bedding and clothing.
Plasmodium spp	See Malaria earlier in this table.	
Pneumocystis	See *Pneumocystis jiroveci* pneumonia in Chapter 5, Table 5B.	
Scabies (*Sarcoptes scabiei*)[75]	Permethrin (5%) cream applied to entire body (including scalp in infants), left on for 8–14 h then washed off, repeat in 1 wk (BII); OR ivermectin 200 mcg/kg PO once weekly for 2 doses (BII); OR crotamiton (10%) applied topically overnight on days 1, 2, 3, and 8, washed off in am (BII).	Launder bedding and clothing. Crotamiton treatment failure has been observed. The FDA has not reviewed data on the safety and efficacy of ivermectin in children who weigh <15 kg, although for individual infants, the benefits of treatment are likely to outweigh risks. Reserve lindane for patients >10 y who do not respond to other therapy; concern for toxicity. Itching may continue for weeks after successful treatment; can be managed with antihistamines.

Schistosomiasis (*Schistosoma haematobium, Schistosoma intercalatum, Schistosoma japonicum, Schistosoma mansoni, Schistosoma mekongi*)[76–78]	Praziquantel 40 (for *S haematobium, S mansoni,* and *S intercalatum*) or 60 (for *S japonicum* and *S mekongi*) mg/kg/day PO div bid (if 40 mg/day) or tid (if 60 mg/day) for 1 day (AI)	Take praziquantel with food and liquids. Oxamniquine (not available in United States) 20 mg/kg PO div bid for 1 day (Brazil) or 40–60 mg/kg/day for 2–3 days (most of Africa) (BII). Re-treat with the same dose if eggs still present 6–12 wk after initial treatment.
Strongyloidiasis (*Strongyloides stercoralis*)[79,80]	Ivermectin 200 mcg/kg PO qd for 1–2 days (BI); OR albendazole 400 mg PO bid for 7 days (or longer for disseminated disease) (BII)	Albendazole is less effective but may be adequate if longer courses used. For immunocompromised patients (especially with hyperinfection syndrome), veterinary SQ formulations of ivermectin may be lifesaving. The SQ formulation may be used under a single-patient IND protocol request to the FDA. Rectal administration may also be used for those unable to tolerate oral administration. The FDA has not reviewed data on the safety and efficacy of ivermectin in children who weigh <15 kg, although for individual infants, the benefits of treatment are likely to outweigh risks.
Tapeworms – *Taenia saginata, Taenia solium, Hymenolepis nana, Diphyllobothrium latum, Dipylidium caninum*	Praziquantel 5–10 mg/kg PO once (for *H nana:* 25 mg/kg once; may repeat 10 days later) (BII); OR niclosamide (not available in United States) 50 mg/kg (max 2 g) PO once, chewed thoroughly (for *H nana*: weight 11–34 kg: 1 g in a single dose on day 1, then 500 mg/day PO for 6 days; weight >34 kg: 1.5 g in a single dose on day 1, then 1 g/day PO for 6 days; adults: 2 g in a single dose for 7 days)	Nitazoxanide may be effective (published clinical data limited) 500 mg PO bid for 3 days for age >11 y; 200 mg PO bid for 3 days for ages 4–11 y; 100 mg PO bid for 3 days for ages 1–3 y. Albendazole may be an alternative.

B. PREFERRED THERAPY FOR SPECIFIC PARASITIC PATHOGENS *(continued)*

Disease/Organism	Treatment (evidence grade)	Comments
Toxocariasis[81] (*Toxocara canis* [dog roundworm] and *Toxocara cati* [cat roundworm])	Visceral larval migrans: albendazole 400 mg PO bid for 5 days (BII) Ocular larva migrants: albendazole 400 mg PO bid for 5 days with prednisone (0.5–1 mg/kg/day with slow taper)	Mild disease often resolves without treatment. Corticosteroids may be used for severe symptoms in visceral larval migrans. Mebendazole (100–200 mg/day PO bid for 5 days) is an alternative. May need up to 2 wk of albendazole for ocular *Toxocara* with sight-threatening inflammation.
Toxoplasmosis (*Toxoplasma gondii*)[82–84]	See Chapter 2 for congenital infection. Severe acute toxoplasmosis: Pyrimethamine 2 mg/kg/day PO div bid for 2 days (max 100 mg), then 1 mg/kg/day (max 50 mg/day) PO qd AND sulfadiazine 100–200 mg/kg/day PO div qid (max 4–6 g/day for severe disease); with supplemental folinic acid (leucovorin) 10–25 mg with each dose of pyrimethamine (AI) for 2–4 wk. Active toxoplasmic chorioretinitis: Pyrimethamine 2 mg/kg/day PO div bid for 2 days (max 100 mg), then 1 mg/kg/day (max 50 mg/day) PO qd AND sulfadiazine 75 mg/kg/dose 1 dose PO followed in 12 h by 50 mg/kg PO bid (max 4 g/day) AND folinic acid (leucovorin) 10–20 mg/day PO. For treatment in pregnancy, spiramycin 50–100 mg/kg/day PO div qid (available as investigational therapy through the FDA at 301/796-1400) (CII). Treatment is most effective if initiated within 8 wk of seroconversion.	Acute toxoplasmosis in immunocompetent, nonpregnant individuals is typically self-limited and may not require treatment. For acute disease clindamycin, azithromycin, or atovaquone plus pyrimethamine may be effective for patients intolerant of sulfa-containing drugs. Experienced ophthalmologic consultation (retinal specialist with experience treating toxoplasmic chorioretinitis) encouraged for treatment of ocular disease. Treatment of ocular disease with TMP/SMX can be done until first-line therapy is available; 15–20 mg TMP/kg; 75–100 mg/kg SMX qd div q6h–q8h. Treatment continued for 2 wk after resolution of illness (about 3–6 wk); concurrent corticosteroids given for ocular or CNS infection. Prolonged therapy if HIV positive. Compounded pyrimethamine may be obtained from specialized pharmacies; consult your local pharmacist for information on which pharmacies are approved for creating these products. Take pyrimethamine with food to decrease GI adverse effects; sulfadiazine should be taken on an empty stomach with water.

		Consult expert advice for treatment during pregnancy, management of congenital infection, management of chorioretinitis, and management of toxoplasmosis in immunocompromised individuals.
Travelers diarrhea[37,85–87]	Azithromycin 10 mg/kg qd for 1–3 days (AII); OR rifaximin 200 mg PO tid for 3 days (age ≥12 y) (BIII); OR ciprofloxacin (BII)	See 2017 guidelines from International Society of Travel Medicine: https://academic.oup.com/jtm/article/24/suppl_1/S63/3782742 (accessed September 30, 2022). Azithromycin preferable to ciprofloxacin for travelers to Southeast Asia and India given high prevalence of fluoroquinolone-resistant *Campylobacter.* Do not use rifaximin for *Campylobacter, Salmonella, Shigella*, and other causes of invasive diarrhea or bloody diarrhea that may be associated with bacteremia. Antibiotic regimens may be combined with loperamide (≥2 y). Rifamycin evaluated by the FDA in adults ≥18 y for treatment of TD caused by noninvasive strains of *Escherichia coli* (388 mg [2 tabs] bid for 3 days).
Trichinellosis (*Trichinella spiralis*)[88]	Albendazole 400 mg PO bid for 8–14 days (BII) OR mebendazole 200–400 mg PO tid for 3 days, then 400–500 mg PO tid for 10 days	Therapy ineffective for larvae already in muscles Anti-inflammatory drugs, steroids for CNS or cardiac involvement or severe symptoms
Trichomoniasis (*Trichomonas vaginalis*)[89]	Tinidazole 50 mg/kg (max 2 g) PO for 1 dose (BII) OR metronidazole 500 mg PO bid for 7 days (preferred for women) (BII) OR metronidazole 2 g PO for 1 dose	Treat sex partners simultaneously. Higher rates of treatment failure have been shown to occur with a single dose compared to a 7-day course of treatment with metronidazole. Metronidazole resistance occurs and may be treated with higher-dose metronidazole or tinidazole.
Trichuris trichiura	See Whipworm later in this table.	

B. PREFERRED THERAPY FOR SPECIFIC PARASITIC PATHOGENS *(continued)*

Disease/Organism	Treatment (evidence grade)	Comments
– Chagas disease[26–28] (*Trypanosoma cruzi*)	Benznidazole PO: age <2 y, 5.0–7.5 mg/kg/day div bid for 60 days; ages 2–12 y, 5–8 mg/kg/day div bid for 60 days; age ≥12 y, 5–7 mg/kg/day div bid for 60 days (BIII); OR nifurtimox PO age birth–<18 y, 2.5 kg–<40 kg: 10–20 mg/kg/day, PO, in 3 div doses for 60 days; age ≥17 y, 8–10 mg/kg/day div tid for 60 days (BIII)	Therapy recommended for acute and congenital infection, reactivated infection, and chronic infection in children and teens <18 y; consider in those up to 50 y with chronic infection without advanced cardiomyopathy. Benznidazole has been evaluated by the FDA for use in children aged 2–12 y (www.benznidazoletablets.com; accessed September 30, 2022); data have not been submitted for review for children aged <2 y. Some experts use 300 mg/day for 60 days for adults regardless of body weight. Nifurtimox has been reviewed and approved by the FDA for children and teens up to 17 y. Side effects are common but occur less often in younger patients. Both drugs contraindicated in pregnancy.
– Human African trypanosomiasis[90–95] Acute (hemolymphatic) stage (*Trypanosoma brucei gambiense* [West African]; *Trypanosoma brucei rhodesiense* [East African])	*Tb gambiense:* pentamidine isethionate 4 mg/kg/day IM or IV for 7 days *Tb rhodesiense:* suramin (from CDC); after test dose of 2 mg/kg (max 100 mg) IV, 10–20 mg/kg (max 1 g) IV on days 1, 3, 7, 14, and 21	Consult with the CDC (www.cdc.gov/parasites/sleepingsickness/index.html; accessed September 30, 2022), an infectious disease specialist, or a tropical medicine specialist, if unfamiliar with trypanosomiasis. CSF examination required for all patients to assess CNS involvement. Examination of the buffy coat of peripheral blood may be helpful. *Tb gambiense* may be found in lymph node aspirates. Fexinidazole is an oral second-line alternative drug for *Tb gambiense* hemolymphatic stage and CNS involvement, a nitroimidazole antimicrobial that is FDA approved for the treatment of both first- and second-stage human African trypanosomiasis due to

		Tb gambiense in patients aged ≥6 y and weighing at least 20 kg. Due to the decreased efficacy observed in patients with severe second-stage human African trypanosomiasis with CSF white blood cell counts >100/µL, fexinidazole should be used only if there are no other available treatment options.
Late (CNS) stage (*Trypanosoma brucei gambiense* [West African]; *Trypanosoma brucei rhodesiense* [East African])	*Tb gambiense*: nifurtimox 15 mg/kg/day PO, div tid, for 10 days and eflornithine (from CDC) 400 mg/kg/day IV in two 2-h infusions (each dose diluted in 250 mL of water for injection) for 7 days (NECT); OR nifurtimox 15 mg/kg/day PO, div tid, for 10 days and eflornithine 400 mg/kg/day IV in four 2-h infusions (each dose diluted in 100 mL of water for injection) for 14 days (NECT) over the long term *Tb rhodesiense*: melarsoprol, 2.2 mg/kg/day IV (max 180–200 mg/day) for 10 days; corticosteroids often given with melarsoprol to decrease risk of CNS toxicity	CSF examination needed for management (double-centrifuge technique recommended); repeat CSF examinations q6mo for 2 y to detect relapse. Eflornithine: children weighing <10 kg, dilute in 50 mL of water for injection; children weighing 10–25 kg, dilute in 100 mL of water for injection. If water for injection is unavailable, eflornithine can be diluted in 5% dextrose or saline. See above regarding fexinidazole.
Uncinaria stenocephala	See Cutaneous larva migrans earlier in this table.	
Whipworm (trichuriasis) *Trichuris trichiura*	Albendazole 400 mg PO qd for 3 days; OR mebendazole 100 mg PO bid for 3 days; OR ivermectin 200 mcg/kg/day PO qd for 3 days (BII)	Treatment can be given for 5–7 days for heavy infestation.
Wuchereria bancrofti	See Filariasis earlier in this table.	
Yaws	Azithromycin 30 mg/kg, max 2 g once (also treats bejel and pinta)	Alternative regimens include IM benzathine penicillin and second-line agents doxycycline, tetracycline, and erythromycin.

10. Choosing Among Antiparasitic Agents: Antimalarial Drugs, Nitroimidazoles, Benzimidazoles, and Neglected Tropical Diseases

Antimalarial Drugs

Prevention of Malaria

Seven drugs are available in the United States for prevention of malaria; one (tafenoquine) is licensed only for adults 18 years and older. Another (doxycycline) is not suitable for children younger than 8 years due to the duration it must be taken. Two (primaquine and tafenoquine) require testing for glucose-6-phosphate dehydrogenase (G6PD) deficiency before use. Five of these drugs are taken weekly (chloroquine, hydroxychloroquine, mefloquine, primaquine, and tafenoquine) and the other 2 are taken daily (atovaquone/proguanil and doxycycline). The first consideration in the choice of a drug for prevention of malaria is presence of chloroquine resistance at the destination (from the Centers for Disease Control and Prevention [CDC]: wwwnc.cdc.gov/travel/yellowbook/2020/preparing-international-travelers/yellow-fever-vaccine-and-malaria-prophylaxis-information-by-country#5391; accessed September 30, 2022). If present, neither chloroquine nor hydroxychloroquine can be used. The next factor to consider is preference of caregivers about giving a medication to a child daily or weekly, as antimalarial effectiveness depends primarily on taking the medication, not which medication is prescribed. Potential adverse events factor into the decision families make about antimalarials. Many parents will decline mefloquine as soon as the black box warning about the risk of neuropsychiatric adverse reactions is explained, although taking a weekly medication might increase convenience and adherence, and mefloquine may be less costly. In general, families traveling to destinations where there is chloroquine resistance will be choosing between atovaquone/proguanil (daily medication, possibly more costly) and mefloquine (weekly medication, black box warning). Primaquine is used extremely rarely in children; testing for G6PD deficiency is required, and many clinicians are unfamiliar with the use of this drug. Doxycycline needs to be given for a longer period than ideal for children younger than 8 years and is limited by its adverse events profile. Tafenoquine also requires G6PD testing and is limited to those older than 18 years.

For families traveling to areas where there is chloroquine-susceptible malaria, both chloroquine and hydroxychloroquine are options. These medications may be difficult to find, and it is prudent to be sure a family can obtain them; if not, any of the other drugs may be considered for use.

Our preference for the best tolerated and effective agent for prophylaxis in areas of chloroquine resistance is atovaquone/proguanil; in areas of chloroquine susceptibility, chloroquine.

Treatment of Malaria

Seven drugs are available in the United States for treatment of acute malaria; choice of drug depends on the severity of illness, location where malaria was acquired, and age of the child. When malaria is acquired in a location without chloroquine resistance, chloroquine or hydroxychloroquine can be used if the patient is able to take medications orally and it is available. When malaria is acquired in chloroquine-resistant locations, or when it is acquired in chloroquine-susceptible areas but chloroquine or hydroxychloroquine is not available immediately, and when medications can be taken orally, artemether/lumefantrine is the preferred option, with atovaquone/proguanil (if not used for prophylaxis) also being an option. Mefloquine and quinine (in combination with clindamycin or doxycycline) are available but limited by adverse events profiles. When malaria is severe or the patient is unable to take medications orally, intravenous artesunate should be used. Identification of the species of *Plasmodium* may not be available at the time of choosing the antimalarial drug; in general, treating for *Plasmodium falciparum* is appropriate until more information is available.

The CDC has detailed treatment decision-tree algorithms and tables available at www.cdc.gov/malaria/diagnosis_treatment/treatment.html (accessed September 30, 2022).

Choosing Among Nitroimidazoles (Treatment Option for Some Protozoa, Amoebas)

The choice among nitroimidazoles (metronidazole, tinidazole, triclabendazole, and secnidazole) is based primarily on availability (secnidazole is not available in the United States), cost, convenience, and adverse events. All drugs in this group may produce a disulfiram-like effect when taken with alcohol. Tinidazole has a longer half-life and is better tolerated than metronidazole but may be more costly. Triclabendazole has a narrower spectrum confined to *Fasciola hepatica, Fasciola gigantica,* and paragonimiasis.

Choosing Among Benzimidazoles (Treatment Option for Some Helminths)

The choice between the benzimidazoles mebendazole and albendazole depends on the specific organism, availability, and cost. Albendazole is a broader-spectrum antihelminth than mebendazole but may be more costly.

Need is great for effective, affordable, and easily available drugs for diseases known as *neglected tropical diseases,* which include, but are not limited to, the diseases mentioned previously and Chagas disease, leishmaniasis, lymphatic filariasis, and trypanosomiasis. For many of these diseases, options for treatment are limited, include drugs with significant adverse events, or include drugs with limited availability. Additional funding would accelerate research on drug development and implementation of control measures for these diseases such as mass drug distribution, as it has for treatment and prevention of HIV/AIDS, malaria, and tuberculosis. Until additional focus is put on these neglected tropical diseases, which impose large burdens on the health primarily of those living in low-income countries, the "choosing among" section in this book for antiparasitic drugs will continue to be far shorter that the sections on antibacterial, antiviral, and antifungal drugs.

11. How Antibiotic Dosages Are Determined by Use of Susceptibility Data, Pharmacodynamics, and Treatment Outcomes

Factors Involved in Dosing Recommendations

Our view of assessing the optimal dose of antimicrobials is continually changing. As the published literature and our experience with each drug increase, our recommendations for specific dosages evolve as we compare the efficacy, safety, and cost of each drug in the context of current and previous data from adults and children. Virtually every new antibiotic must first demonstrate some degree of efficacy and safety in adults with antibiotic exposures that occur at specific dosages, which are duplicated in children as closely as possible. We keep track of pediatric pharmacokinetics (PK) in all age-groups, reported toxicities, and unanticipated clinical failures, and on occasion, we may end up modifying our initial recommendations for an antibiotic.

Important considerations in any recommendations we make include (1) the susceptibilities of pathogens to antibiotics, which are constantly changing, are different from region to region, and are often hospital and unit specific; (2) the antibiotic concentrations achieved at the site of infection over a 24-hour dosing interval; (3) the mechanism of how antibiotics kill bacteria; (4) how often the dose we select produces a clinical and microbiological cure; (5) how often we encounter toxicity; (6) how likely the antibiotic exposure will lead to antibiotic resistance in the treated child and in the population in general; and (7) the effect on the child's microbiome.

Susceptibility

Susceptibility data for each bacterial pathogen against a wide range of antibiotics are available from the microbiology laboratory of virtually every hospital. This antibiogram can help guide you in antibiotic selection for empiric therapy while you wait for specific susceptibilities to come back from your cultures. Many hospitals can separate the inpatient culture results from the outpatient results, and many can give you the data by hospital ward (eg, pediatric ward vs neonatal intensive care unit vs adult intensive care unit). Susceptibility data are also available by region and by country from reference laboratories or public health laboratories. The recommendations made in *Nelson's Pediatric Antimicrobial Therapy* reflect overall susceptibility patterns present in the United States. Tables A and B in Chapter 3 provide some overall guidance on susceptibility of gram-positive and gram-negative pathogens, respectively. Wide variations may exist for certain pathogens in different regions of the United States and the world. New techniques for rapid molecular diagnosis of a bacterial, mycobacterial, fungal, or viral pathogen based on polymerase chain reaction or next-generation sequencing may quickly give you the name of the pathogen, but with current molecular technology, susceptibility data are not usually available.

Drug Concentrations at the Site of Infection

With every antibiotic, we can measure the concentration of antibiotic present in the serum. We can also directly measure the concentrations in specific tissue sites, such as spinal fluid or middle ear fluid. Because "free," nonprotein-bound antibiotic is required to inhibit and kill pathogens, it is also important to calculate the amount of free drug available at the site of infection. While traditional methods of measuring antibiotics focused just on the peak concentrations in serum and how rapidly the drugs were excreted (the half-life), newer models of drug distribution in both plasma *and* tissue sites (eg, cerebrospinal fluid, urine, peritoneal fluid) and elimination from both plasma and tissue compartments now exist. Antibiotic exposure to pathogens at the site of infection can be described mathematically in many ways: (1) the percentage of time in a 24-hour dosing interval that the antibiotic concentrations are above the minimum inhibitory concentration (MIC; the antibiotic concentration required for inhibition of growth of an organism) at the site of infection (%T>MIC); (2) the mathematically calculated area below the serum concentration-versus-time curve (area under the curve [AUC]); and (3) the maximal concentration of drug achieved in serum and at the tissue site (Cmax). For each of these 3 values, *a ratio of that value to the MIC of the pathogen in question* can be calculated and provides more useful information on specific drug activity against a specific pathogen than a simple look at serum concentrations or the AUC. It allows us to compare the exposure of different antibiotics (that achieve quite different concentrations in tissues) to a pathogen (where the MIC for each drug may be different) and to assess the activity of a single antibiotic that may be used for empiric therapy against the many different pathogens (potentially with many different MICs) that may be causing an infection at that tissue site.

Pharmacodynamics

Pharmacodynamic (PD) descriptions provide the clinician with information on *how* the bacterial pathogens are killed (see Suggested Reading later in this chapter). Beta-lactam antibiotics tend to eradicate bacteria following prolonged exposure of relatively low concentrations of the antibiotic to the pathogen at the site of infection, usually expressed as the percentage of time over a dosing interval that the antibiotic is present at the site of infection in concentrations greater than the MIC (%T>MIC). For example, amoxicillin needs to be present at the site of a pneumococcal infection (such as the middle ear) at a concentration above the MIC for only 40% of a 24-hour dosing interval. Remarkably, neither higher concentrations of amoxicillin nor a more prolonged exposure will substantially increase the cure rate. On the other hand, gentamicin's activity against *Escherichia coli* is based primarily on the absolute concentration of free antibiotic at the site of infection, in the context of the MIC of the pathogen (Cmax:MIC). The more antibiotic you can deliver to the site of infection, the more rapidly you can sterilize the tissue; we are limited only by the toxicities of gentamicin. For fluoroquinolones such as ciprofloxacin, the antibiotic exposure best linked to clinical and microbiological success is, like that of aminoglycosides, concentration dependent. However, the best mathematical correlate to assess microbiological (and clinical) outcomes for fluoroquinolones is the AUC:MIC, rather than the Cmax:MIC. Each of the 3 PD metrics of antibiotic exposure should be linked to the MIC of the pathogen to best understand how well the antibiotic will eradicate a particular pathogen causing an infection.

Assessment of Clinical and Microbiological Outcomes

In clinical trials of anti-infective agents, most adults and children will hopefully be cured, but the therapy of a few will fail. For those few, we may note unanticipated treatment failure, due to inadequate drug exposure (eg, more rapid drug elimination in a particular patient; the inability of a particular antibiotic to penetrate to the site of infection) or due to a pathogen with a particularly high MIC. By analyzing the successes and the failures based on the appropriate exposure parameters outlined previously (%T>MIC, AUC:MIC, or Cmax:MIC), we can often observe a particular value of exposure, above which we observe a higher rate of cure and below which the cure rate drops quickly. Knowing this target value in adults (the "antibiotic exposure break point") allows us to calculate the dosage that will create treatment success in most children. We do not evaluate antibiotics in children with study designs that have failure rates sufficient to calculate a pediatric exposure break point, of course. It is the adult *exposure value* that leads to success that we all (including the US Food and Drug Administration [FDA] and pharmaceutical companies) subsequently share with you, a pediatric health care practitioner, as one likely to cure your patient. FDA-approved break points that are reported by microbiology laboratories (S, I, and R) are now determined by outcomes linked to drug PK and exposure, the MIC, and the PD parameter for that agent. Recommendations to the FDA for break points for the United States often come from "break point organizations," such as the Clinical and Laboratory Standards Institute Subcommittee on Antimicrobial Susceptibility Testing (https://clsi.org) or the US Committee on Antimicrobial Susceptibility Testing (www.uscast.org).

Physiologic-Based Pharmacokinetic Modeling

Just to keep everyone informed about where the field of antibiotic exposure modeling is going, the next advance is physiologic-based PK (PBPK) modeling. Currently, we use PK/PD modeling, described by Monte Carlo simulation software using the overall observed distribution of PK values in a specific pediatric population (eg, neonates, infants, children, adolescents), the range of MICs observed in pathogens of interest, and the PD description for inhibition of bacteria growth (discussed previously) for each antibiotic/pathogen pair. We can then find the likelihood that a certain dose will treat a certain pathogen at a certain tissue site, by using a specific dose. What PBPK adds to the equation is additional information about the physicochemical properties of drugs (some diffuse well into adipose tissues; others, not so much), about ongoing organ function development through childhood, and about blood flow/organ perfusion throughout the entire body, to allow better prediction of how drugs move through tissue compartments of the body during absorption, distribution, metabolism, and excretion for each age-group in pediatrics. In that sense, PK/PD modeling can describe by observation, but PBPK modeling can better predict how an antibiotic will "behave" in a child for both efficacy and toxicity. The FDA is encouraging PBPK modeling, and the more data we have on drug behavior, the better the PBPK models become for children. The Verscheijden review listed in Suggested Reading gives a nice overview of PBPK modeling in pediatrics.

Suggested Reading

Le J, et al. *J Clin Pharmacol.* 2018;58(suppl 10):S108–S122 PMID: 30248202

Onufrak NJ, et al. *Clin Ther.* 2016;38(9):1930–1947 PMID: 27449411

Trang M, et al. *Curr Opin Pharmacol.* 2017;36:107–113 PMID: 29128853

Verscheijden LFM, et al. *Pharmacol Ther.* 2020;211:107541 PMID: 32246949

12. Approach to Antibiotic Therapy for Drug-Resistant Gram-negative Bacilli and Methicillin-Resistant *Staphylococcus aureus*

Multidrug-Resistant Gram-negative Bacilli

Increasing antibiotic resistance in gram-negative bacilli, primarily the enteric bacilli (eg, *Escherichia coli, Klebsiella, Enterobacter, Serratia, Citrobacter*), *Pseudomonas aeruginosa*, and *Acinetobacter* species, has caused profound difficulties in treatment of patients around the world; some of the pathogens now resist all available agents. *Stenotrophomonas*, with profound intrinsic antibiotic resistance, is increasing as a cause of nosocomial infections and of infection in those with chronic recurrent infection (eg, cystic fibrosis). At this time, only a limited number of pediatric tertiary care centers in North America have reported outbreaks of multidrug-resistant (MDR) pathogens, but *sustained* transmission of completely resistant organisms is quite uncommon in pediatric health care institutions, likely due to the critical infection control strategies in place to identify and prevent the spread of these pathogens. Antibiotic resistance in pathogens, particularly the non-fermenting gram-negative rods, is not new but, rather, the result of more than 100 million years of exposure to antibiotics elaborated by other organisms in their environment. Inducible enzymes to cleave antibiotics and modify binding sites, efflux pumps, and gram-negative cell wall alterations to prevent antibiotic penetration may all be present. Some mechanisms of resistance, if not intrinsic, can be acquired from other bacilli. By using antibiotics, we "awaken" resistance; therefore, using antibiotics only when appropriate limits the selection, or induction, of resistance for pathogens in the treated child and for all children (see Chapter 17). Community prevalence, as well as health care institution prevalence, of extended-spectrum beta-lactamase (ESBL)–containing enteric bacilli that are resistant to ceftriaxone is increasing. Carbapenemase-containing pathogens that are meropenem resistant are now beginning to spread in neonates, infants, and children. Two major classes of carbapenemases exist: serine beta-lactamases (SBLs), named for a serine at the active site, and metallo-beta-lactamases (MBLs), having a zinc at the active site. Antibiotic resistance patterns differ for the 2 classes. The most prominent carbapenemases in the United States are SBLs, most often *Klebsiella pneumoniae* carbapenemase (KPC)–related enzymes and increasingly OXA-48–like enzymes. Globally, MBLs are often the most prominent classes in circulation (eg, VIM [Verona integron-encoded], NDM [New Delhi], IMP [imipenemase]), with ongoing spread within the United States. Some SBLs and MBLs are now being addressed by new, active antibiotics and new beta-lactamase inhibitors (BLIs). However, as we have found in the past, as soon as new drugs are available, resistance develops quickly. We cannot win, but we can usually stay in the fight against these pathogens.

In **Figure 12-1,** we assume that the clinician has the antibiotic susceptibility report in hand (or at least a local antibiogram). Each tier provides increasingly broader-spectrum activity, from the narrowest of the gram-negative agents to the broadest (and most toxic), colistin. Tier 1 is ampicillin, safe and widely available but not active against *Klebsiella, Enterobacter*, or *Pseudomonas* and only active against about half of *E coli* in the community setting. Tier 2 contains antibiotics that not only have a broader spectrum

Figure 12-1. Enteric Bacilli: Bacilli and *Pseudomonas* With Known Susceptibilities (See Text for Interpretation)

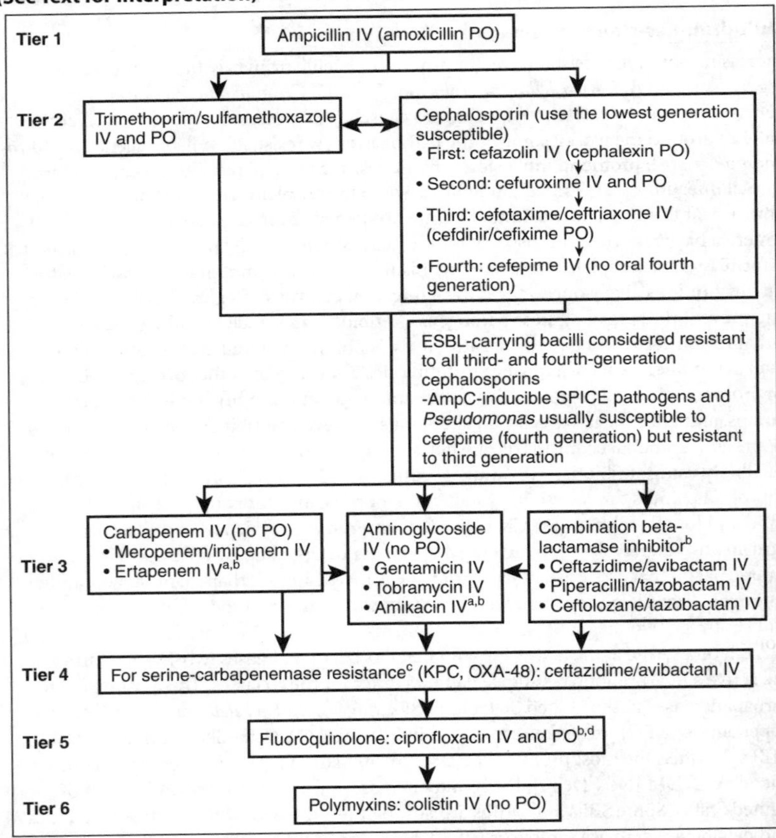

Abreviations: ESBL, extended-spectrum beta-lactamase; IM, intramuscular; IV, intravenous; *Klebsiella pneumoniae* carbapenemase; PO, orally; SPICE, *Serratia*, indole-positive *Proteus, Citrobacter, Enterobacter*.

[a] Ertapenem is the only carbapenem *not* active against *Pseudomonas*. Ertapenem and amikacin can be given once daily as outpatient IV/IM therapy for infections where these drugs achieve therapeutic concentrations (eg, urinary tract). Some use once-daily gentamicin or tobramycin.

[b] For mild to moderate ESBL infections caused by organisms susceptible only to IV/IM beta-lactam or aminoglycoside therapy but also susceptible to fluoroquinolones, oral fluoroquinolone therapy is preferred over IV/IM therapy if the infection is amenable to treatment by oral therapy.

[c] Not active against metallo-carbapenemases; for metallo-carbapenemases, use fluoroquinolones, aminoglycosides, or aztreonam PLUS ceftazidime/avibactam.

[d] If you have susceptibility to only a few remaining agents, consider combination therapy to prevent the emergence of resistance to your last-resort antibiotics (no prospective, controlled data in these situations).

but also have a very safe and effective profile (trimethoprim/sulfamethoxazole [TMP/SMX] and cephalosporins) with decades of experience. In general, use an antibiotic from tier 2 before turning to broader-spectrum agents. The first-through-fifth generation cephalosporins are not reliably active against ESBL-containing pathogens. Please also be aware that many enteric bacilli (the "SPICE" bacteria, *Serratia,* indole-positive *Proteus, Citrobacter,* and *Enterobacter,* and a few others) have inducible, chromosomal beta-lactam resistance (ampC beta-lactamases, which are active against all cephalosporins except cefepime, a fourth-generation cephalosporin). Resistance usually develops only after exposure of the pathogen to the antibiotic. Tier 3 is made up of very broad-spectrum antibiotics (ie, carbapenems, ceftazidime/avibactam, piperacillin/tazobactam, ceftolozane/tazobactam). Ceftolozane is more active against *P aeruginosa* than ceftazidime or piperacillin, and it is paired with tazobactam, allowing for additional activity again ESBL-producing enteric bacilli. Aminoglycosides remain active against many MDR pathogens with resistance to beta-lactams but demonstrate significantly more toxicity than beta-lactam agents, although we have used them safely for decades. Tier 4 is represented by a new broad-spectrum BLI, avibactam, in combination with ceftazidime (ceftazidime/avibactam is US Food and Drug Administration [FDA] approved for children), that demonstrates activity against ESBL-producing enteric bacilli and against the KPC and OXA-48 serine carbapenemases but *lacks* stability against the metallo-carbapenemases present most commonly in enteric bacilli (including *E coli*) worldwide.[1] With substantial data on safety with widespread use, ceftazidime/avibactam is preferred over fluoroquinolones. Tier 5 is fluoroquinolones, to be used only when lower-tier antibiotics cannot be used due to potential cartilage/tendon toxicities (not yet reported in children for fluoroquinolones available in the United States). Tier 6 is colistin, one of the broadest-spectrum agents available. Colistin was FDA approved in 1962 with significant toxicity and limited clinical experience in children.

Some of the newer-generation tetracyclines have activity against MBL-producing enteric bacilli (ie, tigecycline, eravacycline, omadacycline) but are not discussed in this book.

Many additional drugs for MDR gram-negative organisms are currently moving from animal models into adult clinical trials. Stay tuned.

Investigational Agents Recently Approved for Adults and Being Studied in Children

Cefiderocol. Represents a new class of beta-lactam antibiotics as a siderophore cephalosporin (eg, binding to iron) that defies the "generation" categories with respect to spectrum of activity. The cefiderocol-iron complex allows for pathogens to actively transport the complex across the cell wall into the periplasmic space, thus allowing the antibiotic access to the transpeptidases not as easily achievable with standard beta-lactams. It is stable to ESBLs, SBLs and MBLs, ampC, and OXA-48 enzymes, with activity that includes *Pseudomonas, Acinetobacter,* and *Stenotrophomonas.* Pediatric treatment studies are well underway.

Imipenem and relebactam. Imipenem was the first carbapenem approved for use in children and is now paired with relebactam, a BLI with similar structure to that of avibactam, providing stability for the combination against KPC-containing enteric bacilli, thus extending the aerobic/anaerobic broad spectrum of carbapenems that already includes ESBLs and ampC beta-lactamases. Pediatric treatment studies are well underway.

Meropenem and vaborbactam. Meropenem, a familiar broad-spectrum aerobic/anaerobic coverage carbapenem that is already stable to ESBLs and ampC beta-lactamases, is now paired with vaborbactam, allowing for activity against the KPC serine carbapenemases but not metallo-carbapenemases. Pediatric pharmacokinetic studies are underway.

Plazomicin. Represents a new aminoglycoside antibiotic that is active against many of the gentamicin-, tobramycin-, and amikacin-resistant enteric bacilli and *Pseudomonas*. Not currently available in the United States.

Investigational Agents Under Study in Adults We Are Following

Aztreonam and avibactam. This antibiotic is being developed to address metallo-carbapenemases, for which avibactam and relebactam do not provide protection. Aztreonam, a monobactam antibiotic first approved in 1986, is stable to many MBLs but susceptible to cleavage from virtually all the other beta-lactamases; *however,* when it is paired with avibactam, the combination becomes stable to a vast array of beta-lactamases.

Cefepime and taniborbactam. Represents another older antibiotic, cefepime, that is now paired with taniborbactam, a broad-spectrum, borate-based BLI, stable against ESBLs, SBLs and MBLs, and ampC beta-lactamases.

Fosfomycin. Is available in the United States in oral form for uncomplicated cystitis, with new studies in the United States having been conducted in adults with an intravenous (IV) formulation. Interferes with the synthesis of cell walls (inhibits linking of glycan and peptide to form peptidoglycan cross-linked structures that form cell walls) and demonstrates stability to MBLs carried by *E coli.* Pharmacokinetic studies are underway in children.

Community-Associated Methicillin-Resistant *Staphylococcus aureus*

Community-associated methicillin-resistant *Staphylococcus aureus* (CA-MRSA) is a community pathogen for children (that can also spread from child to child in hospitals) that first developed in the United States in the mid-1990s and currently represents 10% to 30% of all community isolates in various regions of the United States (check your hospital microbiology laboratory for your local rate); it is present in many areas of the world, with some strain variation documented. Notably, we have begun to see a decrease in invasive MRSA infections in multiple locations in the United States.[2,3] CA-MRSA resists beta-lactam antibiotics, with the notable exception of ceftaroline, a fifth-generation cephalosporin antibiotic that was FDA approved for pediatrics in June 2016 (see Chapter 1).

There are an undetermined number of pathogenicity factors that make CA-MRSA strains more aggressive than methicillin-susceptible *S aureus* (MSSA) strains. CA-MRSA seems to cause greater tissue necrosis, an increased host inflammatory response, an increased rate of complications, and an increased rate of recurrent infections, compared with MSSA. Response of MRSA to therapy with non–beta-lactam antibiotics (eg, vancomycin) seems to be inferior, compared with response of MSSA to oxacillin/nafcillin or cefazolin, but it is unknown whether poorer outcomes are due to a hardier, better-adapted, more aggressive strain of *S aureus* or alternative agents are just not as effective against MRSA as beta-lactam agents are against MSSA. In children, studies using ceftaroline to treat skin infections (many caused by MRSA) were conducted by way of a non-inferiority clinical trial design, comparing ceftaroline with vancomycin, with the finding that ceftaroline was equivalent to vancomycin. Guidelines for management of MRSA infections (2011) and management of skin and soft tissue infections (2014) have been published by the Infectious Diseases Society of America (IDSA)[4] and are available at www.idsociety.org, as well as in *Red Book: 2021–2024 Report of the Committee on Infectious Diseases.*

Antimicrobials for CA-MRSA

Vancomycin (IV) has been the mainstay of parenteral therapy for MRSA infections for the past 4 decades and continues to have activity against more than 98% of strains isolated from children. New guidelines on the use of vancomycin for MRSA infections have recently been published through a collaboration among the American Society of Health-System Pharmacists, IDSA, Pediatric Infectious Diseases Society, and Society of Infectious Diseases Pharmacists.[5] A few cases of intermediate resistance and "heteroresistance" (transient moderately increased resistance likely to be caused by thickened staphylococcal cell walls) have been reported, most commonly in adults who are receiving long-term therapy or who have received multiple exposures to vancomycin. Unfortunately, the response to therapy using standard vancomycin dosing of 40 mg/kg/day in the treatment of many CA-MRSA strains has not been as predictably successful as in the past with MSSA. For vancomycin efficacy, the ratio of the area under the curve (the mathematically calculated area below the serum concentration-versus-time curve) to minimum inhibitory concentration (AUC:MIC) seems to be the best exposure metric to predict a successful outcome. Better outcomes are likely to be achieved with an AUC:MIC of about 400 or greater, rather than with a serum trough value in the range of 15 to 20 mcg/mL, which is associated with greater renal toxicity (see Chapter 11 for more on the AUC:MIC). This ratio of 400:1 is achievable for CA-MRSA strains with in vitro MIC values of 1 mcg/mL or less but difficult to achieve for strains with values of 2 mcg/mL or greater.[6] Recent data suggest that vancomycin MICs may actually be decreasing in children for MRSA causing bloodstream infections as they increase for MSSA.[7] Strains with MIC values of 4 mcg/mL or greater should be considered resistant to vancomycin. When using higher "meningitis" treatment dosages of 60 mg/kg/day (or higher) to achieve a 400:1 vancomycin exposure, one needs to follow renal function carefully for the development of toxicity and the possible subsequent need to switch classes of antibiotics.

Dalbavancin is a glycopeptide, structurally very similar to vancomycin but with enhanced in vitro activity against MRSA and a much longer serum half-life, allowing once-weekly dosing, or even just a single dose, to treat skin infections. Approved for pediatrics from birth to age 18 years in 2021, it is an important option for outpatient parenteral therapy once-weekly IV injection, when outpatient *IV* therapy and *oral* therapy are not feasible.

Clindamycin (oral [PO] or IV) is active against about 70% to 90% of strains of either MRSA or MSSA, with great geographic variability (again, check with your hospital laboratory).[8] The dosage for moderate to severe infections is 30 to 40 mg/kg/day, in 3 divided doses, with the same milligram per kilogram dose PO or IV. Clindamycin is not as bactericidal as vancomycin but achieves higher concentrations in abscesses (because of high intracellular concentrations in neutrophils). Some CA-MRSA strains are susceptible to clindamycin on testing but have inducible clindamycin resistance (methylase-mediated) that is usually assessed by the "D-test" and can now be assessed by multi-well microtiter plates. Within each population of CA-MRSA organisms, a rare organism (between 1 in 10^9 and 10^{11} organisms) will have a mutation that allows for *constant,* rather than induced, resistance.[9] Although still somewhat controversial, clindamycin should be effective therapy for infections that have a relatively low organism load (eg, cellulitis, small or drained abscesses) and are unlikely to contain a significant population of these constitutive methylase-producing mutants that are truly resistant; in fact, staphylococcal methylase is poorly induced by clindamycin. Infections with a high organism load (empyema) may have a greater risk of failure, as a large population is more likely to have a significant number of truly resistant organisms and clindamycin should not be used as the preferred agent for these infections. Many laboratories no longer report D-test results but simply call the organisms "resistant," prompting the use of alternative therapy that may not be needed.

Clindamycin is used to treat most CA-MRSA infections that are not life-threatening, and if the child responds, therapy can be switched from IV to PO (although the PO solution is not very well tolerated). *Clostridium difficile* enterocolitis is a concern; however, despite a great increase in the use of clindamycin in children during the past decade, recent published data do not document a clinically significant increase in the rate of this complication in children.

Trimethoprim/sulfamethoxazole (PO, IV), Bactrim/Septra, is active against CA-MRSA in vitro. Prospective, comparative data on treatment of skin or skin structure infections in adults and children document efficacy equivalent to clindamycin.[10] Given our current lack of prospective, comparative information in MRSA bacteremia, pneumonia, and osteomyelitis (in contrast to skin infections), TMP/SMX should not be used routinely to treat these more serious infections at this time.

Linezolid (PO, IV), active against virtually 100% of CA-MRSA strains, is another reasonable alternative but is considered bacteriostatic and has relatively frequent hematologic toxicity in adults (ie, neutropenia, thrombocytopenia) and some infrequent neurologic toxicity (ie, peripheral neuropathy, optic neuritis), particularly when used for courses of 2 weeks or longer. A complete blood cell count should be checked every week or two in children receiving prolonged linezolid therapy. The cost of generic linezolid is still substantially more than of clindamycin or vancomycin.

Daptomycin (IV) is FDA approved for adults with skin infections and bacteremia/endocarditis and was approved for use in children with skin infections in April 2017. It is a unique class of antibiotic, a lipopeptide, and is highly bactericidal. Daptomycin became generic in 2017 and should be considered for treatment of skin infection and bacteremia when other, better-studied antibiotics fail. **Daptomycin should not be used to treat pneumonia,** as it is inactivated by pulmonary surfactant. Pediatric studies for skin infections and bacteremia have been completed and published.[11,12] Studies in pediatric osteomyelitis[13] are now published, showing that daptomycin was not statistically different than comparator standard-of-care antibiotics for all *S aureus* (few subjects with MRSA were enrolled in the global study). However, based on a complex, early time point evaluation at day 5, daptomycin was not found to be statistically non-inferior to comparators. We believe that daptomycin should still be considered an option for treatment of MRSA osteomyelitis, but it may not provide better outcomes for MSSA osteomyelitis. Some newborn animal neurologic toxicity data suggest additional **caution for the use of daptomycin in infants younger than 1 year,** prompting a warning in the package label. Routine pediatric clinical trial investigations in young infants were not pursued due to these concerns.

Tigecycline and fluoroquinolones, both of which may show in vitro activity, are not generally recommended for children if other agents are available and are tolerated, due to potential toxicity issues and rapid emergence of resistance with fluoroquinolones (except for delafloxacin, which is investigated and approved only in adults at this time).

Ceftaroline, a fifth-generation cephalosporin antibiotic, the first FDA-approved beta-lactam antibiotic to be active against MRSA, was approved for children in June 2016. The gram-negative coverage is like that of ceftriaxone, with no activity against *Pseudomonas*. Published data are available for pediatric pharmacokinetics, as well as for prospective, randomized comparative treatment trials of skin and skin structure infections,[14] community-acquired pneumonia,[15,16] and neonatal sepsis.[17] The efficacy and toxicity profile for adults is what one would expect from most cephalosporins. Based on these published data, ceftaroline should be effective and safer than vancomycin for treatment of MRSA infections for all age-groups, including neonates. Just as beta-lactams are preferred over vancomycin for MSSA infections, ceftaroline is now considered by the editors to be the preferred treatment of MRSA infections over vancomycin, except for central nervous system infections/endocarditis only due to lack of clinical data for these infections. Neither renal function nor drug levels need to be followed with ceftaroline therapy. Since pediatric approval in mid-2016, there have been no serious postmarketing adverse experiences in children reported; recommendations may change should unexpected clinical data on lack of efficacy or unexpected toxicity beyond what may be expected with beta-lactams be presented.

Combination therapy for serious infections, with vancomycin and rifampin (for deep abscesses) or vancomycin and gentamicin (for bacteremia), is often used, but no prospective, controlled human clinical data exist on improved efficacy over single antibiotic therapy. Some experts use vancomycin and clindamycin in combination, particularly for children with a toxic-shock clinical manifestation. Ceftaroline has also been used in combination therapy with other agents, including daptomycin in adults, but no prospective, controlled clinical data exist to assess benefits.

Investigational Gram-positive Agents Recently Approved for Adults and Being Studied in Children

Oritavancin. Represents an IV glycopeptide, structurally very similar to vancomycin but with enhanced in vitro activity against MRSA and a much longer serum half-life, allowing once-weekly dosing. A very similar antibiotic, dalbavancin, was just approved for children in 2021.

Telavancin. A glycolipopeptide with mechanisms of activity that include cell wall inhibition and cell membrane depolarization, telavancin is administered once daily.

Tedizolid. A second-generation oxazolidinone like linezolid, tedizolid is more potent in vitro against MRSA than linezolid, with somewhat decreased toxicity to bone marrow in adult clinical studies.

Recommendations for Empiric Therapy for Suspected MRSA Infections

Life-threatening and serious infections. If any CA-MRSA is present in your community, empiric therapy for presumed staphylococcal infections that are life-threatening or infections for which any risk of failure is unacceptable should follow the recommendations for CA-MRSA and include ceftaroline OR *high-dose* vancomycin, clindamycin, or linezolid, *in addition to nafcillin or oxacillin* (beta-lactam antibiotics are considered better than vancomycin or clindamycin for MSSA).

Moderate infections. If you live in a location with greater than 10% methicillin resistance, consider using the CA-MRSA recommendations for hospitalized children with presumed staphylococcal infections of any severity, and start empiric therapy with clindamycin (usually active against >80% of CA-MRSA), ceftaroline, vancomycin, or linezolid IV.

In skin and skin structure abscess treatment, antibiotics may be unnecessary following incision and drainage, which may, in fact, be curative.

Mild infections. For nonserious, presumed staphylococcal infections in regions with significant CA-MRSA, topical empiric therapy with mupirocin (Bactroban) or retapamulin (Altabax) ointment, or PO therapy with TMP/SMX or clindamycin, is preferred. For older children, doxycycline and minocycline are also options based on data in adults.

Prevention of Recurrent Infections

For children with problematic, recurrent infections, no well-studied, prospectively collected data provide a solution. Bleach baths (½ cup of bleach in a full bathtub)[18] seemed to be able to transiently decrease the number of colonizing organisms but were not shown to decrease the number of infections in a prospective, controlled study in children with eczema. Similarly, a regimen to decolonize with twice-weekly bleach baths in an attempt to prevent recurrent infection did not lead to a statistically significant decrease.[19,20] Bathing with chlorhexidine (Hibiclens, a preoperative antibacterial skin disinfectant) daily or 2 to 3 times each week should provide topical anti-MRSA activity for several hours following a bath. Treating the entire family with decolonization regimens will additionally decrease risk for recurrence for the index child.[21] Nasal mupirocin ointment (Bactroban) designed to eradicate colonization may also be used. All these measures have advantages and disadvantages and need to be used together with environmental measures (eg, washing towels frequently, using hand sanitizers, not sharing items of clothing). Helpful advice can be found on the Centers for Disease Control and Prevention website (www.cdc.gov/mrsa; accessed September 30, 2022).

Vaccines are being investigated but are not likely to be available for several years.

13. Antibiotic Therapy for Children With Obesity

When prescribing an antimicrobial for a child with obesity or overweight, selecting a dose based on milligrams per kilograms of total body weight (TBW) may overexpose the child if the drug does not freely distribute into fat tissue. Conversely, underexposure can occur when a dosage is reduced for obesity for drugs without distribution limitations.

Table 13-1 lists major antimicrobial classes and our suggestions on how to calculate an appropriate dose. The evidence to support these recommendations is Level II to III (pharmacokinetic studies in children, extrapolations from adult studies, and expert opinion). Whenever a dose is used that is greater than one prospectively investigated for efficacy and safety, the clinician must weigh the benefits with potential risks. Data are not available on all agents.

TABLE 13-1. DOSING RECOMMENDATIONS

Drug Class	By EBW[a]	By Adjusted BW	By TBW[b]
Antibacterials			
Beta-lactams			
Piperacillin/tazobactam			X
Cephalosporins			X
Meropenem			X
Ertapenem	X		
Clindamycin			X (no max)
Vancomycin		1,500–2,000 mg/m²/day	20 mg/kg LD, then 60 mg/kg/day div q6–8h
Aminoglycosides		0.7 × TBW	
Fluoroquinolones		EBW + 0.45 (TBW–EBW)	
Miscellaneous			
TMP/SMX			X
Metronidazole			X
Linezolid			X
Daptomycin			X (See max doses in comments below.)

TABLE 13-1. DOSING RECOMMENDATIONS *(continued)*

Drug Class	By EBW[a]	By Adjusted BW	By TBW[b]
Antifungals			
Amphotericin B			X (max 150 mg for AmB-D, max 500 mg for L-AmB)
Fluconazole			X (max 1,200 mg/day)
Flucytosine	X		
Anidulafungin			X (max 250 mg LD, max 125 mg/day)
Caspofungin			X (max 150 mg/day)
Micafungin			X (max 300 mg/day)
Voriconazole	X		
Antivirals (Non-HIV)			
Nucleoside analogues (acyclovir, ganciclovir)	X		
Oseltamivir	X		
Antimycobacterials			
Isoniazid	X		
Rifampin			X
Pyrazinamide			X
Ethambutol			X

Abbreviations: AmB-D, amphotericin B deoxycholate; BMI, body mass index; BW, body weight; div, divided; EBW, expected body weight; L-AmB, liposomal amphotericin B; LD, loading dose; max, maximum; q, every; TBW, total body weight; TMP/SMX, trimethoprim/sulfamethoxazole.

[a] EBW (kg) = BMI 50th percentile for age × actual height (in meters)^2; from Le Grange D, et al. *Pediatrics*. 2012;129(2):e438–e446 PMID: 22218841.

[b] Dose up to adult max (see Chapter 18) if not otherwise specified.

For **gentamicin**, using the child's fat-free mass, an approximate 30% reduction in dosing weight, has been recommended. When you are performing this empiric dosing strategy with aminoglycosides in children with obesity, we recommend closely following serum concentrations.

Vancomycin is traditionally dosed based on TBW in adults with obesity due to increases in kidney size and glomerular filtration rate. In children with obesity, weight-adjusted distribution volume and clearance are slightly lower than in their counterparts without obesity. An empiric maximum dose of 60 mg/kg/day based on TBW, or dosing using body surface area, may be more appropriate. We recommend closely following serum concentrations.

In the setting of **cefazolin** for surgical prophylaxis (see Chapter 15), adult studies of patients with obesity have generally shown that distribution to the subcutaneous fat tissue target can be subtherapeutic when standard doses are used. Higher single doses are recommended in adults with obesity (eg, 2 g instead of the standard 1 g) with re-dosing at 4-hour intervals for longer cases. In children with obesity, we recommend dosing cephalosporins for surgical prophylaxis based on TBW up to the adult maximum.

In critically ill adults with obesity treated with **carbapenems** or **piperacillin/tazobactam,** extended infusion times (over 2–3 hours, instead of 30 minutes) have been shown to increase the likelihood of achieving therapeutic bloodstream antibiotic exposures, particularly against bacteria with higher minimum inhibitory concentrations (MICs). With availability of rapid beta-lactam antibiotic assays by commercial laboratories with high-performance liquid chromatography/mass spectrometry technology, clinicians now have the opportunity to assess adequacy of serum concentrations in critically ill children with obesity.

Daptomycin dosing can be performed by using TBW, but the maximum dose should be 500 mg for skin infections and 750 mg for bloodstream infections. Bolus administration over 2 minutes can improve the likelihood of achieving target concentrations when the maximum dose is less than the calculated dose in an adolescent with obesity.

Adult maximum doses of **linezolid** may be inadequate to achieve target plasma concentrations to treat susceptible methicillin-resistant *Staphylococcus aureus* infections with high MICs. However, higher doses should be attempted only with the aid of concentration monitoring to avoid hematologic toxicity.

Bibliography

Camaione L, et al. *Pharmacotherapy.* 2013;33(12):1278–1287 PMID: 24019205

Chambers J, et al. *Eur J Clin Pharmacol.* 2019;75(4):511–517 PMID: 30511329

Chung EK, et al. *J Clin Pharmacol.* 2015;55(8):899–908 PMID: 25823963

Donoso FA, et al. *Arch Argent Pediatr*. 2019;117(2):e121–e130 PMID: 30869490

Hall RG. *Curr Pharm Des.* 2015;21(32):4748–4751 PMID: 26112269

Harskamp-van Ginkel MW, et al. *JAMA Pediatr.* 2015;169(7):678–685 PMID: 25961828

Maharaj AR, et al. *Paediatr Drugs*. 2021;23(5):499–513 PMID: 34302290

Meng L, et al. *Pharmacotherapy*. 2017;37(11):1415–1431 PMID: 28869666

Moffett BS, et al. *Ther Drug Monit.* 2018;40(3):322–329 PMID: 29521784

Natale S, et al. *Pharmacotherapy.* 2017;37(3):361–378 PMID: 28079262

Pai MP. *Clin Ther.* 2016;38(9):2032–2044 PMID: 27524636

Pai MP, et al. *Antimicrob Agents Chemother.* 2011;55(12):5640–5645 PMID: 21930881

Payne KD, et al. *Expert Rev Anti Infect Ther.* 2016;14(2):257–267 PMID: 26641135

Smith MJ, et al. *Antimicrob Agents Chemother*. 2017;61(4):e02014-16 PMID: 28137820

Wasmann RE, et al. *Antimicrob Agents Chemother.* 2018;62(7):e00063-18 PMID: 29712664

Wasmann RE, et al. *Clin Infect Dis*. 2020;70(10):2213–2215 PMID: 31588493

Wasmann RE, et al. *J Antimicrob Chemother*. 2019;74(4):978–985 PMID: 30649375

Xie F, et al. *J Antimicrob Chemother*. 2019;74(3):667–674 PMID: 30535122

14. Sequential Parenteral-Oral Antibiotic Therapy (Oral Step-down Therapy) for Serious Infections

The concept of oral *step-down* or "oral switch" therapy is not new; evidence-based recommendations from Nelson and colleagues appeared over 40 years ago in the *Journal of Pediatrics*.[1,2] Bone and joint infections,[3–5] complicated bacterial pneumonia with empyema,[6] deep-tissue abscesses, and appendicitis,[7,8] as well as cellulitis or pyelonephritis,[9] may require initial parenteral therapy to control the growth and spread of pathogens and minimize injury to tissues. For abscesses in soft tissues, joints, bones, and empyema, most organisms are removed by surgical drainage, and presumably, many are killed by the initial parenteral therapy. When the signs and symptoms of infection begin to resolve, often within 2 to 4 days, continuing intravenous (IV) therapy may not be required, as a normal host neutrophil response begins to assist in clearing the infection when the pathogen load drops below a certain critical density, as has been demonstrated in an animal model.[10] In addition to following the clinical response before oral switch, following objective laboratory markers, such as C-reactive protein (CRP) or procalcitonin (PCT), during the hospitalization may also help the clinician better assess the response to antibacterial therapy, particularly in the infant or child who is difficult to examine.[11,12] The benefits of oral step-down therapy over prolonged parenteral therapy are substantial and well-documented in treatment of acute osteomyelitis, including a decrease in both emergency department visits and rehospitalizations, with equivalent treatment success outcomes.[13] For many children who have successful drainage of their intra-abdominal abscesses and recover quickly, either short-course oral therapy (7 days' total) or no additional antibiotic treatment following clinical and laboratory recovery may be appropriate.[14] However, defining those children with intra-abdominal abscesses who may benefit from oral step-down therapy (versus no additional antibiotic therapy) is difficult, as the extent of a deep infection, the adequacy of source control (surgical drainage and the variety of techniques involved), and the susceptibility of pathogen(s) involved are not always known.[15]

For the beta-lactam class of antibiotics, absorption of orally administered antibiotics in *standard* dosages originally studied by companies during clinical trials provides peak serum concentrations that are routinely only 5% to 20% of those achieved with IV or intramuscular administration. However, *high-dose* oral beta-lactam therapy provides the tissue antibiotic exposure thought to be required to eradicate the remaining pathogens at the infection site as the tissue perfusion improves. For most oral antibiotics, prospectively collected data on safety and efficacy at higher dosages have not been systematically collected and presented to the US Food and Drug Administration (FDA) for approval; most of the data to support high-dose oral beta-lactam often come from retrospectively reviewed data or small prospective studies. Without FDA review and formal approval, these dosages are, by definition, off-label. High-dose oral beta-lactam antibiotic therapy for osteoarticular infections has been associated with treatment success since 1978.[3] For beta-lactams, begin with a dosage 2 to 3 times the normal dosage (eg, 75–100 mg/kg/day of amoxicillin or 100 mg/kg/day of cephalexin). It is reassuring that high-quality retrospective cohort data have recently confirmed similar outcomes achieved in those treated with oral step-down therapy compared with those treated with IV.[13] High-dose prolonged oral beta-lactam therapy may be associated with reversible neutropenia; checking for hematologic toxicity every few weeks during therapy is suggested.[16] Retrospective reviews of oral step-down therapy in adults suggest that the use of this standard of pediatric care may be increasing in the treatment of certain infections in adults.[17]

Clindamycin and many antibiotics of the fluoroquinolone class (eg, ciprofloxacin, levofloxacin) and oxazolidinone class (eg, linezolid, tedizolid) have excellent absorption of their oral formulations and provide virtually the same tissue antibiotic exposure at a particular milligram per kilogram dose, compared with that dose given intravenously; therefore, higher dosages are not needed for oral therapy. Trimethoprim/sulfamethoxazole and metronidazole are also very well absorbed.

One must also assume that the parent and child are adherent to the administration of each antibiotic dose, that the oral antibiotic will be absorbed from the gastrointestinal tract into the systemic circulation (no vomiting or diarrhea), and that the parents will seek medical care if the clinical course does not continue to improve for their child.

Monitor the child clinically for a continued response on oral therapy; follow CRP or PCT after the switch to oral therapy, and if there are concerns about continued response, make sure the antibiotic and dosage you selected are appropriate and the family is adherent. In one of the first published series of oral step-down therapy for osteoarticular infection by Syrogiannopoulos and Nelson, failures caused by presumed nonadherence were reported.[18]

15. Antimicrobial Prophylaxis/Prevention of Symptomatic Infection

This chapter summarizes recommendations for prophylaxis of infections, defined as provision of therapy before the onset of clinical signs or symptoms of infection. Prophylaxis can be considered in several clinical scenarios.

A. Postexposure Antimicrobial Prophylaxis to Prevent Symptomatic Infection

Given for a relatively short, specified period (days) after exposure to specific pathogens/organisms, where the risks of acquiring the infection are felt to justify antimicrobial treatment to eradicate a colonizing pathogen or prevent symptomatic infection when the child (healthy or with increased susceptibility to infection) is likely to have been inoculated/exposed (eg, an asymptomatic child closely exposed to meningococcus; a neonate born to a mother with active genital herpes simplex virus [HSV]) but does not yet have signs or symptoms of infection.

B. Long-term Antimicrobial Prophylaxis to Prevent Symptomatic New Infection

Given to a particular, defined population of children with relatively high risk of acquiring a severe infection from a single exposure or multiple exposures (eg, a child post-splenectomy; a child with documented rheumatic heart disease to prevent subsequent streptococcal infection), with prophylaxis provided during the period of risk, potentially for months or years.

C. Prophylaxis of Symptomatic Disease in Children Who Have Asymptomatic Infection/Latent Infection

Where a child has a documented infection but is asymptomatic. Targeted antimicrobials are given to prevent the development of symptomatic disease (eg, latent tuberculosis [TB] infection or therapy of a stem cell transplant patient with documented cytomegalovirus viremia but no symptoms of infection or rejection; to prevent reactivation of HSV). Treatment period is usually defined, particularly when the latent infection can be cured (TB, requiring 6 months of therapy), but other circumstances, such as prevention of reactivation of latent HSV, may require months or years of prophylaxis.

D. Surgical/Procedure Prophylaxis

A child receives a surgical/invasive catheter procedure, planned or unplanned, in which the risk for infection postoperatively or post-procedure may justify prophylaxis to prevent an infection from occurring (eg, prophylaxis to prevent infection following spinal rod placement). **Treatment is usually short-term (hours),** beginning just before the procedure and ending at the conclusion of the procedure, or within 24 hours.

E. Travel-Related Exposure Prophylaxis

Not discussed in this chapter; please refer to information on specific disease entities (eg, travelers diarrhea, chapters 1 and 9) or specific pathogens (eg, malaria, Chapter 9).

Constantly updated, current information for travelers about prophylaxis (often starting just before travel and continuing until return) and current worldwide infection risks can be found on the Centers for Disease Control and Prevention website at www.cdc.gov/travel (accessed September 30, 2022).

NOTE

- **Abbreviations:** AAP, American Academy of Pediatrics; ACOG, American College of Obstetricians and Gynecologists; AHA, American Heart Association; ALT, alanine aminotransferase; amox/clav, amoxicillin/clavulanate; ARF, acute rheumatic fever; bid, twice daily; CDC, Centers for Disease Control and Prevention; CPB, cardiopulmonary bypass; CSF, cerebrospinal fluid; div, divided; DOT, directly observed therapy; GI, gastrointestinal; HSV, herpes simplex virus; IGRA, interferon-γ release assay; IM, intramuscular; INH, isoniazid; IV, intravenous; max, maximum; MRSA, methicillin-resistant *Staphylococcus aureus;* NA, not applicable; PCR, polymerase chain reaction; PO, orally; PPD, purified protein derivative; q, every; qd, once daily; qid, 4 times daily; spp, species; TB, tuberculosis; tid, 3 times daily; TIG, tetanus immune globulin; TMP/SMX, trimethoprim/sulfamethoxazole; UTI, urinary tract infection.

A. POSTEXPOSURE ANTIMICROBIAL PROPHYLAXIS TO PREVENT INFECTION

Prophylaxis Category	Therapy (evidence grade)	Comments
Bacterial		
Bites, animal and human[1–5] (*Pasteurella multocida* [animal], *Eikenella corrodens* [human], *Staphylococcus* spp, and *Streptococcus* spp)	Amox/clav 45 mg/kg/day PO div tid (amox/clav 7:1; see Chapter 4 for amox/clav ratio descriptions) for 3–5 days (AII) OR ampicillin and clindamycin (BII). For penicillin allergy, consider ciprofloxacin (for *Pasteurella*) plus clindamycin (BIII).	Recommended for children who (1) have moderate to severe injuries, especially to the hand or face; (2) are immunocompromised; (3) are asplenic; or (4) have injuries that may have penetrated the periosteum or joint capsule (AII).[3] Consider rabies prophylaxis for at-risk animal bites through state and local rabies consultation contacts (AI)[6]; consider tetanus prophylaxis.[7] Human bites have a very high rate of infection (do not close open wounds routinely). Cat bites have a higher rate of infection than dog bites. *Staphylococcus aureus* coverage is only fair with amox/clav and provides no coverage for MRSA.
Endocarditis prophylaxis[8,9]: Given that (1) endocarditis is rarely caused by dental/GI procedures and (2) prophylaxis for procedures prevents an exceedingly small number of cases, the risks of antibiotics most often outweigh benefits. However, some "highest-risk" conditions are currently recommended for prophylaxis: (1) prosthetic heart valve (or prosthetic material used to repair a valve); (2) previous endocarditis; (3) cyanotic congenital heart disease that is unrepaired (or palliatively repaired with shunts and conduits); (4) congenital heart disease that is repaired but with defects at the site of repair adjacent to prosthetic material; (5) completely repaired congenital heart disease by using prosthetic material, for the first 6 mo after repair; or (6) cardiac transplant patients with valvulopathy. Routine prophylaxis has not been required for children with native valve abnormalities since updated guidelines were published in 2015.[9] Follow-up data in children suggest that following these new guidelines, no increase in endocarditis has been detected.[10–13]		
– In highest-risk patients: dental procedures that involve manipulation of the gingival or periodontal region of teeth	Amoxicillin 50 mg/kg (max 2 g) PO 1 h before procedure OR ampicillin or ceftriaxone or cefazolin, all at 50 mg/kg IM/IV 30–60 min before procedure	If penicillin allergy: clindamycin 20 mg/kg PO (1 h before) or IV (30 min before) OR azithromycin 15 mg/kg or clarithromycin 15 mg/kg (1 h before)

A. POSTEXPOSURE ANTIMICROBIAL PROPHYLAXIS TO PREVENT INFECTION *(continued)*

Prophylaxis Category	Therapy (evidence grade)	Comments
– Genitourinary and GI procedures	None	No longer recommended
Lyme disease (*Borrelia burgdorferi*)[14]	Doxycycline 4.4 mg/kg (max 200 mg), once. Dental staining should not occur with a single course of doxycycline. Amoxicillin prophylaxis is not well studied, and experts recommend a full 14-day course if amoxicillin is used.	ONLY for those in highly Lyme-endemic areas AND the tick has been attached for >36 h (and is engorged) AND prophylaxis started within 72 h of tick removal.
Meningococcus (*Neisseria meningitidis*)[15,16]	For prophylaxis of close contacts, including household members, child care center contacts, and anyone directly exposed to the patient's oral secretions (eg, through kissing, mouth-to-mouth resuscitation, endotracheal intubation, endotracheal tube management) in the 7 days before symptom onset **Rifampin** Infants <1 mo: 5 mg/kg PO q12h for 4 doses Children ≥1 mo: 10 mg/kg PO q12h for 4 doses (max 600 mg/dose) OR **Ceftriaxone** Children <15 y: 125 mg IM once Children ≥16 y: 250 mg IM once OR **Ciprofloxacin** 500 mg PO once (adolescents and adults)	A single dose of ciprofloxacin should not present a significant risk of cartilage damage, but no prospective data exist in children for prophylaxis of meningococcal disease. For a child, an exposure for ciprofloxacin equivalent to that in adults would be 15–20 mg/kg as a single dose (max 500 mg). A few ciprofloxacin-resistant strains have now been reported. Insufficient data to recommend azithromycin at this time. Meningococcal vaccines that target the specific serogroup may also be recommended in case of an outbreak.
Pertussis[17,18]	Same regimen as for treatment of pertussis: azithromycin 10 mg/kg/day qd for 5 days OR clarithromycin (for infants >1 mo) 15 mg/kg/day div bid for 7 days OR erythromycin (estolate preferable) 40 mg/kg/day PO div qid for 14 days (AII) Alternative: TMP/SMX 8 mg/kg/day div bid for 14 days (BIII)	Prophylaxis to family members; contacts defined by the CDC: persons within 21 days of exposure to an infectious pertussis case, who are at high risk for severe illness or who will have close contact with a person at high risk for severe illness (including infants, pregnant women in their third trimester, immunocompromised persons, those who have close contact with infants <12 mo). Close

contact can be considered face-to-face exposure within 3 feet of a symptomatic person; direct contact with respiratory, nasal, or oral secretions; or sharing of the same confined space in close proximity to an infected person for ≥1 h.

Community-wide prophylaxis is not currently recommended.

Azithromycin and clarithromycin are better tolerated than erythromycin (see Chapter 2); azithromycin is preferred in exposed very young infants to reduce pyloric stenosis risk.

Tetanus
(*Clostridium tetani*)[7,19]

Need for Tetanus Vaccine or TIG[a]

	Clean Wound		**Contaminated Wound**	
Number of past tetanus vaccine doses	Need for tetanus vaccine	Need for TIG 500 U IM[a]	Need for tetanus vaccine	Need for TIG 500 U IM[a]
<3 doses	Yes	No	Yes	Yes
≥3 doses	No (if <10 y[b]) Yes (if ≥10 y[b])	No	No (if <5 y[b]) Yes (if ≥5 y[b])	No

[a] IV immune globulin should be used when TIG is not available.
[b] Years since last tetanus-containing vaccine dose.

For deep, contaminated wounds, wound debridement is essential. For wounds that cannot be fully debrided, consider metronidazole 30 mg/kg/day PO div q8h until wound healing is underway and anaerobic conditions no longer exist, as short as 3–5 days (BIII).

A. POSTEXPOSURE ANTIMICROBIAL PROPHYLAXIS TO PREVENT INFECTION *(continued)*

Prophylaxis Category	Therapy (evidence grade)	Comments
Tuberculosis (*Mycobacterium tuberculosis*) "Window prophylaxis" of exposed children <4 y, or immunocompromised patient (high risk for dissemination)[20,21] For treatment of latent TB infection,[21,22] see Tuberculosis in Table 15C.	Scenario 1: Previously uninfected child at high risk for serious infection and dissemination becomes exposed to a person with active disease. Exposed children <4 y, or immunocompromised patient (high risk for dissemination): rifampin 15–20 mg/kg/dose PO qd OR INH 10–20 mg/kg PO qd; for at least 2–3 mo (AIII), at which time cellular immunity is established and the PPD/IGRA may be more accurately assessed. If positive, treatment for latent TB should continue. Children ≥4 y may also begin prophylaxis postexposure, but if exposure is questionable, can wait 2–3 mo after exposure to assess for infection; if not given prophylaxis, and PPD/IGRA at 2–3 mo is positive and child remains asymptomatic at that time, see Scenario 2 below.	If PPD or IGRA remains negative at 2–3 mo and child remains well, consider stopping empiric therapy. However, tests at 2–3 mo may not be reliable in immunocompromised patients. The window prophylaxis regimen is to prevent infection in a young child or compromised host after exposure, rather than to treat latent asymptomatic infection.
	Scenario 2: Asymptomatic child is found to have a positive skin test/IGRA test for TB, documenting latent TB infection; see Tuberculosis in Table 15C. Treat with at least 4 mo of rifampin OR 6 mo of INH, OR, for those ≥2 y, INH and rifapentine.	
Viral		
Herpes simplex virus		
– During pregnancy	For women with recurrent genital herpes, follow ACOG guidelines[23]: acyclovir 400 mg PO tid; valacyclovir 500 mg PO bid from 36 wk of gestation until delivery (CII).	Neonatal HSV disease after unsuccessful maternal suppression has been documented.[24]

– Neonatal: **primary or nonprimary first clinical episode of maternal infection,** neonate exposed at delivery[25]	Asymptomatic, exposed neonate: at 24 h after birth, sample mucosal sites for HSV culture (and PCR if possible) (see Comments), obtain CSF and whole-blood PCR for HSV DNA, obtain ALT, and start preemptive therapeutic acyclovir IV (60 mg/kg/day div q8h) for 10 days (AII). Some experts would evaluate at birth for exposure following presumed maternal primary infection and start preemptive therapy rather than wait 24 h.	*AAP Red Book 2021–2024*[25] provides a management algorithm that determines the type of maternal infection and, thus, the appropriate evaluation and preemptive therapy of the neonate. Mucosal sites for culture: conjunctivae, mouth, nasopharynx, rectum. Infants treated with 10 days of preemptive IV therapy should not subsequently receive oral acyclovir suppression, because their HSV exposure never progressed to infection or disease. Any *symptomatic* baby, at any time, requires a full evaluation for invasive infection and IV acyclovir therapy for 14–21 days, depending on extent of disease.
– Neonatal: **recurrent maternal infection,** neonate exposed at delivery[25]	Asymptomatic, exposed neonate: at 24 h after birth, sample mucosal sites for HSV culture (and PCR if desired) (see Comments) and obtain whole-blood PCR for HSV DNA. Hold on therapy unless cultures or PCRs are positive, at which time the diagnostic evaluation should be completed (CSF PCR for HSV DNA, serum ALT) and preemptive therapeutic IV acyclovir (60 mg/kg/day div q8h) should be administered for 10 days (AIII).	*AAP Red Book 2021–2024*[25] provides a management algorithm that determines the type of maternal infection and, thus, the appropriate evaluation and preemptive therapy of the neonate. Mucosal sites for culture: conjunctivae, mouth, nasopharynx, rectum. Infants treated with 10 days of preemptive IV therapy should not subsequently receive oral acyclovir suppression, because their HSV exposure never progressed to infection or disease. Any *symptomatic* baby, at any time, requires a full evaluation for invasive infection and IV acyclovir therapy for 14–21 days, depending on extent of disease.
– Neonatal: following symptomatic disease, to prevent recurrence	See Neonatal in Table 15C under Herpes Simplex Virus.	
– Keratitis (ocular) in otherwise healthy children	See Keratitis in Table 15C under Herpes Simplex Virus.	

A. POSTEXPOSURE ANTIMICROBIAL PROPHYLAXIS TO PREVENT INFECTION *(continued)*

Prophylaxis Category	Therapy (evidence grade)	Comments
Influenza virus (A or B)[26]	Oseltamivir prophylaxis (AI) 3–≤8 mo: 3 mg/kg/dose qd for 10 days; 9–11 mo: 3.5 mg/kg/dose PO qd for 10 days[27]; based on body weight for children ≥12 mo: ≤15 kg: 30 mg qd for 10 days; >15–23 kg: 45 mg qd for 10 days; >23–40 kg: 60 mg qd for 10 days; >40 kg: 75 mg qd for 10 days	Not routinely recommended for infants 0–≤3 mo unless exposure judged substantial (single event or ongoing [eg, breastfeeding mother with active influenza]), because of limited reported data on safety/efficacy and variability of drug exposure in this age-group
	Zanamivir prophylaxis (AI) ≥5 y: 10 mg (two 5-mg inhalations) qd for as long as 28 days (community outbreaks) or 10 days (household settings)	
	Baloxavir prophylaxis (AI) <20 kg: single dose PO of 2 mg/kg ≥5 y: 20–79 kg: single dose PO of 40 mg ≥80 kg: single dose PO of 80 mg	
Rabies virus[28]	Rabies immune globulin, 20 IU/kg, infiltrate around wound, with remaining volume injected IM (AII) PLUS Rabies immunization (AII)	For dog, cat, or ferret bite from **symptomatic animal,** immediate rabies immune globulin and immunization; otherwise, can wait 10 days for observation of animal, if possible, before rabies immune globulin or vaccine. PLEASE evaluate the context of the bite. A provoked bite from a threatened or annoyed dog (especially a known dog) is not an indication for rabies prophylaxis. Bites of squirrels, hamsters, guinea pigs, gerbils, chipmunks, rats, mice and other rodents, rabbits, hares, and pikas almost never require anti-rabies prophylaxis. For bites of bats, skunks, raccoons, foxes, most other carnivores, and woodchucks, immediate rabies immune globulin and immunization (regard as rabid unless geographic area is known to be free of rabies or until animal's condition is proven negative by laboratory tests)

Varicella-zoster virus[29]	Acyclovir 20 mg/kg/dose PO qid (max daily dose 3,200 mg) or valacyclovir 20 mg/kg/dose PO tid (max daily dose 3,000 mg) beginning 7 days after exposure and continuing for 7–10 days	Preemptive antiviral therapy in those who have been exposed to varicella, during the incubation period, to prevent symptomatic infection: for immunocompromised patients without evidence of immunity from past infection or vaccine or for immunocompetent, susceptible patients for whom varicella may be severe (eg, adolescents)

B. LONG-TERM ANTIMICROBIAL PROPHYLAXIS TO PREVENT SYMPTOMATIC NEW INFECTION

Prophylaxis Category	Therapy (evidence grade)	Comments
Bacterial otitis media[30,31]	Amoxicillin or other antibiotics can be used in half the therapeutic dose qd or bid to prevent infections if the benefits outweigh the risks of (1) emergence/selection of resistant organisms for that child (and contacts) and (2) antibiotic side effects.	True, recurrent acute bacterial otitis is far less common in the era of conjugate pneumococcal immunization. To prevent recurrent infections, as alternative to antibiotic prophylaxis, also consider the risks and benefits of placing tympanostomy tubes to improve middle ear ventilation.[31] Studies have demonstrated that amoxicillin, sulfisoxazole, and TMP/SMX are effective. However, antimicrobial prophylaxis may alter the nasopharyngeal flora and foster colonization with resistant organisms, compromising long-term efficacy of the prophylactic drug. Continuous PO administered antimicrobial prophylaxis should be reserved for control of recurrent acute otitis media, only when defined as ≥3 distinct and well-documented episodes during a period of 6 mo or ≥4 episodes during a period of 12 mo, which is now uncommon in the era of conjugate pneumococcal vaccines.
Rheumatic fever	For >27.3 kg (>60 lb): 1.2 million U penicillin G benzathine, q4wk (q3wk for high-risk children) For <27.3 kg: 600,000 U penicillin G benzathine, q4wk (q3wk for high-risk children) OR Penicillin V (phenoxymethyl), 250 mg PO bid	AHA policy statement at www.ahajournals.org/doi/epub/10.1161/CirculationAHA.109.191959 (accessed September 30, 2022). Doses studied many years ago, with no new data; ARF is an uncommon disease currently in the United States. Alternatives to penicillin include amoxicillin, sulfisoxazole, or macrolides, including erythromycin, azithromycin, and clarithromycin.
Urinary tract infection, recurrent[32–38]	TMP/SMX 3 mg/kg/dose of TMP PO qd OR nitrofurantoin 1–2 mg/kg PO qd at bedtime; more rapid resistance may develop by using beta-lactams (BII).	Only for those with grade III–V reflux or with recurrent febrile UTI: prophylaxis no longer recommended for patients with grade I–II (some also exclude grade III) reflux. Prophylaxis prevents infection but may not prevent scarring. Early treatment of new infections is recommended for children not given prophylaxis. Resistance eventually develops to every antibiotic; follow resistance patterns for each patient.

Fungal: For detailed information on prevention of candidiasis in the neonate, see Chapter 2; for detailed information on prevention of fungal infection (*Candida* spp, *Aspergillus* spp, *Rhizopus* spp) in children undergoing chemotherapy, see Chapter 5.

Pneumocystis jiroveci (previously *Pneumocystis carinii*)[39–42]	Non-HIV infection regimens (stem cell transplants, solid-organ transplants, many malignancies, and T-cell immunodeficiencies [congenital or secondary to treatment]). Duration of prophylaxis depends on the underlying condition. TMP/SMX 5–10 mg/kg/day of TMP PO, in 2 div doses, q12h, either qd or 2 times/wk or 3 times/wk, on consecutive days or alternating days (AI); OR TMP/SMX 5–10 mg/kg/day of TMP PO as a *single dose,* qd, given 3 times/wk on consecutive days (AI) (once-weekly regimens have also been successful); OR dapsone 2 mg/kg (max 100 mg) PO qd, or 4 mg/kg (max 200 mg) once weekly; OR atovaquone 30 mg/kg/day for infants 1–3 mo; 45 mg/kg/day for infants/children 4–24 mo; and 30 mg/kg/day for children ≥24 mo.	Prophylaxis in specific populations based on degree of immunosuppression. For children with HIV, please see the ClinicalInfo.HIV.gov for information on pediatric opportunistic infections: https://clinicalinfo.hiv.gov/en/guidelines/pediatric-opportunistic-infection/pneumocystis-jirovecii-pneumonia?view=full (updated October 6, 2013; accessed September 30, 2022). Inhaled pentamidine only for those who cannot tolerate the regimens noted above.

C. PROPHYLAXIS OF SYMPTOMATIC DISEASE IN CHILDREN WHO HAVE ASYMPTOMATIC INFECTION/LATENT INFECTION

Prophylaxis Category	Therapy (evidence grade)	Comments
Herpes simplex virus		
Neonatal: following symptomatic disease, to prevent recurrence[25]	Acyclovir 300 mg/m^2/dose PO tid for 6 mo, following cessation of IV acyclovir treatment of acute disease (AI)	Follow absolute neutrophil counts at 2 and 4 wk, then monthly during prophylactic/suppressive therapy. Oral acyclovir suppression is not indicated for patients who received IV acyclovir as postexposure antimicrobial prophylaxis to prevent infection.
Keratitis (ocular) in otherwise healthy children	Suppressive acyclovir therapy for frequent recurrence (no pediatric data): long-term suppression (≥1 y) of recurrent infection with oral acyclovir 80 mg/kg/day in 3 div doses (max dose 800 mg) (AIII)	Decisions to continue suppressive therapy should be revisited annually. The frequency of dosing may need to be increased to qid or the drug may need to be changed to valacyclovir, if breakthrough ocular infection occurs. Potential risks must balance potential benefits to vision (BIII). Check for acyclovir resistance for those who relapse while on appropriate therapy. Suppression oftentimes required for many years. Watch for severe recurrence at conclusion of suppression.
Tuberculosis[20–22] (latent TB infection [asymptomatic, true infection], defined by a positive skin test or IGRA, with no clinical or radiographic evidence of active disease)	Rifampin 15–20 mg/kg/dose qd, preferably the entire daily dose given qd (max 600 mg) for 4 mo, OR For children ≥2 y, once-weekly DOT for 12 wk using BOTH INH 15 mg/kg/dose (max 900 mg) AND rifapentine: 10.0–14.0 kg: 300 mg; 14.1–25.0 kg: 450 mg; 25.1–32.0 kg: 600 mg; 32.1–49.9 kg: 750 mg; ≥50.0 kg: 900 mg (max)	Alternative regimens: INH 10–20 mg/kg PO qd AND rifampin 15–20 mg/kg/dose daily (max 600 mg) for 3 mo, OR INH 10–20 mg/kg PO qd for 9 mo (≥12 mo for an immunocompromised child), OR INH 20–40 mg/kg PO DOT twice weekly for 9 mo For exposure to drug-resistant strains, consult with TB specialist.

D. SURGICAL/PROCEDURE PROPHYLAXIS[43–54]

The CDC National Healthcare Safety Network uses a classification of surgical procedure-related wound infections based on an estimation of the load of bacterial contamination: Class I, clean; Class II, clean-contaminated; Class III, contaminated; and Class IV, dirty/infected.[44,54] Other major factors creating risk for postoperative surgical site infection include the duration of surgery (a longer-duration operation, defined as one that exceeded the 75th percentile for a given procedure) and the medical comorbidities of the patient, as determined by an American Society of Anesthesiologists score of III, IV, or V (presence of severe systemic disease that results in functional limitations, is life-threatening, or is expected to preclude survival from the operation). The virulence/pathogenicity of bacteria inoculated and the presence of foreign debris/devitalized tissue/surgical material in the wound are also considered risk factors for infection.

For all categories of surgical prophylaxis, dosing recommendations are derived from (1) choosing agents based on the organisms likely to be responsible for inoculation of the surgical site; (2) giving the agents at an optimal time (<60 min for cefazolin, or <60–120 min for vancomycin and ciprofloxacin) before starting the operation to achieve appropriate serum and tissue exposures at the time of incision; (3) providing additional doses during the procedure at times based on the standard dosing guideline for that agent; and (4) stopping the agents at the end of the procedure or for no longer than 24 h after the end of the procedure. Optimal duration of prophylaxis after delayed sternal or abdominal closure is not well-defined in adults or children.

Bathing with soaps or an antiseptic agent the night before surgery is recommended, based on limited data.[50]

Procedure/Operation	Recommended Agents	Preoperative Dose	Intraoperative Re-dosing Interval (h) for Prolonged Surgery
Cardiovascular			
Cardiac[55] *Staphylococcus epidermidis, Staphylococcus aureus, Corynebacterium* spp	Cefazolin	30 mg/kg	4
	Vancomycin, if MRSA likely	15 mg/kg	8
	Ampicillin/sulbactam if enteric gram-negative bacilli a concern	50 mg/kg of ampicillin	3
Cardiac with CPB[47,56]	Cefazolin	30 mg/kg	15 mg/kg at CPB start and also at rewarming. Begin postoperative prophylaxis 30 mg/kg at 8 h after intraoperative rewarming dose.

D. SURGICAL/PROCEDURE PROPHYLAXIS[43–54] *(continued)*

Procedure/Operation	Recommended Agents	Preoperative Dose	Intraoperative Re-dosing Interval (h) for Prolonged Surgery
Cardiovascular			
Vascular *S epidermidis, S aureus, Corynebacterium* spp, gram-negative enteric bacilli, particularly for procedures in the groin	Cefazolin, OR	30 mg/kg	4
	Vancomycin, if MRSA likely	15 mg/kg	8
Thoracic (noncardiac)			
Lobectomy, video-assisted thoracoscopic surgery, thoracotomy (but no prophylaxis needed for simple chest tube placement for pneumothorax)	Cefazolin, OR	30 mg/kg	4
	Ampicillin/sulbactam if enteric gram-negative bacilli a concern	50 mg/kg of ampicillin	3
	Vancomycin or clindamycin if drug allergy or MRSA likely	15 mg/kg vancomycin	8
		10 mg/kg clindamycin	6
Gastrointestinal			
Gastroduodenal Enteric gram-negative bacilli, respiratory tract gram-positive cocci	Cefazolin	30 mg/kg	4
Biliary procedure, open Enteric gram-negative bacilli, enterococci, *Clostridia*	Cefazolin, OR	30 mg/kg	4
	Cefoxitin	40 mg/kg	2
Appendectomy, non-perforated (no prophylaxis needed postoperatively if appendix is intact)[57]	Cefoxitin, OR	40 mg/kg	2
	Cefazolin and metronidazole	30 mg/kg cefazolin, 10 mg/kg metronidazole	4 for cefazolin 8 for metronidazole

Complicated appendicitis or other ruptured colorectal viscus[58] Enteric gram-negative bacilli, enterococci, anaerobes. For complicated appendicitis, antibiotics provided to treat ongoing infection, rather than prophylaxis.	Cefazolin and metronidazole, OR	30 mg/kg cefazolin, 10 mg/kg metronidazole	4 for cefazolin 8 for metronidazole
	Cefoxitin, OR	40 mg/kg	2
	Ceftriaxone and metronidazole, OR	50 mg/kg ceftriaxone, 10 mg/kg metronidazole	12 for ceftriaxone 8 for metronidazole
	Ertapenem, OR	15 mg/kg (max 500 mg) for children 3 mo–12 y; 1 g for children ≥13 y	8
	Meropenem, OR	20 mg/kg	4
	Imipenem	20 mg/kg	4
Genitourinary			
Cystoscopy (requires prophylaxis only for children with suspected active UTI or those having foreign material placed) Enteric gram-negative bacilli, enterococci	Cefazolin, OR	30 mg/kg	4
	TMP/SMX (if low local resistance), OR Select a second- (cefuroxime) or third-generation cephalosporin or fluoroquinolone (ciprofloxacin) if the child is known to be colonized with cefazolin-resistant, TMP/SMX-resistant strains.	4–5 mg/kg	NA
Open or laparoscopic surgery Enteric gram-negative bacilli, enterococci	Cefazolin	30 mg/kg	4

D. SURGICAL/PROCEDURE PROPHYLAXIS[43–54] *(continued)*

Procedure/Operation	Recommended Agents	Preoperative Dose	Intraoperative Re-dosing Interval (h) for Prolonged Surgery
Head and neck surgery			
Assuming incision through respiratory tract mucosa Anaerobes, enteric gram-negative bacilli, *S aureus*	Clindamycin, OR	10 mg/kg	6
	Cefazolin and metronidazole	30 mg/kg cefazolin, 10 mg/kg metronidazole	4 for cefazolin 8 for metronidazole
	Ampicillin/sulbactam if enteric gram-negative bacilli a concern	50 mg/kg of ampicillin	3
Neurosurgery			
Craniotomy, ventricular shunt placement *S epidermidis, S aureus*	Cefazolin, OR	30 mg/kg	4
	Vancomycin, if MRSA likely	15 mg/kg	8
Orthopedic			
Internal fixation of fractures, spinal rod placement, prosthetic joints *S epidermidis, S aureus*	Cefazolin, OR	30 mg/kg	4
	Vancomycin, if MRSA likely	15 mg/kg	8

Trauma			
Exceptionally varied; no prospective, comparative data in children; agents should focus on skin flora (*S epidermidis, S aureus*) as well as the flora inoculated into the wound, based on the trauma exposure, that may include enteric gram-negative bacilli, anaerobes (including *Clostridia* spp), and fungi. Cultures at time of wound exploration are critical to focus therapy for potential pathogens inoculated into the wound.	Cefazolin (for skin), OR	30 mg/kg	4
	Vancomycin (for skin), if MRSA likely, OR	15 mg/kg	8
	Meropenem OR imipenem (for anaerobes, including *Clostridia* spp, and non-fermenting gram-negative bacilli), OR	20 mg/kg for either	4
	Gentamicin and metronidazole (for non-fermenting gram-negative bacilli and anaerobes, including *Clostridia* spp), OR	2.5 mg/kg gentamicin, 10 mg/kg metronidazole	6 for gentamicin 8 for metronidazole
	Piperacillin/tazobactam	100 mg/kg piperacillin component	2

16. Approach to Antibiotic Allergies

Introduction

Antibiotics are a common cause of drug reactions. Beta-lactam antibiotics are most commonly implicated, with about 10% of the US population reporting a history of penicillin allergy. However, antibiotic allergies are frequently mislabeled and, even if present, are often outgrown over time. In such cases, unnecessary use of broad-spectrum antibiotics may result in suboptimal therapy, medication-related side effects, the development of antibiotic resistance, and increased health care costs. More than 90% of those with a positive history of an antibiotic allergy are ultimately able to safely tolerate the antibiotic. Thus, it is important to use a systematic approach to children with reported antibiotic allergies, including the routine evaluation of reported penicillin allergy.

American Academy of Allergy, Asthma and Immunology (AAAAI); American College of Allergy, Asthma, and Immunology; and Joint Council of Allergy, Asthma and Immunology practice parameters provide an excellent overview of drug allergies; the following information summarizes recommendations with respect to antibiotic allergies from these guidelines and other resources listed in Suggested Reading later in this chapter.

Classification of Antibiotic Allergies

Antibiotic allergies are immune-mediated reactions to a drug that occur in a previously sensitized child. More commonly, adverse drug reactions are not immune mediated and do not represent a true antibiotic allergy (but are often mislabeled as such). It is important to distinguish between clinically relevant categories of adverse antibiotic reactions (**Table 16-1**).

TABLE 16-1. CLASSIFICATION OF ADVERSE ANTIBIOTIC REACTIONS

Classification	Mechanism	Characteristics	Examples	Future Use of Antibiotic
Immediate hypersensitivity reactions	Type I IgE mediated	Anaphylactic May be life-threatening Occur within minutes of exposure to the antibiotic Uncommon	Immediate urticaria Angioedema Laryngeal edema/stridor Bronchospasm/wheezing Cardiorespiratory symptoms	Future use of antibiotic *contraindicated.* If no alternative, administer via desensitization protocol (see **Table 16-3**).
Delayed drug-induced exanthems	Type IV Cell mediated	Non-anaphylactic Not life-threatening Typically occur after several days of antibiotic exposure More common	Delayed maculopapular rash (typically fixed/nonmobile, non-pruritic) Delayed urticaria	Future use of antibiotic *may be considered.*
Severe cutaneous adverse reactions	Type IV T-cell mediated	Severe delayed hypersensitivity reactions May be life-threatening Rare	SJS/TEN DRESS AGEP	Future use of antibiotic *contraindicated*
Serum sickness	Type III Immune-complex mediated (drug-antibody complex)	Delayed reaction at 1–3 wk after exposure May occur earlier if preformed antibody present Uncommon	Classic symptoms: fever, rash, polyarthralgia, or polyarthritis May also have urticaria and lymphadenopathy	Future use of antibiotic *contraindicated*
Nonimmune drug reaction	Nonallergic response to a drug	Multiple types; examples include • Drug intolerance • Pseudoallergic reaction Do not require prior sensitization Common, frequently mislabeled as allergy	Drug intolerance • GI symptoms • Headache Pseudoallergic reaction • Vancomycin glycopeptide flushing syndrome	Future use of antibiotic *may be considered* by using prevention/management strategies.

Abbreviations: AGEP, acute generalized exanthematous pustulosis; DRESS, drug rash with eosinophilia and systemic symptoms; GI, gastrointestinal; SJS, Stevens-Johnson syndrome; TEN, toxic epidermal necrolysis.

General Approach

Table 16-2 describes a modified stepwise approach to the workup and management of potential antibiotic allergies.

TABLE 16-2. STEPWISE APPROACH TO REPORTED ANTIBIOTIC ALLERGIES

Steps	Components	Notes
Step 1	Perform a thorough history and physical examination; review available clinical data.	Attempt to classify the reaction. • Timing in relation to antibiotic administration • Review of previous antibiotic administration history and other medications • Review of associated signs and symptoms • Physical manifestations (examination and/or review of photos, if available) • Review of imaging/laboratory results (if available)
Step 2	Determine if the adverse reaction is likely due to antibiotic.	If yes, determine type of suspected reaction (eg, immediate hypersensitivity reaction vs delayed drug-induced exanthem vs nonimmune adverse drug reaction). If no, consider removing antibiotic allergy label.
Step 3	If possible immediate hypersensitivity reaction • Perform confirmatory testing (if available); consider referral to allergist.	Testing typically performed ≥4–6 wk after symptom resolution. Penicillin skin testing can be used to test for IgE-mediated penicillin allergy. Although not standardized, most allergy clinics will also perform ampicillin and cefazolin skin testing.
	If suspected delayed drug-induced exanthem (not SCAR) or nonimmune drug reaction • Consider strategies for evaluation and/or de-labeling.	Depending on type of suspected reaction • Consider management/prevention strategies if nonimmune. • May consider skin testing. • May consider observed challenge. • May be able to remove antibiotic allergy label.
Step 4	Review available results.	Confirmed not allergic • OK to give antibiotic. • Remove antibiotic allergy label. Confirmed allergic • Choose alternative antibiotic. • Perform desensitization procedure if need to give antibiotic. Possibly allergic • Choose alternative antibiotic. • Perform observed challenge before giving antibiotic.

Abbreviation: SCAR, severe cutaneous adverse reaction.

Adapted from Joint Task Force on Practice Parameters; American Academy of Allergy, Asthma and Immunology; American College of Allergy, Asthma, and Immunology; Joint Council of Allergy, Asthma and Immunology. Drug allergy: an updated practice parameter. *Ann Allergy Asthma Immunol.* 2010;105(4):259–273 PMID: 20934625 https://doi.org/10.1016/j.anai.2010.08.002.

Table 16-3 details protocols.

TABLE 16-3. OBSERVED CHALLENGE AND DESENSITIZATION PROTOCOLS

Protocol	Details	Notes
Observed challenge	Test dosing of antibiotic. Perform controlled administration of single dose or divided increasing doses (graded challenge) until full dose reached. Example graded challenge: give 10%–25% of therapeutic dose and observe for 15–30 min (about 75% will react within 20 min), then give rest of dose and observe for another 30–60 min (up to 2 h; about 100% will react within 2 h).	Used when low likelihood of IgE-mediated allergy Can verify child will not have immediate hypersensitivity reaction Does not alter immune response or induce tolerance
Desensitization procedure	Rapid induction of antibiotic tolerance Administration of incremental doses Performed under the guidance of an allergist in a controlled setting	Used when high likelihood of IgE-mediated allergy and no alternative antibiotics available Alters immune response by providing *temporary* tolerance

Adapted from Joint Task Force on Practice Parameters; American Academy of Allergy, Asthma and Immunology; American College of Allergy, Asthma, and Immunology; Joint Council of Allergy, Asthma and Immunology. Drug allergy: an updated practice parameter. *Ann Allergy Asthma Immunol.* 2010;105(4):259–273 PMID: 20934625 https://doi.org/10.1016/j.anai.2010.08.002.

Specific Antibiotic Allergies and Allergic Cross-reactivity

Beta-lactam Antibiotics

Penicillin

An AAAAI position statement recommends routine evaluation of reported penicillin allergies by skin testing. Penicillin skin testing has a negative predictive value near 100%. If negative, the child may receive penicillin with minimal risk (depending on the severity of the prior reaction, the first dose may be given via observed challenge). The positive predictive value of penicillin skin testing appears to be high. If positive, penicillin should be avoided (if no acceptable alternatives are available, desensitization should be performed).

Some physicians screen for children with low-risk histories who may bypass penicillin skin testing and proceed directly to an observed challenge to confirm tolerance. Of note, in vitro serum testing for penicillin-specific IgE has an undefined predictive value and should not be used in lieu of skin testing and/or an observed challenge.

Penicillin allergic cross-reactivity: The rate of allergic cross-reactivity between penicillin and cephalosporins was traditionally reported to be about 10%, although more recent studies suggest a rate of less than 2%. Cross-reactivity is more common with some first-generation cephalosporins (as these antibiotics may have similar R-group side chains; see Cephalosporins later in this chapter). Most children with a history of penicillin allergy tolerate cephalosporins, particularly if the reaction was not severe. If a child has a negative penicillin skin test result, the child may safely receive cephalosporins. Of children who have a positive penicillin skin test result, about 2% will react to some cephalosporins. **Table 16-4** details various approaches to cephalosporin administration in children with a reported history of penicillin allergy.

TABLE 16-4. APPROACHES TO CEPHALOSPORIN ADMINISTRATION IN CHILDREN WITH REPORTED HISTORY OF PENICILLIN ALLERGY

Skin Test	Options for Cephalosporin Administration
Penicillin skin test	Negative result • OK to give Positive result • Choose alternative (non–beta-lactam) antibiotic. • Administer via observed challenge or desensitization (depending on severity of prior reaction).
Cephalosporin skin test (not standardized)	Negative result • Administer via observed challenge. Positive result • Choose alternative (non–beta-lactam) antibiotic. • Choose alternative cephalosporin (with dissimilar R-group side chain) and administer via cautious observed challenge or desensitization (depending on severity of prior reaction). • Administer via desensitization if no alternative antibiotic.
Skin testing unavailable	Administer via cautious observed challenge or desensitization (depending on severity of prior reaction).

Adapted from Joint Task Force on Practice Parameters; American Academy of Allergy, Asthma and Immunology; American College of Allergy, Asthma, and Immunology; Joint Council of Allergy, Asthma and Immunology. Drug allergy: an updated practice parameter. *Ann Allergy Asthma Immunol.* 2010;105(4):259–273 PMID: 20934625 https://doi.org/10.1016/j.anai.2010.08.002.

Cephalosporins

The rate of allergic reactions to cephalosporins is significantly lower than of penicillin. Cephalosporin skin testing is not standardized, although many allergists will perform cefazolin skin testing by using a nonirritating concentration of the antibiotic. While a positive skin test result suggests the presence of specific IgE antibodies, a negative skin test result does not definitively rule out an allergy, and an observed challenge should be considered before administration.

Cephalosporin allergic cross-reactivity: Most immediate hypersensitivity reactions with cephalosporins are directed at the R-group side chains (rather than the core beta-lactam ring). Tables are available that detail the beta-lactam antibiotics that share similar R-group side chains (see Suggested Reading later in this chapter and **Table 16-5**). If there is a history of an immediate hypersensitivity reaction to a given cephalosporin, beta-lactams with similar R-group side chains should be avoided. However, beta-lactams with non-similar R-group side chains may be considered, with the first dose given via observed challenge or desensitization (depending on severity of the prior reaction). For children with a history of cephalosporin allergy, penicillin skin testing should be considered before administering penicillins. If negative, the child may receive penicillins; if positive, penicillins should be avoided (if no acceptable alternatives are available, desensitization should be performed). If penicillin skin testing is unavailable, a cautious observed challenge should be performed before administration.

TABLE 16-5. CLINICALLY RELEVANT BETA-LACTAM ANTIBIOTICS WITH SIMILAR R-GROUP SIDE CHAINS

Antibiotics in *italics* are in different classes and/or generations.

Antibiotic	Beta-lactam Antibiotics Sharing Similar R-group Side Chains
Penicillins	Penicillin G, penicillin VK
Aminopenicillins	Amoxicillin, *cefadroxil, cefprozil* Ampicillin, *cefaclor, cephalexin*
First-generation cephalosporins	Cefaclor, cefadroxil, cephalexin, *cefprozil, amoxicillin, ampicillin* Cephalothin, *cefoxitin* **NOTE:** Cefazolin has unique R-group side chains.
Second-generation cephalosporins	Cefoxitin, *cephalothin* Cefuroxime, cefoxitin Cefprozil, *cefaclor, cefadroxil, cephalexin, amoxicillin, ampicillin* **NOTE:** Cefotetan and cefamandole have unique R-group side chains.
Third-, fourth-, and fifth-generation cephalosporins	Ceftriaxone, cefotaxime, cefepime Cefdinir, cefixime Ceftaroline, ceftobiprole, ceftolozane/tazobactam Cefditoren, cefpodoxime Ceftazidime, *aztreonam*
Monobactams	Aztreonam, *ceftazidime*

Adapted from Norton AE, Konvinse K, Phillips EJ, Broyles AD. Antibiotic allergy in pediatrics. *Pediatrics.* 2018;141(5):e20172497 PMID: 29700201 https://doi.org/10.1542/peds.2017-2497.

Aminopenicillins

Immediate hypersensitivity reactions to amoxicillin or ampicillin are less common than to penicillins. Skin testing with aminopenicillins is not as standardized as penicillin, although many allergists will perform testing by using a nonirritating concentration of ampicillin along with the major determinants for penicillin. It should be noted that the negative predictive value is not known, so an observed challenge may be considered in the setting of negative aminopenicillin skin testing results. Some physicians will identify children with low-risk histories who may bypass skin testing and proceed directly to an observed challenge.

Delayed drug-induced exanthems are relatively common with aminopenicillin use in children. The reaction is hypothesized to occur in the setting of a concomitant viral illness, with the classic example being an amoxicillin-induced rash in the setting of a child with acute Epstein-Barr virus infection (occurs in nearly 100%). In such cases, skin testing or an observed challenge may be considered before a future course is given.

Aminopenicillin allergic cross-reactivity: Immediate hypersensitivity reactions to aminopenicillins may be directed at either the core penicillin determinants or the R-group side chains. If the reaction is due to IgE antibodies versus the R-group side chains, children will have a negative penicillin skin test result and will be able to tolerate other penicillins. If there is a history of an immediate hypersensitivity reaction to an aminopenicillin, beta-lactams with the same R-group side chains should be avoided (see **Table 16-5**). If there is no alternative antibiotic, desensitization should be performed.

Monobactams

Allergic reactions to aztreonam are much less common than those to other beta-lactam antibiotics.

Monobactam allergic cross-reactivity: Monobactams do not exhibit allergic cross-reactivity with other beta-lactams, except for ceftazidime (which shares an R-group side chain with aztreonam).

Carbapenems

Immediate hypersensitivity reactions to carbapenems appear to be rare. Carbapenem skin testing is not standardized and has unknown predictive value.

Carbapenem allergic cross-reactivity: Allergic cross-reactivity between other beta-lactams and carbapenems is extremely low (<1%). One approach for children with a history of penicillin allergy is to perform a penicillin skin test. If negative, it is safe to use carbapenems; if positive, the child should receive carbapenems via observed challenge. If no penicillin skin test is performed, consider giving carbapenems via observed challenge.

Non–beta-lactam Antibiotics

Immediate hypersensitivity reactions to non–beta-lactam antibiotics are uncommon (**Table 16-6**). There are no validated tests to evaluate IgE-mediated reactions for these antibiotic classes (eg, skin testing is not standardized and lacks adequate predictive value). If the prior reaction to a non–beta-lactam antibiotic is consistent with an immediate hypersensitivity reaction, that antibiotic should be used only if there is no alternative agent and then only via desensitization.

TABLE 16-6. NON–BETA-LACTAM ANTIBIOTIC REACTIONS

Antibiotic Class	Frequency of Immediate Hypersensitivity Reactions	Other Antibiotic Reaction Notes
Aminoglycoside	Rare	None
Glycopeptide	Rare	Vancomycin frequently causes non–IgE-mediated histamine release (pseudoallergic reaction), often related to the rapidity of infusion, which is now called "vancomycin glycopeptide flushing syndrome." This syndrome is not a contraindication; premedicate with antihistamines and slow the infusion rate.
Lincosamide	Rare	None
Macrolide	Rare	Delayed drug-induced exanthems more common
Quinolone	Increasingly reported with expanded use	Delayed drug-induced exanthems in about 2%
Sulfonamide	Rare	Delayed drug-induced exanthems more common Severe cutaneous adverse reactions possible
Tetracyclines	Rare	None

Non–beta-lactam antibiotics allergic cross-reactivity: Importantly, there is no reported allergic cross-reactivity with beta-lactam antibiotics (or with alternative classes of non–beta-lactam antibiotics). There may be allergic cross-reactivity within the same antibiotic class (eg, some quinolone or macrolide groups).

Alternative Antibiotic Options for Common Infections

As detailed previously, it is important to identify children who are mislabeled or who have outgrown a reported allergy and can safely receive the antibiotic. For children with documented allergies, alternative antibiotic selection should be as narrow in spectrum as possible while balancing the effectiveness, rate of resistance, side effects, and potential allergic cross-reactivity of the medication. **Table 16-7** details alternative antibiotic options for select common infections. Consider the susceptibilities of the pathogens for each infection category, as all alternatives may not cover the required antibacterial spectrum equally well.

TABLE 16-7. ALTERNATIVE ANTIBIOTIC OPTIONS FOR SELECT COMMON INFECTIONS

Infection Category (Antibiotic Allergy)	Alternative Antibiotic Options
Acute otitis media (Amoxicillin allergy)	Third-generation cephalosporin (IV: ceftriaxone, cefotaxime; PO: cefdinir, cefixime, cefpodoxime) Azithromycin (Rate of macrolide resistance in *Pneumococcus* is high.) Clindamycin (does not cover *Haemophilus influenzae*) Levofloxacin
GAS pharyngitis (Penicillin/amoxicillin allergy)	Macrolides (azithromycin, erythromycin) Clindamycin Cephalosporins (5-day course is FDA approved for some oral cephalosporins.) ***NOTE:*** *Not TMP/SMX (does not reliably prevent rheumatic fever).*
Community-acquired pneumonia (Amoxicillin/ampicillin allergy)	Cephalosporins active against *Pneumococcus* (IV: ceftriaxone, cefotaxime, ceftaroline; PO: cefdinir, cefixime, cefpodoxime) Vancomycin IV Levofloxacin IV or PO Linezolid IV or PO
Atypical pneumonia (Macrolide allergy)	Doxycycline IV or PO Levofloxacin IV or PO
Skin and soft tissue/osteoarticular infections (due to *Staphylococcus aureus* or *Streptococcus* spp) (Varied allergies)	Penicillinase-resistant penicillins (IV: oxacillin, nafcillin; PO: dicloxacillin) First-generation cephalosporins (IV: cefazolin; PO: cephalexin) Ceftaroline IV (will cover MRSA) Clindamycin IV or PO TMP/SMX (skin) IV or PO Linezolid IV or PO Vancomycin IV Daptomycin IV ***NOTE:*** *When choosing option, consider if MRSA coverage needed.*

Abbreviations: FDA, US Food and Drug Administration; GAS, group A streptococcus; IV, intravenous; MRSA, methicillin-resistant *Staphylococcus aureus;* PO, oral; spp, species; TMP/SMX, trimethoprim/sulfamethoxazole.

Suggested Reading

Blumenthal KG, et al. *Lancet*. 2019;393(10167):183–198 PMID: 30558872

Collins C. *J Pediatr*. 2019;212:216–223 PMID: 31253408

Collins CA, et al. *Ann Allergy Asthma Immunol*. 2019;122(6):663–665 PMID: 30878624

Joint Task Force on Practice Parameters, et al. *Ann Allergy Asthma Immunol*. 2010;105(4):259–273 PMID: 20934625

Norton AE, et al. *Pediatrics*. 2018;141(5):e20172497 PMID: 29700201

Penicillin Allergy in Antibiotic Resistance Workgroup. *J Allergy Clin Immunol Pract*. 2017;5(2):333–334 PMID: 28283158

17. Antibiotic Stewardship

Antibiotic therapy is one of the most important advances in health care, along with the development of vaccines and the improvements in environmental health at the beginning of the 20th century. Appropriate use of antibiotics can be lifesaving. However, the use of antibiotics is also associated with increased microbial resistance, toxicity to the child, and cost. Therefore, antibiotic prescribing should be done carefully and responsibly to maximize benefit while minimizing adverse or unintended consequences. It is this need for balance on which the term *antibiotic stewardship* is based. *Merriam-Webster* defines *stewardship* as "the careful and responsible management of something entrusted to one's care."[1] It is not the purpose of antibiotic stewardship to drive antibiotic use inexorably toward a hypothetical zero, denying the benefit of treatment to those in need. It is, instead, the role of the steward to ensure that the right drug, at the right dose, for the right duration, is administered the right way to the right host for a particular infection caused by the "right" pathogen. In so doing, the steward maximizes the effect of the antibiotic while ensuring its continued availability and efficacy for the patients who follow.

To optimize use, there are 7 principles that should be followed (**Table 17-1**). These include infection prevention, diagnostic stewardship, effective empiric therapy for suspected infections, narrowing or stopping of therapy as additional information becomes available and the infection resolves, avoidance of unnecessary therapy by treating only infections, optimization of administration, and multidisciplinary accountability.

Infection Prevention

Infection prevention is a key component of antibiotic stewardship. Put simply, each infection that does not occur is one less that will require antibiotic treatment. Effective infection prevention strategies vary by site and by pathogen, and a full discussion of infection prevention is beyond the scope of this book. We direct the interested reader to the Centers for Disease Control and Prevention library.[2] The single most effective strategy for infection prevention remains adherence to hand hygiene. Effective hand hygiene can reduce person-to-person spread of pathogens that are spread by contact and droplet transmission, and studies have shown that infection rates correlate closely with hand hygiene performance regardless of other strategies that may be in place.

Diagnostic Stewardship

As discussed later in this chapter, selecting an appropriate antibiotic regimen for a patient depends largely on obtaining the proper test results for infection. Samples for culture or molecular diagnostic tests should be obtained before antibiotic therapy whenever possible, and the samples should be collected in a manner that will maximize the likelihood ratio of a positive or negative test result. For example, it matters if a urine culture that yields *Escherichia coli* was obtained via catheterization or by bag collection, just as it matters if a sterile urine culture was obtained before administering antibiotics or 48 hours after administration. Culture of non-sterile sites, such as the skin, mucous membranes, and trachea, may be useful in specific scenarios, but positive culture results from non-sterile sites must be interpreted with caution in the context of the pretest probability of

TABLE 17-1. OPTIMIZING ANTIBIOTIC USE

Facets of Stewardship	Examples for Implementation
Infection prevention	• Effective infection control and prevention • Close attention to hand hygiene
Diagnostic stewardship	• Obtain appropriate cultures before antibiotic therapy. • Avoid culturing non-sterile sites, and interpret cultures from those sites carefully. • Consider molecular diagnostics when appropriate. • Use ancillary laboratory tests for infection, but remember that positive predictive value may be poor.
Empiric therapy	• Use the narrowest-spectrum agents that cover the likely pathogens to achieve the necessary cure rate for your patient, infection site, severity of infection, and underlying comorbid conditions. • Use an antibiotic that penetrates the infected compartment (eg, achieves effective exposure at the site of infection) (see Chapter 11). • Use local epidemiology (including antibiogram) and previous patient cultures to guide therapy.
Reevaluation of therapy	• Discontinue empiric antibiotics when infection is no longer suspected. • For proven infection, adjust antibiotics once speciation and susceptibilities are available. • Treat for the shortest effective duration, and follow up to ensure a successful outcome.
Treatment only of infections	• Avoid treating – Colonization – Contaminants – Noninfectious conditions
Optimization of administration	• Closely collaborate with pharmacists. • Use protocols that maximize pharmacodynamics of agent. • Perform therapeutic drug monitoring where appropriate.
Accountability	• Multidisciplinary team • Prospective audit and feedback • Guarantee of representation and buy-in by including "champions"

infection. Similarly, molecular diagnostic test results from nucleic acid amplification or next-generation sequencing (usually obtained from blood and infected tissue sites) are frequently positive even after antibiotics have been given to children and sensitivity of cultures decreases quickly.[3] Next-generation sequencing has not been prospectively studied in children; is likely to pick up a low signal by colonization of commensal organisms that may not represent invasive infection. Those with mucositis may have DNA from multiple organisms detected, which does not necessarily indicate invasive infection by all detected bacteria. Finally, abnormal values of ancillary tests, such as white blood cell count, C-reactive protein (CRP), and procalcitonin, may lead to unnecessary antibiotic use when the likelihood of infection is low. A careful diagnostic approach is needed to optimize antibiotic use.

Empiric Therapy

Appropriate therapy for a suspected infection should be administered once the appropriate diagnostic test results have been obtained. This empiric therapy should be based on a variety of factors, including the organisms most likely to cause the suspected infection, the body compartment(s) infected, host characteristics including renal and hepatic clearance, drug-drug interactions, and local antibiotic susceptibilities. Ideally, empiric therapy would be the narrowest-possible regimen that penetrates the infected space and covers the most likely organisms. These parameters may change over time; for example, in the setting of a local methicillin-resistant *Staphylococcus aureus* (MRSA) outbreak, clinicians might consider different empiric therapy for skin and soft tissue infection than they would otherwise. Similarly, prior antibiotic susceptibilities of a recurrent infection should be used to guide empiric treatment. For example, therapy for a child with a first occurrence of *E coli* pyelonephritis will be guided by local rates of susceptibility, but past susceptibility information should guide empiric therapy in the same child experiencing a recurrence. It is also important to assess the need to achieve a certain level of success in selecting empiric therapy antibacterial coverage. For the child with mild impetigo, perhaps using drugs that provide 70% coverage of the suspected pathogens is acceptable, and the clinician can follow the treatment progress to see if changes need to be made. On the other hand, for the child who has leukemia and is neutropenic, with bacterial meningitis associated with gram-negative bacilli on stains of cerebrospinal fluid, we strive to start empiric therapy with antibiotic(s) as close to covering 100% of suspected pathogens as we can get, quickly reevaluating therapy (see the next section in this chapter). Clinicians should assess their willingness to accept some degree of treatment failure for any given infection, acknowledging that 100% coverage is not required for less severe infections.

Reevaluation of Therapy

Empiric therapy is just that, and it should change once additional information is available. In most cases, this means stopping therapy if infection is no longer suspected (eg, if cultures are sterile after 36–48 hours; if molecular tests for pathogens show no significant pathogen signal) or narrowing therapy if an organism is identified (eg, narrowing from ceftriaxone to ampicillin for susceptible *E coli* recovered from urine). However, therapy should also be reevaluated and possibly broadened if the clinical situation dictates (eg, if a child's condition becomes clinically unstable; if new physical examination findings or radiographic changes are seen; if a culture yields an organism that is unlikely to be covered by the empiric antimicrobials).

Treatment Only of Infections

Antibiotics are powerful tools, but they treat *only* fever and other local and systemic signs and symptoms of infection if those are caused by bacteria, fungi, or mycobacteria. If a stable patient has fever and a careful, systematic evaluation and diagnostic workup have not identified a treatable organism, it is reasonable in many cases to continue to evaluate that patient without prolonged antibiotic therapy. Many noninfectious diseases can develop with signs and symptoms that are consistent with infection, including numerous rheumatologic and oncologic conditions. Anchoring to a diagnosis of infection in the absence of evidence for infection may not only drive unnecessary antibiotic use but also delay time to diagnosis of another significant health condition. Similarly, clinicians should strive to avoid treating organisms that are colonizing commensals or contaminants. For example, prolonged vancomycin therapy for a *Corynebacterium* species recovered from blood culture after 58 hours of incubation is not an appropriate use of antibiotics. Culture from non-sterile sites is particularly challenging to interpret in this context, and those cultures should be obtained only when the likelihood of infection at those sites is high. Often, tests for inflammation are elevated when true, invasive infection is present. A normal CRP level after 3 to 4 days of high fever suggests a diagnosis other than bacterial infection, particularly when supported by negative culture and negative molecular test results. Next-generation sequencing tests do not require prior knowledge of a specific pathogen to make a diagnosis; they assess the presence of nucleic acid sequences from any of a thousand pathogens in a gene library.

Optimization of Administration

The dose, route, and frequency of antibiotics can be manipulated to optimize their pharmacodynamics and efficacy and minimize toxicity. Close collaboration with pharmacology is critical to ensure that dosing is optimal. Examples of strategies include continuous infusion of beta-lactam antibiotics to maximize time above minimum inhibitory concentration (MIC) for a resistant *Pseudomonas aeruginosa* infection in a child with cystic fibrosis, vancomycin clearance calculations to ensure adequate area under the serum concentration-versus-time curve to MIC ratio for a complex MRSA infection, or therapeutic drug monitoring to minimize toxicity of aminoglycosides or voriconazole. Dosing strategies can be protocolized, but such strategies should be reviewed periodically, as approaches designed to optimize pharmacokinetics and pharmacodynamics are constantly evolving.

Accountability

Effective antibiotic stewardship cannot be accomplished in a vacuum. Effective stewardship programs require multidisciplinary buy-in and support as well as effective and continuous closed-loop communication. At a minimum, these teams usually consist of pharmacists, physicians including infectious disease (ID) specialists, designated clinicians for representative service lines (eg, a "unit champion"), nurses and nursing leadership, and hospital administrators. Clinical microbiologists, infection control and prevention specialists, information technology specialists, and hospital epidemiologists are key resources even if they do not participate directly in stewardship activities. Antibiotic stewardship programs have myriad tools available (**Table 17-2**), including prospective audit and feedback, prior authorization, clinical practice guidelines, electronic decision support, antibiotic time-outs, electronic hard stops, and intravenous-to-oral conversion. Use of some or all of these interventions must be coupled to education and reporting to staff to demonstrate the utility of the program.

TABLE 17-2. ANTIBIOTIC STEWARDSHIP INTERVENTIONS

Intervention	Description	Advantages and Disadvantages
Prospective audit and feedback	Antibiotic use is monitored prospectively, and information about use is shared with clinicians via continuous or intermittent reports. Specific areas of antibiotic misuse and overuse are targeted for education and feedback.	Staple of stewardship Can be time-consuming if not automated Should be combined with education to maximize effect
Prior authorization	Specific antibiotics are restricted without prior approval of ID team or stewardship team.	Extremely effective in curtailing specific antibiotic usage but extremely unpopular; clinicians may develop work-arounds to circumvent restrictions.
Clinical practice guidelines	Antibiotic use for a given clinical scenario is built into a protocol or guideline.	Can reduce time to effective therapy, but may not allow flexibility if certain aspects of case are different from usual (eg, if patient has a history of ESBL-producing *Escherichia coli* infection but gets ceftriaxone because of UTI guideline)
Electronic decision support	Language built into electronic medical records to recognize specific conditions (eg, suspected sepsis) and trigger decision support	Can increase awareness of specific conditions, but may contribute to "alert fatigue"
Antibiotic time-outs	Scheduled reevaluation of empiric therapy at a set time point, usually 48 or 72 h after initiation	Important role in ensuring that empiric therapy is reevaluated as new information comes in. Timing may differ based on clinical scenario.
Electronic hard stops	More automated time-out in which antibiotic therapy is automatically discontinued at a set time point	Very effective in limiting empiric therapy, but must be implemented and monitored carefully to ensure antibiotic therapy is not inadvertently discontinued without notice
IV-to-PO conversion	Periodic or automated review by stewardship team to determine if antibiotics can be changed to PO administration	Particularly useful at hospital discharge to avoid unnecessary outpatient parenteral antibiotic therapy. John Nelson first documented success almost 50 years ago for osteomyelitis.

Abbreviations: ESBL, extended-spectrum beta-lactamase; ID, infectious disease; IV, intravenous; PO, oral; UTI, urinary tract infection.

Historically, many of us opposed antibiotic stewardship programs that reported outcomes only in reduced antibiotic costs and volume and did not consider the adverse effects of the inappropriate use of inexpensive narrow-spectrum antibiotics for serious infection (eg, empiric ampicillin treatment of severe pyelonephritis). However, clinicians are generally more concerned with the outcome of their patients than they are on abstract purchasing data. As a result, stewardship programs have moved toward reporting more patient-centered outcomes, including adverse drug reactions, antibiotic resistance rates, length of stay, and failure of initial therapy. Clinicians are also more inclined to participate in and adhere to stewardship program interventions if they have a seat at the table and can contribute to shared decision-making. This is the role of the unit champion. For example, neonatologists, pulmonologists, and ambulatory pediatricians might each designate a faculty member to attend the monthly stewardship meeting to ensure that their perspectives are considered. Finally, pediatricians should consider including parents or family members in shared decision-making about antibiotic use.

In conclusion, antibiotics are critically important for treatment of infections. However, overuse or misuse of antibiotics will drive antimicrobial resistance and adverse patient outcomes. We have learned that there is no "new antibiotic" against which bacteria do not develop resistance. It is the role of the antibiotic steward to maximize the benefit of antibiotics, minimize their toxicity, and preserve their use for subsequent children. There are many resources available to achieve these goals—for example, antibiotic stewardship programs, pharmacists, ID physicians, and prescribing guides such as *Nelson's Pediatric Antimicrobial Therapy.* However, at the end of the day, every health care worker who cares for children is also charged with being a steward of antibiotics—to optimize their use for the patient at hand, while safeguarding their efficacy for all the children yet to come.

18. Systemic and Topical Antimicrobial Dosing and Dose Forms

NOTES

- Higher dosages in a dose range are generally indicated for more serious infections. For pathogens with higher minimal inhibitory concentrations against beta-lactam antibiotics, a more prolonged infusion of the antibiotic will allow increased antibacterial effect (see Chapter 11).
- Maximum dosages for adult-sized children (≥40 kg) are based on US Food and Drug Administration (FDA)–approved product labeling or postmarketing data.
- See also Chapter 7 for HIV and SARS-CoV-2 antiviral agents not listed in this chapter.
- Antiviral monoclonal antibodies and immunomodulators are not listed.
- Dose Levels of Evidence:

  Level I: FDA-approved pediatric dosing or based on randomized clinical trials

  Level II: data from noncomparative trials or small comparative trials

  Level III: expert or consensus opinion or case reports
- If no oral liquid form is available, round the child's dose to a combination of available solid dosage forms. Consult a pediatric pharmacist for recommendations on the availability of extemporaneously compounded liquid formulations.
- Cost estimates are in US dollars per course, or per month for maintenance regimens. Estimates are based on wholesale acquisition costs at the editor's institution. These may differ from those of the reader. Legend: $ = <$100, $$ = $100–$400, $$$ = $401–$1,000, $$$$ = >$1,000, $$$$$ = >$10,000.
- There are some agents that we do not recommend even though they may be available. We believe they are significantly inferior to those we do recommend in chapters 1 through 12 and could possibly lead to poor outcomes if used. Such agents are not listed.
- **Abbreviations:** AOM, acute otitis media; ARC, augmented renal clearance; AUC:MIC, area under the curve (the mathematically calculated area under the serum concentration-versus-time curve) to minimum inhibitory concentration; bid, twice daily; BSA, body surface area; CABP, community-acquired bacterial pneumonia; CA-MRSA, community-associated methicillin-resistant *Staphylococcus aureus;* cap, capsule or caplet; CF, cystic fibrosis; CMV, cytomegalovirus; CNS, central nervous system; CrCl, creatinine clearance; div, divided; DOT, directly observed therapy; DR, delayed-release; EC, enteric-coated; ER, extended release; FDA, US Food and Drug Administration; GI, gastrointestinal; hs, bedtime; HBV, hepatitis B virus; HSV, herpes simplex virus; IBS-d, irritable bowel syndrome with diarrhea; IM, intramuscular; INH, isoniazid; IV, intravenous; IVesic, intravesical; IVPB, intravenous piggyback (premixed bag); LD, loading dose; MAC, *Mycobacterium avium* complex; max, maximum;

MDR, multidrug-resistant; MIC, minimum inhibitory concentration; MRSA, methicillin-resistant *S aureus;* NS, normal saline (physiologic saline solution); oint, ointment; OPC, oropharyngeal candidiasis; ophth, ophthalmic; PEG, pegylated; PIP, piperacillin; PJP, *Pneumocystis jiroveci* pneumonia; PMA, postmenstrual age; PO, oral; pwd, powder; q, every; qd, once daily; qhs, every bedtime; qid, 4 times daily; RSV, respiratory syncytial virus; RTI, respiratory tract infection; SIADH, syndrome of inappropriate antidiuretic hormone; SMX, sulfamethoxazole; soln, solution; SPAG-2, small particle aerosol generator model-2; SQ, subcutaneous; SSSI, skin and skin structure infection; STI, sexually transmitted infection; susp, suspension; tab, tablet; TB, tuberculosis; TBW, total body weight; tid, 3 times daily; TMP, trimethoprim; top, topical; UTI, urinary tract infection; vag, vaginal; VZV, varicella-zoster virus; WHO, World Health Organization.

A. SYSTEMIC ANTIMICROBIALS WITH DOSAGE FORMS AND USUAL DOSAGES

Generic and Trade Names	Dosage Form (cost estimate)	Route	Dose (evidence level)	Interval
Acyclovir,[a] Zovirax (See also Valacyclovir later in this table.)	500-, 1,000-mg vials ($)	IV	15–45 mg/kg/day (I) (See chapters 2 and 7.) Max 1,500 mg/m²/day (II) (See Chapter 13.)	q8h
	200-mg/5-mL susp ($–$$) 200-mg cap ($) 400-, 800-mg tab ($)	PO	900 mg/m²/day (I) 60–80 mg/kg/day, max 3,200 mg/day (I) Adult max 4 g/day for VZV (I) (See chapters 2 and 7.)	q8h q6–8h
Albendazole,[a] Albenza	200-mg tab ($–$$$)	PO	15 mg/kg/day for cysticercosis or echinococcosis (I) (See Chapter 9 for other indications.)	q12h
Amikacin,[a] Amikin	500-mg/2-mL, 1,000-mg/4-mL vials ($)	IV, IM	15–22.5 mg/kg/day[b] (I) (See Chapter 4.) 30–35 mg/kg/day[b] for CF (II)	q8–24h q24h
		IVesic	50–100 mL of 0.5 mg/mL in NS (III)	q12h
Amoxicillin,[a] Amoxil	125-, 200-, 250-, 400-mg/5-mL susp ($) 125-, 250-mg chew tab ($) 250-, 500-mg cap ($) 500-, 875-mg tab ($)	PO	Standard dose: 40–45 mg/kg/day (I) High dose: 80–90 mg/kg/day (I) 150 mg/kg/day for penicillin-resistant *Streptococcus pneumoniae* otitis media (III) Max 4,000 mg/day (III)	q8–12h q12h q8h

A. SYSTEMIC ANTIMICROBIALS WITH DOSAGE FORMS AND USUAL DOSAGES *(continued)*

Generic and Trade Names	Dosage Form (cost estimate)	Route	Dose (evidence level)	Interval
Amoxicillin/clavulanate,[a] Augmentin	16:1 Augmentin XR: 1,000/62.5-mg tab ($$)	PO	16:1 formulation: ≥40 kg and adults, 4,000-mg amoxicillin/day (not per kg) (I)	q12h
	14:1 Augmentin ES: 600/42.9-mg/5-mL susp ($)	PO	14:1 formulation: 90-mg amoxicillin/kg/day (I), max 4,000 mg amoxicillin/day (III)	q12h
	7:1 Augmentin ($): 875/125-mg tab 200/28.5-, 400/57-mg chew tab 200/28.5-, 400/57-mg/5-mL susp	PO	7:1 formulation: 25- or 45-mg amoxicillin/kg/day, max 1,750 mg amoxicillin/day (I)	q12h
	4:1 Augmentin: 500/125-mg tab ($) 250/62.5-mg/5-mL susp ($)	PO	4:1 formulation: 20- or 40-mg amoxicillin/kg/day, max 1,500 mg amoxicillin/day (I)	q8h
	2:1 Augmentin: 250/125-mg tab ($)	PO	2:1 formulation: ≥40 kg: 750-mg amoxicillin/day (not per kg) (I)	q8h
Amphotericin B deoxycholate,[a] Fungizone	50-mg vial ($–$$)	IV	1–1.5 mg/kg (I), max 150 mg (II) 0.5 mg/kg for *Candida* esophagitis or cystitis (II)	q24h
		IVesic	50–100 mcg/mL in sterile water × 50–100 mL (III)	q8h
Amphotericin B, lipid complex, Abelcet	100-mg/20-mL vial ($$$)	IV	5 mg/kg (I), max 10 mg/kg or 500 mg (II)	q24h
Amphotericin B, liposomal, AmBisome	50-mg vial ($$$)	IV	5 mg/kg (I), max 10 mg/kg or 500 mg (II)	q24h
Ampicillin sodium[a]	125-, 250-, 500-mg vial ($) 1-, 2-, 10-g vial ($)	IV, IM	50–200 mg/kg/day, max 8 g/day (I) 300–400 mg/kg/day, max 12 g/day endocarditis/meningitis (III)	q6h q4–6h

Ampicillin trihydrate[a]	500-mg cap ($)	PO	50–100 mg/kg/day if <20 kg (I) ≥20 kg and adults: 1–2 g/day (I)	q6h
Ampicillin/sulbactam,[a] Unasyn	1/0.5-, 2/1-, 10/5-g vial ($–$$)	IV, IM	200-mg ampicillin/kg/day (I) ≥40 kg and adults: 4–max 8 g/day (I)	q6h
Anidulafungin, Eraxis	100-mg vial ($$–$$$)	IV	3 mg/kg LD, then 1.5 mg/kg (I) Max 200-mg LD, then 100 mg (I)	q24h
Artemether and lumefantrine, Coartem	20/120-mg tab ($–$$)	PO	5–<15 kg: 1 tab/dose (I) ≥15–<25 kg: 2 tabs/dose (I) ≥25–<35 kg: 3 tabs/dose (I) ≥35 kg: 4 tabs/dose (I)	6 doses over 3 days at 0, 8, 24, 36, 48, 60 h
Artesunate	110-mg vial ($$$$$)	IV	2.4 mg/kg (I) See Malaria in Chapter 9, Table 9B.	q12h × 3, then q24h
Atovaquone,[a] Mepron	750-mg/5-mL susp ($$–$$$)	PO	30 mg/kg/day if 1–3 mo or >24 mo (I) 45 mg/kg/day if >3–24 mo (I) Max 1,500 mg/day (I)	q12h q24h for prophylaxis
Atovaquone and proguanil,[a] Malarone	62.5/25-mg pediatric tab ($–$$) 250/100-mg adult tab ($–$$)	PO	Prophylaxis for malaria: 11–20 kg: 1 pediatric tab, 21–30 kg: 2 pediatric tabs, 31–40 kg: 3 pediatric tabs, >40 kg: 1 adult tab (I) Treatment: 5–8 kg: 2 pediatric tabs, 9–10 kg: 3 pediatric tabs, 11–20 kg: 1 adult tab, 21–30 kg: 2 adult tabs, 31–40 kg: 3 adult tabs, >40 kg: 4 adult tabs (I)	q24h

A. SYSTEMIC ANTIMICROBIALS WITH DOSAGE FORMS AND USUAL DOSAGES *(continued)*

Generic and Trade Names	Dosage Form (cost estimate)	Route	Dose (evidence level)	Interval
Azithromycin,[a] Zithromax	250-, 500-, 600-mg tab ($) 100-, 200-mg/5-mL susp ($) 1-g packet for susp ($)	PO	Otitis: 10 mg/kg/day for 1 day, then 5 mg/kg for 4 days; or 10 mg/kg/day for 3 days; or 30 mg/kg once (I). Pharyngitis: 12 mg/kg/day for 5 days, max 2,500-mg total dose (I). Sinusitis: 10 mg/kg/day for 3 days, max 1.5-g total dose (I). CABP: 10 mg/kg for 1 day, then 5 mg/kg/day for 4 days (max 1.5-g total dose), or 60 mg/kg once of ER (Zmax) susp, max 2 g (I). MAC prophylaxis: 20 mg/kg, max 1.2 g weekly (III). Adult dosing for RTI: 500 mg day 1, then 250 mg daily for 4 days or 500 mg for 3 days. Adult and adolescent dosing for STI: non-gonorrhea: 1 g once. Gonorrhea: 2 g once. (See other indications in chapters 1, 3, and 9.)	q24h
	500-mg vial ($)	IV	10 mg/kg, max 500 mg (II)	q24h
Aztreonam,[a] Azactam	1-, 2-g vial ($$–$$$)	IV, IM	90–120 mg/kg/day, max 8 g/day (I)	q6–8h
Baloxavir, Xofluza	40-, 80-mg tab ($$) 40-mg/20-mL susp ($$)	PO	≥5 y (I) <20 kg: 2 mg/kg 20–79 kg: 40 mg per dose ≥80 kg: 80 mg per dose	Once
Bedaquiline, Sirturo	20-mg dispersible tab, 100-mg tab Available from Metro Medical specialty distributor 855/691-0963	PO	≥5 y + ≥15 kg: 200 mg (not per kg), then 100 mg (I) ≥30 kg + adults: 400 mg, then 200 mg (I); in combination with other agents for MDR TB (See Chapter 1, Table 1F.)	q24h for 2 wk, then the lower dose 3 times/wk

Benznidazole	12.5-, 100-mg tab Contact 877/303-7181.	PO	2–12 y: 5–8 mg/kg/day (I) (See also Trypanosomiasis in Chapter 9.)	q12h
Bezlotoxumab, Zinplava	1-g vial ($$$$)	IV	Adults: 10 mg/kg (I)[c]	One time
Capreomycin, Capastat	1-g vial ($$$$)	IV, IM	15–30 mg/kg (III), max 1 g (I)	q24h
Caspofungin,[a] Cancidas	50-, 70-mg vial ($$)	IV	Load with 70 mg/m^2 once, then 50 mg/m^2, max 70 mg (I).	q24h
Cefaclor,[a] Ceclor	250-, 500-mg cap ($) 500-mg ER tab ($)	PO	20–40 mg/kg/day, max 1 g/day (I)	q12h
Cefadroxil,[a] Duricef	250-, 500-mg/5-mL susp ($) 500-mg cap ($) 1-g tab ($)	PO	30 mg/kg/day, max 2 g/day (I)	q12–24h
Cefazolin,[a] Ancef	0.5-, 1-, 10-g vial ($)	IV, IM	25–100 mg/kg/day (I)	q8h
			100–150 mg/kg/day for serious infections (III), max 12 g/day	q6h
Cefdinir,[a] Omnicef	125-, 250-mg/5-mL susp ($) 300-mg cap ($)	PO	14 mg/kg/day, max 600 mg/day (I)	q12–24h
Cefepime,[a] Maxipime	1-, 2-g vial ($)	IV, IM	100 mg/kg/day, max 4 g/day (I)	q12h
			150 mg/kg/day empiric therapy for fever with neutropenia, max 6 g/day (I)	q8h
Cefiderocol, Fetroja	1-g vial ($$$$)	IV	Adults 2 g/day (I)[c]	q8h
Cefixime,[a] Suprax	100-, 200-mg/5-mL susp ($$) 400-mg cap ($$)	PO	8 mg/kg/day, max 400 mg/day (I)	q24h
			For convalescent PO therapy for serious infections, up to 20 mg/kg/day (III)	q12h
Cefotaxime,[a] Claforan	0.5-, 1-, 2-, 10-g vial Not currently manufactured in the United States	IV, IM	150–180 mg/kg/day, max 8 g/day (I) 200–225 mg/kg/day for meningitis, max 12 g/day (I)	q8h q6h

A. SYSTEMIC ANTIMICROBIALS WITH DOSAGE FORMS AND USUAL DOSAGES *(continued)*

Generic and Trade Names	Dosage Form (cost estimate)	Route	Dose (evidence level)	Interval
Cefotetan,[a] Cefotan	1-, 2-g vial ($) 1-, 2-g/50-mL IVPB ($$)	IV, IM	60–100 mg/kg/day (II), max 6 g/day (I)	q12h
Cefoxitin,[a] Mefoxin	1-, 2-, 10-g vial ($)	IV, IM	80–160 mg/kg/day, max 12 g/day (I)	q6–8h
Cefpodoxime,[a] Vantin	100-mg/5-mL susp ($) 100-, 200-mg tab ($)	PO	10 mg/kg/day, max 400 mg/day (I)	q12h
Cefprozil,[a] Cefzil	125-, 250-mg/5-mL susp ($) 250-, 500-mg tab ($)	PO	15–30 mg/kg/day, max 1 g/d (I)	q12h
Ceftaroline, Teflaro	400-, 600-mg vial ($$$$)	IV	0–<2 mo: 18 mg/kg/day (I) ≥2 mo–<2 y: 24 mg/kg/day (I) ≥2 y: 36 mg/kg/day (I) >33 kg: 1.2 g/day (I) Adults: 1.2 g/day (I) 45–60 mg/kg/day, max 3 g/day ± prolonged infusion for CF (II)	q8h q8h q8h q12h q12h q8h
Ceftazidime[a]; Tazicef, Fortaz	0.5-, 1-, 2-, 6-g vial ($)	IV, IM	90–150 mg/kg/day, max 6 g/day (I), max 8 g/day div q6h in children with obesity (II)	q8h
		IV	200–300 mg/kg/day for serious *Pseudomonas* infection, max 12 g/day (II)	q8h
Ceftazidime/avibactam, Avycaz	2-g/0.5-g vial ($$$$)	IV	3–5 mo: 120 mg ceftazidime/kg/day (I) ≥6 mo: 150 mg ceftazidime/kg/day, max 6 g (not per kg)/day (I)	q8h infused over 2 h
Ceftolozane/tazobactam, Zerbaxa	1.5-g (1-g/0.5-g) vial ($$$$)	IV	Adults: 4.5 g (3 g/1.5 g)/day (I) <12 y: 60/30 mg/kg/day (II)[c]	q8h

Ceftriaxone,[a] Rocephin	0.25-, 0.5-, 1-, 2-, 10-g vial ($)	IV, IM	50–75 mg/kg/day, max 2 g/day (I) Meningitis: 100 mg/kg/day, max 4 g/day (I) AOM: 50 mg/kg, max 1 g, 1–3 doses (II)	q24h q12h q24h
Cefuroxime,[a] Ceftin	250-, 500-mg tab ($)	PO	20–30 mg/kg/day, max 1 g/day (I) For bone and joint infections, up to 100 mg/kg/day, max 3 g/day (III)	q12h q8h
Cefuroxime,[a] Zinacef	0.75-, 1.5-g vial ($)	IV, IM	100–150 mg/kg/day, max 6 g/day (I)	q8h
Cephalexin,[a] Keflex	125-, 250-mg/5-mL susp ($) 250-, 500-mg cap, tab ($) 750-mg cap ($-$$)	PO	25–50 mg/kg/day (I)	q12h
			75–100 mg/kg/day for bone and joint, or severe, infections (II); max 4 g/day (I)	q6–8h
Chloroquine phosphate,[a] Aralen	250-, 500-mg (150-, 300-mg base) tabs ($–$$)	PO	See Malaria in Chapter 9, Table 9B.	
Cidofovir,[a] Vistide	375-mg vial ($$$)	IV	5 mg/kg (III) (See Adenovirus in Chapter 7, Table 7C.)	Weekly
Ciprofloxacin,[a] Cipro	250-, 500-mg/5-mL susp ($$) 250-, 500-, 750-mg tab ($)	PO	20–40 mg/kg/day, max 1.5 g/day (I). Do not administer susp via feeding tubes.	q12h
	100-mg tab ($)	PO	Adult women with uncomplicated acute cystitis: 200 mg/day for 3 days (I)	
	200-mg/100-mL, 400-mg/200-mL IVPB ($)	IV	20–30 mg/kg/day, max 1.2 g/day (I)	q12h
Clarithromycin,[a] Biaxin	125-, 250-mg/5-mL susp ($–$$) 250-, 500-mg tab ($)	PO	15 mg/kg/day, max 1 g/day (I)	q12h
Clarithromycin ER,[a] Biaxin XL	500-mg ER tab ($)	PO	Adults 1 g (I)	q24h

A. SYSTEMIC ANTIMICROBIALS WITH DOSAGE FORMS AND USUAL DOSAGES *(continued)*

Generic and Trade Names	Dosage Form (cost estimate)	Route	Dose (evidence level)	Interval
Clindamycin,[a] Cleocin	75-mg/5-mL soln ($) 75-, 150-, 300-mg cap ($)	PO	10–25 mg/kg/day, max 1.8 g/day (I) 30–40 mg/kg/day for CA-MRSA, intra-abdominal infection, or AOM (III)	q8h
	150-mg/mL vial in 2-, 4-, 6-, and 60-mL sizes ($) 0.3-, 0.6-, 0.9-g/50-mL IVPB ($)	IV, IM	20–40 mg/kg/day, max 2.7 g/day (I)	q8h
Clotrimazole,[a] Mycelex	10-mg lozenge ($)	PO	≥3 y: dissolve lozenge in mouth (I).	5 times daily
Colistimethate,[a] Coly-Mycin M	150-mg (colistin base) vial ($). 1-mg base = 2.7-mg colistimethate = 30,000 IU.	IV, IM	2.5- to 5-mg base/kg/day (I) Max 360 mg/day[b] (III)	q8h
Cycloserine, Seromycin	250-mg cap ($$$$)	PO	10–20 mg/kg/day (III) Adults max 1 g/day (I)	q12h
Dalbavancin, Dalvance	500-mg vial ($$$$)	IV	Birth–<6 y: 22.5 mg/kg (I) 6–<18 y: 18 mg/kg, max 1,500 mg (I) Adults: 1,500 mg (I)	One time
Dapsone[a]	25-, 100-mg tab ($)	PO	2 mg/kg, max 100 mg (I)	q24h
			4 mg/kg, max 200 mg (I)	Once weekly
Daptomycin,[a] Cubicin	350-, 500-mg vial ($$)	IV	For SSSI (I): 1–2 y: 10 mg/kg, 2–6 y: 9 mg/kg, 7–11 y: 7 mg/kg, 12–17 y: 5 mg/kg. For *Staphylococcus aureus* bacteremia (I): 1–6 y: 12 mg/kg, 7–11 y: 9 mg/kg, 12–17 y: 7 mg/kg. For other indications, see Chapter 1. Adults: 4–6 mg/kg TBW (I).	q24h

Delafloxacin, Baxdela	450-mg tab ($$$$)	PO	Adults 450 mg (I)	q12h
	300-mg vial ($$$)	IV	Adults 300 mg (I)	q12h
Demeclocycline,[a] Declomycin	150-, 300-mg tab ($)	PO	≥8 y: 7–13 mg/kg/day, max 600 mg/day (I). Dosage differs for SIADH.	q6–12h
Dicloxacillin,[a] Dynapen	250-, 500-mg cap ($)	PO	12–25 mg/kg/day (adults 0.5–1 g/day) (I) For bone and joint infections, up to 100 mg/kg/day, max 2 g/day (III)	q6h
Doxycycline, Vibramycin	25-mg/5-mL susp[a] ($) 50-mg/5-mL syrup ($$) 20-, 40-, 50-, 75-, 100-, 150-mg tab/cap[a] ($–$$) 200-mg tab[a] ($$$)	PO	4.4 mg/kg/day LD day 1, then 2.2–4.4 mg/kg/day, max 200 mg/day (I)	q12–24h
	100-mg vial[a] ($$)	IV		
Elbasvir/grazoprevir, Zepatier	50-mg/100-mg tab ($$$$)	PO	Aged ≥12 y or weighing ≥30 kg: 1 tab (I)	q24h
Entecavir, Baraclude (See Hepatitis B virus in Chapter 7.)	0.05-mg/mL soln ($$$) 0.5-, 1-mg tab[a] ($)	PO	2–<16 y (I) (double the following doses if previous lamivudine exposure): 10–11 kg: 0.15 mg >11–14 kg: 0.2 mg >14–17 kg: 0.25 mg >17–20 kg: 0.3 mg >20–23 kg: 0.35 mg >23–26 kg: 0.4 mg >26–30 kg: 0.45 mg >30 kg: 0.5 mg ≥16 y: 0.5 mg (I)	q24h
Eravacycline, Xerava	50-mg vial ($$$)	IV	≥18 y: 1 mg/kg	q12h

A. SYSTEMIC ANTIMICROBIALS WITH DOSAGE FORMS AND USUAL DOSAGES *(continued)*

Generic and Trade Names	Dosage Form (cost estimate)	Route	Dose (evidence level)	Interval
Ertapenem,[a] Invanz	1-g vial ($$)	IV, IM	30 mg/kg/day, max 1 g/day (I) ≥13 y and adults: 1 g/day (I)	q12h q24h
Erythromycin base[a]	250-, 500-mg tab ($–$$) 250-mg DR cap ($) 250-, 333-, 500-mg DR tab (Ery-Tab) ($$)	PO	50 mg/kg/day, max 4 g/day (I). Dose differs for GI prokinesis.	q6–8h
Erythromycin ethylsuccinate[a]; EES, EryPed	200-, 400-mg/5-mL susp ($$–$$$) 400-mg tab ($$)	PO	50 mg/kg/day, max 4 g/day (I). Dose differs for GI prokinesis.	q6–8h
Erythromycin lactobionate, Erythrocin	0.5-g vial ($$–$$$)	IV	20 mg/kg/day, max 4 g/day (I)	q6h
Ethambutol,[a] Myambutol	100-, 400-mg tab ($)	PO	15–25 mg/kg, max 2.5 g (I)	q24h
Ethionamide, Trecator	250-mg tab ($$)	PO	15–20 mg/kg/day, max 1 g/day (I)	q12–24h
Famciclovir,[a] Famvir	125-, 250-, 500-mg tab ($)	PO	Adults 0.5–2 g/day (I)	q8–12h
Fexinidazole	600-mg tab available from WHO. Contact by email: neglected.diseases@who.int	PO	See Trypanosomiasis in Chapter 9.	q24h
Fidaxomicin, Dificid	200-mg tab ($$$$) 200-mg/5-mL susp ($$$$)	PO	≥6 mo (I) (per dose, not per kg): 4–<7 kg: 80 mg 7–<9 kg: 120 mg 9–<12.5 kg: 160 mg ≥12.5 kg: 200 mg Adults: 200 mg (I)	q12h

Fluconazole,[a] Diflucan	50-, 100-, 150-, 200-mg tab ($) 50-, 200-mg/5-mL susp ($)	PO	6–12 mg/kg, max 800 mg (I). 800–1,000 mg/day may be used for some CNS fungal infections (see Chapter 5).	q24h
	100-mg/50-mL, 200-mg/100-mL, 400-mg/200-mL IVPB ($)	IV		
Flucytosine,[a] Ancobon	250-, 500-mg cap ($$$$)	PO	100 mg/kg/day (I)[b]	q6h
Foscarnet, Foscavir	6-g/250-mL vial ($$$$)	IV	CMV/VZV: 180 mg/kg/day (I)	q8–12h
			CMV suppression: 90–120 mg/kg (I)	q24h
			HSV: 120 mg/kg/day (I)	q8–12h
Fosfomycin, Contepo	6-g vial (not yet commercially available)	IV	Adults: 18 g/day (I)[c]	q8h
Fosfomycin, Monurol	3-g PO granules ($)	PO	Adult women with uncomplicated acute cystitis: 3 g (I)	Once
Ganciclovir,[a] Cytovene	500-mg vial ($$)	IV	CMV treatment: Non-neonate: 10 mg/kg/day (I). Neonate: See Chapter 2.	q12h
			CMV suppression: 5 mg/kg (I)	q24h
			VZV: 10 mg/kg/day (III)	q12h
Gentamicin[a]	10-mg/mL vial ($) 40-mg/mL vial ($)	IV, IM	3–7.5 mg/kg/day (I), CF and oncology 7–10 mg/kg/day (II)[b] (See Chapter 4 for q24h dosing.)	q8–24h
		IVesic	0.5 mg/mL in NS × 50–100 mL (III)	q12h

A. SYSTEMIC ANTIMICROBIALS WITH DOSAGE FORMS AND USUAL DOSAGES *(continued)*

Generic and Trade Names	Dosage Form (cost estimate)	Route	Dose (evidence level)	Interval
Glecaprevir/pibrentasvir, Mavyret Doses given in glecaprevir	50-mg/20-mg pellet packet 100-mg/40-mg tab ($$$$$)	PO	≥12 y or ≥45 kg: glecaprevir 300 mg with pibrentasvir 120 mg qd 3–11 y: <20 kg: glecaprevir 150 mg with pibrentasvir 60 mg qd 20–<30 kg: glecaprevir 200 mg with pibrentasvir 80 mg qd 30–<45 kg: glecaprevir 250 mg with pibrentasvir 100 mg qd (I)	q24h
Griseofulvin microsize,[a] Grifulvin V	125-mg/5-mL susp ($) 500-mg tab ($$)	PO	20–25 mg/kg (II), max 1 g (I)	q24h
Griseofulvin ultramicrosize,[a] Gris-PEG	125-, 250-mg tab ($$)	PO	10–15 mg/kg (II), max 750 mg (I)	q24h
Ibrexafungerp, Brexafemme	150-mg tab ($$)	PO	Post-menarchal females 300 mg/day (not per kg) (I)	q12h × 2 doses
Imipenem/cilastatin,[a] Primaxin	250/250-, 500/500-mg vial ($)	IV, IM	60–100 mg/kg/day, max 4 g/day (I) IM form not approved for <12 y	q6h
Imipenem/cilastatin/ relebactam, Recarbrio	500/500/250-mg vial ($$$$)	IV	Adults 2 g/day of imipenem (I)[c]	q6h
Interferon-PEG alfa-2a, Pegasys	All ($$$$) 180-mcg vials, prefilled	SQ	See Hepatitis B virus and Hepatitis C virus in Chapter 7.	Weekly
Isavuconazonium (isavuconazole), Cresemba Dosing in isavuconazole base	186-mg cap (100-mg base) ($$$$)	PO	Adults: 200-mg base per *dose* PO/IV (I) ≥2 y and <13 y: 10-mg base/kg/dose, max 200 mg (III)[b,c]	q8h × 6 doses, then q24h
	372-mg vial (200-mg base) ($$$$)	IV		

Isoniazid,[a] Nydrazid	50-mg/5-mL soln ($$) 100-, 300-mg tab ($) 1,000-mg vial ($$)	PO IV, IM	10–15 mg/kg/day, max 300 mg/day (I)	q12–24h
			With biweekly DOT, dosage is 20–30 mg/kg, max 900 mg/dose (I).	Twice weekly
			In combination with rifapentine (see Rifapentine later in this table): ≥12 y: 15 mg/kg rounded up to the nearest 50 or 100 mg; 900 mg max 2–<12 y: 25 mg/kg; 900 mg max	Once weekly
Itraconazole,[a] Sporanox	50-mg/5-mL soln ($$) (Preferred over caps; see Chapter 5.) 100-mg cap ($)	PO	10 mg/kg/day (II), max 200 mg/day[b]	q12h
			5 mg/kg/day for chronic mucocutaneous *Candida* (II)	q24h
Itraconazole, Tolsura	65-mg cap ($$$$)	PO	Adults 130 mg (not per kg) (I)	q12h–q24h
Ivermectin,[a] Stromectol	3-mg tab ($)	PO	0.15–0.2 mg/kg, no max (I)	1 dose
Ketoconazole,[a] Nizoral	200-mg tab ($)	PO	≥2 y: 3.3–6.6 mg/kg, max 400 mg (I)	q24h
Lefamulin, Xenleta	150-mg vial ($$$) 600-mg tab ($$$$)	 IV PO	Adults (I)[c] 300 mg/day 1,200 mg/day	q12h
Letermovir, Prevymis	240-, 480-mg tab ($$$$)	PO	Adults 480 mg (I), 240 mg if concomitant cyclosporine therapy (I) (See Cytomegalovirus in Chapter 7.)	q24h
	240-, 480-mg vial ($$$$)	IV		
Levofloxacin,[a] Levaquin	125-mg/5-mL soln ($) 250-, 500-, 750-mg tab ($) 500-, 750-mg vial ($) 250-mg/50-mL, 500-mg/100-mL, 750-mg/150-mL IVPB ($)	PO, IV	For postexposure anthrax prophylaxis (I): <50 kg: 16 mg/kg/day, max 500 mg/day ≥50 kg: 500 mg For respiratory infections: <5 y: 20 mg/kg/day (II), ≥5 y: 10 mg/kg/day; max 500 mg/day (II), up to 1,000 mg/dose in children with obesity (III)	 q12h q24h q12h q24h

A. SYSTEMIC ANTIMICROBIALS WITH DOSAGE FORMS AND USUAL DOSAGES *(continued)*

Generic and Trade Names	Dosage Form (cost estimate)	Route	Dose (evidence level)	Interval
Linezolid,[a] Zyvox	100-mg/5-mL susp ($$$) 600-mg tab ($) 200-mg/100-mL, 600-mg/300-mL IVPB ($$)	PO, IV	Birth–11 y (I): 30 mg/kg/day 45 mg/kg/day for MIC 2 (II) >11 y (I): 1.2 g/day	q8h q8h q12h
Maribavir, Livtencity	200-mg tab ($$$$$)	PO	≥12 y: 400 mg (not per kg) (I)	q12h
Mebendazole, Emverm	100-mg chew tab ($$$–$$$$)	PO	≥2 y: 100 mg (not per kg) (I) See parasitic nematodes and helminths (worms) and other indications in Chapter 9, Table 9B.	See Chapter 9.
Mefloquine,[a] Lariam	250-mg tab ($)	PO	See Malaria in Chapter 9, Table 9B.	
Meropenem,[a] Merrem	0.5-, 1-g vial ($)	IV	60 mg/kg/day, max 3 g/day (I) 120 mg/kg/day meningitis (I) or pediatric intensive care unit sepsis with suspected ARC (II), max 6 g/day	q8h
Meropenem/vaborbactam, Vabomere	2-g vial (contains 1-g each meropenem + vaborbactam) ($$$$)	IV	Adults 6 g meropenem/day (I)[c]	q8h
Methenamine hippurate,[a] Hiprex	1-g tab ($)	PO	6–12 y: 1–2 g/day (I) >12 y: 2 g/day (I)	q12h
Methenamine mandelate[a]	0.5-, 1-g tab ($)		<6 y: 75 mg/kg/day (I) 6–12 y: 2 g/day (I) >12 y: 4 g/day (I)	q6h
Metronidazole,[a] Flagyl	250-, 500-mg tab ($) 250-, 500-mg/5-mL susp compounding kit ($) 375-mg cap ($$)	PO	30–50 mg/kg/day, max 2,250 mg/day (I)	q8h

	500-mg/100-mL IVPB ($)	IV	22.5–40 mg/kg/day (II), max 4 g/day (I)	q6–8h
Micafungin,[a] Mycamine	50-, 100-mg vial ($$)	IV	Neonates: 10 mg/kg (II) (See Chapter 2.) 1–<4 mo (I): 4 mg/kg ≥4 mo (I): 2 mg/kg, max 100 mg (I) Esophageal candidiasis ≥4 mo (I): ≤30 kg: 3 mg/kg >30 kg: 2.5 mg/kg, max 150 mg/day Prophylaxis: 1 mg/kg q24h (I) or 3 mg q48h (II)	q24h
Miltefosine, Impavido	50-mg cap Available at www.impavido.com (accessed September 30, 2022)	PO	<12 y: 2.5 mg/kg/day (II) ≥12 y (I): 30–44 kg: 50 mg (not per kg) ≥45 kg: 50 mg (not per kg) (See Leishmaniasis and Amebic meningoencephalitis in Chapter 9, Table 9B.)	bid bid tid
Minocycline, Minocin	50-, 75-, 100-mg cap[a] ($) 50-, 75-, 100-mg tab[a] ($) 100-mg vial ($$$$)	PO, IV	≥8 y: 4 mg/kg/day, max 200 mg/day (I)	q12h
Minocycline ER; Solodyn,[a] Ximino	45-, 55-, 65-, 80-, 90-, 105-, 115-, 135-mg ER tab[a] ($–$$) 45-, 90-, 135-mg ER cap ($$$)	PO	≥12 y: 1 mg/kg/day for acne (I). Round dose to nearest strength tab or cap.	q24h
Moxidectin	2-mg tab Available from Medicines Development for Global Health (info@medicinesdevelopment.com)	PO	≥12 y: 8 mg (I)[c]	Once

A. SYSTEMIC ANTIMICROBIALS WITH DOSAGE FORMS AND USUAL DOSAGES *(continued)*

Generic and Trade Names	Dosage Form (cost estimate)	Route	Dose (evidence level)	Interval
Moxifloxacin,[a] Avelox	400-mg tab ($) 400-mg/250-mL IVPB ($$)	PO, IV	Adults 400 mg/day (I)	q24h
			Studied in but not FDA approved for children (II) IV: 3 mo–<2 y: 12 mg/kg/day 2–<6 y: 10 mg/kg/day ≥6–<12 y: 8 mg/kg/day, max 400 mg/day ≥12–<18 y (weight <45 kg): 8 mg/kg/day	q12h
			≥12–<18 y (weight >45 kg) IV or PO: 400 mg	q24h
Nafcillin,[a] Nallpen	1-, 2-, 10-g vial ($–$$)	IV, IM	150–200 mg/kg/day (II) Max 12 g/day div q4h (I)	q6h
Neomycin[a]	500-mg tab ($)	PO	50–100 mg/kg/day (II), max 12 g/day (I)	q6–8h
Nifurtimox, Lampit	30-, 120-mg tab ($$)	PO	<40 kg: 10–20 mg/kg/day (I) ≥40 kg: 8–10 mg/kg/day (I)	q8h
Nirmatrelvir/ritonavir, Paxlovid		PO	≥12 y and ≥40 kg: 300 mg nirmatrelvir with 100 mg ritonavir	q12h
Nitazoxanide, Alinia	100-mg/5-mL susp ($$$) 500-mg tab[a] ($$$)	PO	1–3 y: 200 mg/day (I) 4–11 y: 400 mg/day (I) 12 y–adults: 1 g/day (I) (See Giardiasis in Chapter 9, Table 9B.)	q12h
Nitrofurantoin,[a] Furadantin	25-mg/5-mL susp ($$$)	PO	5–7 mg/kg/day, max 400 mg/day (I)	q6h
			1–2 mg/kg for UTI prophylaxis (I)	q24h
Nitrofurantoin macrocrystals,[a] Macrodantin	25-, 50-, 100-mg cap ($)	PO	Same as susp	

Nitrofurantoin monohydrate and macrocrystalline,[a] Macrobid	100-mg cap ($)	PO	>12 y: 200 mg/day (I)	q12h
Nystatin,[a] Mycostatin	500,000-U/5-mL susp ($) 500,000-U tabs ($)	PO	Infants 2 mL/dose, children 4–6 mL/dose; to coat PO mucosa (I) Tabs: 3–6 tabs/day	q6h
Obiltoxaximab, Anthim	600-mg/6-mL vial Available from the Strategic National Stockpile	IV	≤15 kg: 32 mg/kg (I) >15–40 kg: 24 mg/kg (I) >40 kg and adults: 16 mg/kg (I)	Once
Omadacycline, Nuzyra	150-mg tab ($$$$)	PO	Adults: 450 mg qd for 2 days, then 300 mg (not per kg) (I)	q24h
	100-mg vial ($$$$)	IV	Adults: 200 mg once, then 100 mg (not per kg) (I)	q24h
Oritavancin, Orbactiv	400-mg vial ($$$$)	IV	Adults: 1.2 g/day (I)[c]	One time
Oseltamivir,[a] Tamiflu (See Influenza in chapters 2 and 7.)	30-mg/5-mL susp ($) 30-, 45-, 75-mg cap ($)	PO	Neonates (II) (See also Chapter 2.) Preterm <38 wk PMA: 2 mg/kg/day Preterm 38–40 wk PMA: 3 mg/kg/day Preterm >40 wk PMA, and full-term, birth–8 mo (I): 6 mg/kg/day 9–11 mo (II): 7 mg/kg/day ≥12 mo (I): (not per kg) ≤15 kg: 60 mg/day >15–23 kg: 90 mg/day >23–40 kg: 120 mg/day >40 kg: 150 mg/day (I)	q12h
			Prophylaxis: Give half the daily dose (I).	q24h
Oxacillin,[a] Bactocill	1-, 2-, 10-g vial ($–$$)	IV, IM	100 mg/kg/day, max 12 g/day (I) 150–200 mg/kg/day for meningitis (III)	q4–6h

A. SYSTEMIC ANTIMICROBIALS WITH DOSAGE FORMS AND USUAL DOSAGES *(continued)*

Generic and Trade Names	Dosage Form (cost estimate)	Route	Dose (evidence level)	Interval
Palivizumab, Synagis	50-, 100-mg vial ($$$$)	IM	15 mg/kg (I) (See Chapter 7 for indications.)	Monthly during RSV season
Penicillin G IM				
– Penicillin G benzathine, Bicillin L-A	600,000 U/mL in 1-, 2-, 4-mL prefilled syringes ($$)	IM	Infants: 50,000 U/kg (I) Children <60 lb: 300,000–600,000 U, ≥60 lb: 900,000 U (not per kg) (I) (FDA approved in 1952 for dosing by pounds) Adults: 1.2–2.4 million U (I) (See also Syphilis in chapters 1 and 2.)	1 dose
– Penicillin G procaine	600,000 U/mL in 1-, 2-mL prefilled syringes ($$)	IM	Infants: 50,000 U/kg (I) (See also Syphilis in Chapter 2.) Children (I): <60 lb: 300,000 U (not per kg) ≥60 lb or >12 y: 600,000 U Adults: 600,000–1,200,000 U (I)	q24h
Penicillin G IV				
– Penicillin G K,[a] Pfizerpen	5-, 20-million U vial ($)	IV, IM	100,000–300,000 U/kg/day (I) Max daily dose 24 million U	q4–6h
– Penicillin G sodium[a]	5-million U vial ($–$$)	IV, IM	100,000–300,000 U/kg/day (I) Max daily dose 24 million U	q4–6h
Penicillin V PO				
– Penicillin V K[a]	125-, 250-mg/5-mL soln ($) 250-, 500-mg tab ($)	PO	25–50 mg/kg/day, max 2 g/day (I)	q6h

Pentamidine; Pentam, Nebupent	300-mg vial[a] ($$$)	IV, IM	4 mg/kg/day (I), max 300 mg	q24h
	300-mg vial ($)	Inhaled	300 mg for prophylaxis (I)	Monthly
Peramivir, Rapivab	200-mg vial ($$$) Available from Optime Care specialty pharmacy	IV	≥6 mo: 12 mg/kg, max 600 mg (I)	One time
Piperacillin/tazobactam,[a] Zosyn	2/0.25-, 3/0.375-, 4/0.5-, 12/1.5-, 36/4.5-g vial ($)	IV	<40 kg: 240–300 mg PIP/kg/day, max 16 g PIP/day (I) Adults 8–12 g/day	q8h
Plazomicin, Zemdri	500-mg vial ($$$$)	IV	Adults 15 mg/kg (I)	q24h
Polymyxin B[a]	500,000-U vial ($). 1 mg = 10,000 U.	IV	2.5 mg/kg/day (I) Adults 2 mg/kg LD, then 2.5–3 mg/kg/day, dose based on TBW, no max (II)	q12h

A. SYSTEMIC ANTIMICROBIALS WITH DOSAGE FORMS AND USUAL DOSAGES *(continued)*

Generic and Trade Names	Dosage Form (cost estimate)	Route	Dose (evidence level)	Interval
Posaconazole,[b] Noxafil	300-mg DR susp packet ($$$$)	PO	*Candida* or *Aspergillus* prophylaxis ≥2 y (I): (not per kg) 10–<12 kg: 90 mg 12–<17 kg: 120 mg 17–<21 kg: 150 mg 21–<26 kg: 180 mg 26–<36 kg: 210 mg 36–40 kg: 240 mg	q12h × 1 day, then q24h
	200-mg/5-mL susp ($$$$)	PO	≥13 y (I): *Candida* or *Aspergillus* prophylaxis: 600 mg/day OPC treatment: 100 mg q12h for 1 day, then 100 mg/day Refractory OPC: 800 mg/day	 q8h q24h q12h
	100-mg DR tab[a] ($$–$$$)	PO	*Candida* or *Aspergillus* prophylaxis ≥2 y (I): ≤40 kg IV: 6 mg/kg q12h for 1 day, then 6 mg/kg >40 kg IV or DR tab (I): 300 mg (not per kg) q12h for 1 day, then 300 mg	q24h
	300-mg/16.7-mL vial ($$$$)	IV		
Praziquantel,[a] Biltricide	600-mg tab ($$)	PO	20–25 mg/kg/dose, no max (I). Round dose to nearest 200 mg (1/3 tab).	q4–6h for 3 doses
Pretomanid	200-mg tab ($$)	PO	Adults: 200 mg (I) In combination with other agents for MDR TB	q24h
Primaquine phosphate[a]	15-mg base tab ($) (26.3-mg primaquine phosphate)	PO	0.5 mg (base)/kg, max 30 mg (III) (See Malaria in Chapter 9, Table 9B.)	q24h
Pyrantel pamoate[a]	250-mg base/5-mL susp ($) (720-mg pyrantel pamoate/5-mL)	PO	11 mg (base)/kg, max 1 g (I)	Once

Pyrazinamide[a]	500-mg tab ($)	PO	30 mg/kg/day, max 2 g/day (I)	q24h
			Biweekly DOT, 50 mg/kg (I), no max	Twice weekly
Quinupristin/dalfopristin, Synercid	150/350-mg vial (500-mg total) ($$$$)	IV	22.5 mg/kg/day (II) Adults 15–22.5 mg/kg/day, no max (I)	q8h q8–12h
Raxibacumab	1,700-mg/35-mL vial Available from the Strategic National Stockpile	IV	≤15 kg: 80 mg/kg (I) >15–50 kg: 60 mg/kg (I) >50 kg: 40 mg/kg (I)	Once
Remdesivir, Veklury	100-mg vial ($$$$)	IV	Aged ≥28 days or weighing 3.0 kg through <40 kg: 5 mg/kg LD, then 2.5 mg/kg (I) ≥40 kg: 200 mg LD, then 100 mg (not per kg) (I)	q24h
Ribavirin,[a] Rebetol	200-mg cap/tab ($)	PO	15 mg/kg/day (I) 12–17 y (not per kg) (I): 47–59 kg: 800 mg/day 60–73 kg: 1,000 mg/day 74–105 kg: 1,200 mg/day >105 kg: 1,400 mg/day Given as combination therapy with other agents (See Hepatitis C virus in Chapter 7.)	q12h
Ribavirin,[a] Virazole	6-g vial ($$$$$)	Inhaled	1 vial by SPAG-2 (See Respiratory syncytial virus in Chapter 7, Table 7C.)	q24h
Rifabutin,[a] Mycobutin	150-mg cap ($$)	PO	5 mg/kg for MAC prophylaxis (II) 10–20 mg/kg for MAC or TB treatment (I) Max 300 mg/day	q24h

A. SYSTEMIC ANTIMICROBIALS WITH DOSAGE FORMS AND USUAL DOSAGES *(continued)*

Generic and Trade Names	Dosage Form (cost estimate)	Route	Dose (evidence level)	Interval
Rifampin,[a] Rifadin	150-, 300-mg cap ($) 600-mg vial ($$–$$$)	PO, IV	15–20 mg/kg, max 600 mg for active TB (in combination) (I) or as single-drug therapy for latent TB	q24h
			With biweekly DOT, dosage is still 15–20 mg/kg/dose, max 600 mg.	Twice weekly
			20 mg/kg/day for 2 days for meningococcus prophylaxis, max 1.2 g/day (I)	q12h
Rifampin/INH/pyrazinamide	75-/50-/150-mg dispersible tab available from the Stop TB Partnership global drug facility (www.stoptb.org/buyers; accessed September 30, 2022)	PO	4–7 kg: 1 tab 8–11 kg: 2 tab 12–15 kg: 3 tabs 16–24 kg: 4 tab	q24h
Rifamycin, Aemcolo	194-mg tab ($$)	PO	Adults: 2 tabs for travelers diarrhea (I)	q12h for 3 days
Rifapentine, Priftin	150-mg tab ($$)	PO	≥12 y and adults: 600 mg/dose (I)	Twice weekly
			>2 y, with INH for treatment of latent TB (I): 10–14 kg: 300 mg 14.1–25 kg: 450 mg 25.1–32 kg: 600 mg 32.1–50 kg: 750 mg >50 kg: 900 mg max	Once weekly
Rifaximin, Xifaxan	200-mg tab ($) 550-mg tab ($$$$) used for adults with IBS-d	PO	20–30 mg/kg/day (II) ≥12 y and adults: 600 mg/day (I) for travelers diarrhea	q8h

Sarecycline, Seysara	60-, 100-, 150-mg tabs ($$$)	PO	For acne (I): ≥9 y: 60 mg (not per kg) 55–84 kg: 100 mg >84 kg: 150 mg	q24h
Secnidazole, Solosec	2-g granules ($$)	PO	≥2 y: 30 mg/kg (III)[c] Adults: 2 g (I)	Once
Sofosbuvir, Sovaldi	150-, 200-mg pellet packet 200-, 400-mg tab ($$$$$)	PO	Children ≥3 y (I): <17 kg: 150 mg 17–<35 kg: 200 mg ≥35 kg: 400 mg ≥12 y: 400 mg (See Hepatitis C virus in Chapter 7.)	q24h
Sofosbuvir/ledipasvir,[a] Harvoni Doses given in sofosbuvir	150-/33.75-mg pellet packet 200-/45-mg pellet packet 200-/45-mg tab 400-/90-mg tab All forms ($$$$$)	PO	Children ≥3 y (I): <17 kg: 37.5 mg ledipasvir with 150 mg sofosbuvir qd 17–<35 kg: 200 mg ≥35 kg: 400 mg (See Hepatitis C virus in Chapter 7.)	q24h
Sofosbuvir/velpatasvir,[a] Epclusa Doses given in sofosbuvir	150-/37.5-mg pellet packet 200-/50-mg pellet packet 200-/50-mg tab 400-/100-mg tab All forms ($$$$)	PO	Children ≥3 y (I): <17 kg: 150 mg 17–<30 kg: 200 mg ≥30 kg: 400 mg (See Hepatitis C virus in Chapter 7.)	q24h
Sofosbuvir/velpatasvir/voxilaprevir, Vosevi	400-/100-/100-mg tab ($$$$$)	PO	Adults 1 tab (I) (See Hepatitis C virus in Chapter 7.)	q24h
Streptomycin[a,b]	1-g vial ($$)	IM, IV	20–40 mg/kg/day, max 1 g/day (I)	q12–24h
Sulfadiazine[a]	500-mg tab ($$$)	PO	120–150 mg/kg/day, max 4–6 g/day (I) (See Chapter 9.)	q6h
			Rheumatic fever secondary prophylaxis 500 mg qd if ≤27 kg, 1,000 mg qd if >27 kg (II)	q24h

A. SYSTEMIC ANTIMICROBIALS WITH DOSAGE FORMS AND USUAL DOSAGES *(continued)*

Generic and Trade Names	Dosage Form (cost estimate)	Route	Dose (evidence level)	Interval
Tecovirimat, Tpoxx	*Available from the FDA* under expanded access protocol as an investigational new drug (www.cdc.gov/poxvirus/monkeypox/clinicians/Tecovirimat.html; reviewed September 15, 2022; accessed September 30, 2022) in 200-mg cap and IV formulations. Informed consent required through CDC Human Research Committee. Case report forms required. For assistance, call the CDC 770/488-7100.	PO, IV	For children <13 kg, IV tecovirimat is preferred to ensure that each dose is taken and tolerated. IV, each infusion given over 6h: <35 kg: 6 mg/kg q12h 35–<120 kg: 200 mg (not per kg) q12h ≥120 kg: 300 mg q12h PO: <6 kg: ¼ cap q12h 6–<13 kg: ½ cap q12h 13–<25 kg: 1 cap q12h 25–<40 kg: 2 caps q12h 40–<120 kg: 3 caps q12h ≥120 kg: 3 caps q8h	q12h (except for ≥120 kg)
Tedizolid, Sivextro	200-mg tab ($$$$) 200-mg vial ($$$$)	PO, IV	≥12 y and adults: 200 mg (I)[c]	q24h
Telavancin, Vibativ	250-, 750-mg vial ($$$$)	IV	Adults: 10 mg/kg (I)[c]	q24h
Tenofovir alafenamide, Vemlidy	25-mg tab ($$$$)	PO	Adults: 25 mg (I)	q24h
Tenofovir disoproxil fumarate, Viread	40 mg per scoop pwd for mixing with soft food ($$$) 150-, 200-, 250-mg tab ($$$$) 300-mg tab[a] ($)	PO	≥2 y, PO pwd: 8 mg/kg (rounded to nearest 20 mg [½ scoop]) (I) Tab (I): 17–<22 kg: 150 mg (not per kg) 22–<28 kg: 200 mg 28–<35 kg: 250 mg ≥35 kg: 300 mg (See Chapter 7 for HBV and HIV-HBV coinfection use.)	q24h

Terbinafine,[a] Lamisil	250-mg tab ($)	PO	Adults 250 mg (I)	q24h
Tetracycline[a]	250-, 500-mg cap ($)	PO	≥8 y: 25–50 mg/kg/day (I)	q6h
Tinidazole,[a] Tindamax	250-, 500-mg tab ($)	PO	50 mg/kg, max 2 g (I) (See Giardiasis in Chapter 9, Table 9B.)	q24h
Tobramycin,[a] Nebcin	10-mg/mL vial ($) 40-mg/mL vial ($)	IV, IM	3–7.5 mg/kg/day (CF 7–10)[b] (See Chapter 4 regarding q24h dosing.)	q8–24h
Tobramycin inhalation[a]; Tobi, Bethkis	300-mg ampule ($$$$)	Inhaled	≥6 y: 600 mg/day (I)	q12h
Tobi Podhaler	28-mg cap for inhalation ($$$$)	Inhaled	≥6 y: 224 mg/day via Podhaler device (I)	q12h
Triclabendazole, Egaten	250-mg scored tab available from the WHO fascioliasis partnership (fasciola@who.int)	PO	≥6 y (I): 20 mg/kg/day, given as 2 doses in 1 day (See Flukes in Chapter 9, Table 9B.)	q12h
Trimethoprim/SMX[a]; Bactrim, Septra	80-mg TMP/400-mg SMX tab (single strength) ($) 160-mg TMP/800-mg SMX tab (double strength) ($) 40-mg TMP/200-mg SMX per 5-mL PO susp ($) 16-mg TMP/80-mg SMX per mL injection soln in 5-, 10-, 30-mL vial ($$)	PO, IV	8 mg TMP/kg/day (I) Adults 2 double-strength tabs/day (I) 12 mg TMP/kg/day for bacterial MIC 1, max 640 mg TMP/day (II)	q12h
			2 mg TMP/kg/day for UTI prophylaxis (I)	q24h
			15–20 mg TMP/kg/day for PJP treatment (I), no max	q6–8h
			150 mg TMP/m²/day, OR 5 mg TMP/kg/day for PJP prophylaxis (I), max 160 mg TMP/day	q12h 3 times/wk OR q24h
Valacyclovir,[a] Valtrex	500-mg, 1-g tab ($) Recipe for preparing susp formulation provided in product labeling	PO	VZV: ≥3 mo: 60 mg/kg/day (I, II) HSV: ≥3 mo: 40 mg/kg/day (II) Max single dose 1 g (I)	q8h q12h

A. SYSTEMIC ANTIMICROBIALS WITH DOSAGE FORMS AND USUAL DOSAGES *(continued)*

Generic and Trade Names	Dosage Form (cost estimate)	Route	Dose (evidence level)	Interval
Valganciclovir,[a] Valcyte	250-mg/5-mL soln ($$) 450-mg tab ($$)	PO	Congenital CMV treatment: 32 mg/kg/day (II) (See Chapter 2.)	q12h
			CMV prophylaxis (in mg, not mg/kg): 7 mg × BSA (m^2) × CrCl (mL/min/1.73 m^2 by using the modified Schwartz formula), max 900 mg (I) (See also Chapter 7.)	q24h
Vancomycin, Vancocin	125-, 250-mg/5-mL susp ($–$$) 125-, 250-mg cap[a] ($–$$)	PO	40 mg/kg/day (I), max 500 mg/day (III)	q6h
	0.5-, 0.75-, 1-, 5-, 10-g vial[a] ($) 1.25-, 1.5-g vial ($–$$) 0.5-, 0.75-, 1-, 1.25-, 1.5-, 1.75-, 2-g IVPB ($$)	IV	30–45 mg/kg/day (I) For invasive MRSA infection, 60–80 mg/kg/day adjusted to achieve AUC:MIC 400, max 3,600 mg/day	q6–8h
Voriconazole,[a,b] Vfend (See Aspergillosis in Chapter 5, Table 5B, under Treatment.)	200-mg/5-mL susp ($$$) 50-, 200-mg tab ($$)	PO	≥2 y and <50 kg: 18 mg/kg/day, max 700 mg/day (I) ≥50 kg: 400–600 mg/day (I)	q12h
	200-mg vial ($$)	IV	≥2 y and <50 kg: 18 mg/kg/day LD for 1 day, then 16 mg/kg/day (I) ≥50 kg: 12 mg/kg/day LD for 1 day, then 8 mg/kg/day (I)	q12h
Zanamivir, Relenza	5-mg blister cap for inhalation ($)	Inhaled	Prophylaxis: ≥5 y: 10 mg/day (I)	q24h
			Treatment: ≥7 y: 20 mg/day (I)	q12h

[a] Available in a generic formulation.
[b] Monitor serum or plasma concentrations.
[c] Also currently under investigation in children younger than the age given for the listed dosages.

B. TOPICAL ANTIMICROBIALS (SKIN, EYE, EAR, MUCOSA)

Generic and Trade Names	Dosage Form	Route	Dose	Interval
Acyclovir, Sitavig	50-mg tab	Buccal	Adults 50 mg, for herpes labialis	One time
Azithromycin, AzaSite	1% ophth soln	Ophth	1 drop	bid for 2 days, then qd for 5 days
Bacitracin[a]	Ophth oint	Ophth	Apply to affected eye.	q3–4h
	Oint[b]	Top	Apply to affected area.	bid–qid
Benzyl alcohol, Ulesfia	5% lotion	Top	Apply to scalp and hair.	Once; repeat in 7 days.
Besifloxacin, Besivance	0.6% ophth susp	Ophth	≥1 y: 1 drop to affected eye	tid
Butenafine; Mentax, Lotrimin-Ultra	1% cream	Top	≥12 y: apply to affected area.	qd
Butoconazole, Gynazole-1	2% prefilled cream	Vag	Adults 1 applicatorful	One time
Ciclopirox[a]; Loprox, Penlac	0.77% cream, gel, lotion	Top	≥10 y: apply to affected area.	bid
	1% shampoo		≥16 y: apply to scalp.	Twice weekly
	8% nail lacquer		≥12 y: apply to infected nail.	qd
Ciprofloxacin,[a] Cetraxal	0.2% otic soln	Otic	≥1 y: apply 3 drops to affected ear.	bid for 7 days
Ciprofloxacin, Ciloxan	0.3% ophth soln[a]	Ophth	Apply to affected eye.	q2h for 2 days, then q4h for 5 days
	0.3% ophth oint			q8h for 2 days, then q12h for 5 days
Ciprofloxacin, Otiprio	6% otic susp	Otic	≥6 mo: 0.1 mL each ear intratympanic, 0.2 mL to external ear canal for otitis externa	One time

B. TOPICAL ANTIMICROBIALS (SKIN, EYE, EAR, MUCOSA) *(continued)*

Generic and Trade Names	Dosage Form	Route	Dose	Interval
Ciprofloxacin + dexamethasone, Ciprodex	0.3% + 0.1% otic soln	Otic	≥6 mo: apply 4 drops to affected ear.	bid for 7 days
Ciprofloxacin + fluocinolone, Otovel	0.3% + 0.025% otic soln	Otic	≥6 mo: instill 0.25 mL to affected ear.	bid for 7 days
Ciprofloxacin + hydrocortisone, Cipro HC	0.2% + 1% otic soln	Otic	≥1 y: apply 3 drops to affected ear.	bid for 7 days
Clindamycin				
Cleocin	100-mg ovule	Vag	1 ovule	qhs for 3 days
	2% vag cream[a]		1 applicatorful	qhs for 3–7 days
Cleocin-T[a]	1% soln, gel, lotion	Top	Apply to affected area.	qd–bid
Clindesse	2% cream	Vag	Adolescents and adults 1 applicatorful	One time
Evoclin[a]	1% foam			qd
Xaciato	2% gel			One time
Clindamycin + benzoyl peroxide, BenzaClin	1% gel[a]	Top	≥12 y: apply to affected area.	bid
Acanya	1.2% gel	Top	Apply small amount to face.	q24h
Clindamycin + tretinoin; Ziana, Veltin	1.2% gel	Top	Apply small amount to face.	hs
Clotrimazole,[a,b] Lotrimin	1% cream, lotion, soln	Top	Apply to affected area.	bid
Gyne-Lotrimin-3[a,b]	2% cream	Vag	≥12 y: 1 applicatorful	qhs for 7–14 days
Gyne-Lotrimin-7[a,b]	1% cream			qhs for 3 days
Clotrimazole + betamethasone,[a] Lotrisone	1% + 0.05% cream, lotion	Top	≥12 y: apply to affected area.	bid
Colistin + neomycin + hydrocortisone;	0.3% otic susp	Otic	Apply 3–4 drops to affected ear canal; may use with wick	q6–8h

Cortisporin; bacitracin + neomycin + polymyxin B + hydrocortisone	Oint	Top	Apply to affected area.	bid–qid
Cortisporin; neomycin + polymyxin B + hydrocortisone	Otic soln[a]	Otic	3 drops to affected ear	bid–qid
	Cream	Top	Apply to affected area.	bid–qid
Dapsone,[a] Aczone	5% gel	Top	≥9 y: apply to affected area.	bid
	7.5% gel			qd
Econazole,[a] Spectazole	1% cream	Top	Apply to affected area.	qd–bid
Efinaconazole, Jublia	10% soln	Top	Apply to toenail.	qd for 48 wk
Erythromycin[a]	0.5% ophth oint	Ophth	Apply to affected eye.	q4h
Akne-Mycin	2% oint	Top	Apply to affected area.	bid
Ery Pads	2% pledgets[a]			
Eryderm,[a] Erygel[a]	2% soln, gel			
Erythromycin + benzoyl peroxide,[a] Benzamycin	3% gel	Top	≥12 y: apply to affected area.	qd–bid
Ganciclovir, Zirgan	0.15% ophth gel	Ophth	≥2 y: 1 drop in affected eye	q3h while awake (5 times/day) until healed, then tid for 7 days
Gatifloxacin, Zymar	0.3% ophth soln	Ophth	1 drop in affected eye	q2h for 2 days, then q6h
Gatifloxacin,[a] Zymaxid	0.5% ophth soln	Ophth	≥1 y: 1 drop in affected eye	q2h for 1 day, then q6h

B. TOPICAL ANTIMICROBIALS (SKIN, EYE, EAR, MUCOSA) *(continued)*

Generic and Trade Names	Dosage Form	Route	Dose	Interval
Gentamicin,[a] Garamycin	0.1% cream, oint	Top	Apply to affected area.	tid–qid
	0.3% ophth soln, oint	Ophth	Apply to affected eye.	q1–4h (soln) q4–8h (oint)
Gentamicin + prednisolone, Pred-G	0.3% ophth soln, oint	Ophth	Adults: apply to affected eye.	q1–4h (soln) qd–tid (oint)
Imiquimod,[a] Aldara	5% cream	Top	≥12y: to perianal or external genital warts	3 times/wk
Ivermectin, Sklice	0.5% lotion	Top	≥6 mo: thoroughly coat hair and scalp, rinse after 10 minutes.	Once
Ivermectin,[a] Soolantra	1% cream	Top	Adults: apply to face.	qd
Ketoconazole,[a] Nizoral	2% shampoo	Top	≥12 y: apply to affected area.	qd
	2% cream			qd–bid
Extina, Xolegel	2% foam, gel			bid
Nizoral A-D	1% shampoo			bid
Levofloxacin[a]; Quixin, Iquix	0.5%, 1.5% ophth soln	Ophth	Apply to affected eye.	q1–4h
Luliconazole, Luzu	1% cream	Top	≥12 y: apply to affected area.	q24h for 1–2 wk
Mafenide, Sulfamylon	8.5% cream	Top	Apply to burn.	qd–bid
	5-g pwd for reconstitution		To keep burn dressing wet	q4–8h as needed
Malathion,[a] Ovide	0.5% soln	Top	≥6 y: apply to hair and scalp.	Once
Maxitrol[a]; neomycin + polymyxin + dexamethasone	Susp, oint	Ophth	Apply to affected eye.	q1–4h (susp) q4h (oint)

Metronidazole[a]	0.75% cream, gel, lotion	Top	Adults: apply to affected area.	bid
	0.75% vag gel	Vag	Adults 1 applicatorful	qd–bid
	1% gel	Top	Adults: apply to affected area.	qd
Noritate	1% cream	Top	Adults: apply to affected area.	qd
Nuvessa	1.3% vag gel	Vag	≥12 y: 1 applicatorful	Once
Miconazole				
Fungoid[a,b]	2% tincture	Top	Apply to affected area.	bid
Micatin[a,b] and others	2% cream, pwd, oint, spray, lotion, gel	Top	Apply to affected area.	qd–bid
Monistat-1[a,b]	1.2-g ovule + 2% cream	Vag	≥12 y: insert one ovule (plus cream to external vulva bid as needed).	Once
Monistat-3[a,b]	200-mg ovule, 4% cream			qhs for 3 days
Monistat-7[a,b]	100-mg ovule, 2% cream			qhs for 7 days
Vusion	0.25% oint	Top	To diaper dermatitis	Each diaper change for 7 days
Minocycline, Amzeeq	4% foam	Top	≥9 y: apply to acne.	qd
Moxifloxacin, Vigamox	0.5% ophth soln	Ophth	Apply to affected eye.	tid
Mupirocin, Bactroban	2% oint,[a] cream[a]	Top	Apply to infected skin.	tid
Naftifine,[a] Naftin	1%, 2% cream, gel	Top	Apply to affected area.	qd
Natamycin, Natacyn	5% ophth soln	Ophth	Adults: apply to affected eye.	q1–4h

B. TOPICAL ANTIMICROBIALS (SKIN, EYE, EAR, MUCOSA) *(continued)*

Generic and Trade Names	Dosage Form	Route	Dose	Interval
Neosporin[a]				
bacitracin + neomycin + polymyxin B	Ophth oint	Ophth	Apply to affected eye.	q4h
	Oint[a,b]	Top	Apply to affected area.	bid–qid
gramicidin + neomycin + polymyxin B	Ophth soln	Ophth	Apply to affected eye.	q4h
Nystatin,[a] Mycostatin	100,000 U/g cream, oint, pwd	Top	Apply to affected area.	bid–qid
Nystatin + triamcinolone,[a] Mycolog II	100,000 U/g + 0.1% cream, oint	Top	Apply to affected area.	bid
Ofloxacin[a]; Floxin Otic, Ocuflox	0.3% otic soln	Otic	5–10 drops to affected ear	qd–bid
	0.3% ophth soln	Ophth	Apply to affected eye.	q1–6h
Oxiconazole, Oxistat	1% cream,[a] lotion	Top	Apply to affected area.	qd–bid
Ozenoxacin, Xepi	1% cream	Top	Apply to affected area.	bid for 5 days
Permethrin, Nix[a,b]	1% cream	Top	Apply to hair/scalp.	Once for 10 min
Elimite[a]	5% cream		Apply to all skin surfaces.	Once for 8–14 h
Piperonyl butoxide + pyrethrins,[a,b] Rid	4% + 0.3% shampoo, gel	Top	Apply to affected area.	Once for 10 min
Polysporin,[a] polymyxin B + bacitracin	Ophth oint	Ophth	Apply to affected eye.	qd–tid
	Oint[b]	Top	Apply to affected area.	
Polytrim,[a] polymyxin B + TMP	Ophth soln	Ophth	Apply to affected eye.	q3–4h
Retapamulin, Altabax	1% oint	Top	Apply thin layer to affected area.	bid for 5 days

Selenium sulfide,[a] Selsun	2.5% lotion 2.25% shampoo	Top	Lather into scalp or affected area.	Twice weekly, then q1–2wk
Selsun Blue[a,b]	1% shampoo			qd
Sertaconazole, Ertaczo	2% cream	Top	≥12 y: apply to affected area.	bid
Silver sulfadiazine,[a] Silvadene	1% cream	Top	Apply to affected area.	qd–bid
Spinosad,[a] Natroba	0.9% susp	Top	Apply to scalp and hair.	Once; may repeat in 7 days
Sulconazole, Exelderm	1% soln, cream	Top	Adults: apply to affected area.	qd–bid
Sulfacetamide sodium[a]	10% soln	Ophth	Apply to affected eye.	q1–3h
	10% ophth oint			q4–6h
	10% lotion, wash, cream	Top	≥12 y: apply to affected area.	bid–qid
Sulfacetamide sodium + prednisolone,[a] Blephamide	10% ophth oint, soln	Ophth	Apply to affected eye.	tid–qid
Tavaborole, Kerydin	5% soln	Top	Adults: apply to toenail.	qd for 48 wk
Terbinafine,[b] Lamisil-AT	1% cream,[a] spray, gel	Top	Apply to affected area.	qd–bid
Terconazole,[a] Terazol	0.4% cream	Vag	Adults 1 applicatorful or 1 suppository	qhs for 7 days
	0.8% cream 80-mg suppository			qhs for 3 days
Tioconazole[a,b]	6.5% oint	Vag	≥12 y: 1 applicatorful	One time
Tobramycin, Tobrex	0.3% soln,[a] oint	Ophth	Apply to affected eye.	q1–4h (soln) q4–8h (oint)
Tobramycin + dexamethasone, Tobradex	0.3% soln,[a] oint	Ophth	Apply to affected eye.	q2–6h (soln) q6–8h (oint)

B. TOPICAL ANTIMICROBIALS (SKIN, EYE, EAR, MUCOSA) *(continued)*

Generic and Trade Names	Dosage Form	Route	Dose	Interval
Tobramycin + loteprednol, Zylet	0.3% + 0.5% ophth susp	Ophth	Adults: apply to affected eye.	q4–6h
Tolnaftate,[a,b] Tinactin	1% cream, soln, pwd, spray	Top	Apply to affected area.	bid
Trifluridine,[a] Viroptic	1% ophth soln	Ophth	1 drop (max 9 drops/day)	q2h

[a] Generic available.

[b] Over the counter.

Appendix

Nomogram for Determining Body Surface Area

Based on the nomogram shown below, a straight line joining the patient's height and weight will intersect the center column at the calculated body surface area (BSA). For children of normal height and weight, the child's weight in pounds is used, and then the examiner reads across to the corresponding BSA in meters. Alternatively, the Mosteller formula can be used.

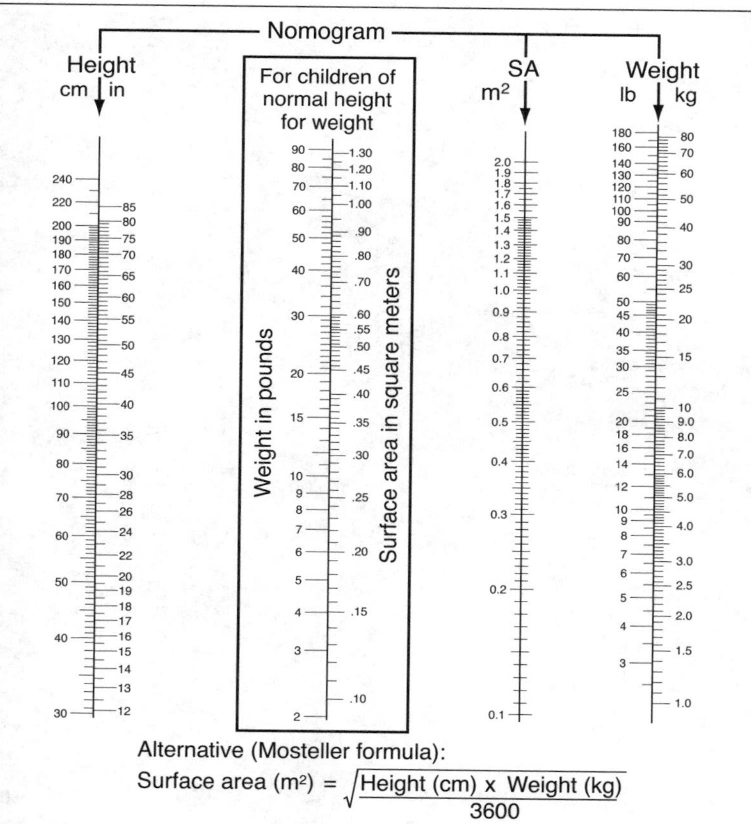

Nomogram and equation to determine body surface area.
From Engorn B, Flerlage J, eds. *The Harriet Lane Handbook*. 20th ed. Elsevier Mosby; 2015. Reproduced with permission from Elsevier.

References

Chapter 1

1. Hultén KG, et al. *Pediatr Infect Dis J.* 2018;37(3):235–241 PMID: 28859018
2. Spaulding AB, et al. *Infect Control Hosp Epidemiol.* 2018;39(12):1487–1490 PMID: 30370879
3. Stevens DL, et al. *Clin Infect Dis.* 2014;59(2):147–159 PMID: 24947530
4. Liu C, et al. *Clin Infect Dis.* 2011;52(3):e18–e55 PMID: 21208910
5. Brown NM, et al. *JAC Antimicrob Resist.* 2021;3(1):dlaa114 PMID: 34223066
6. AAP. *Staphylococcus aureus*. In: Kimberlin DW, et al, eds. *Red Book: 2021–2024 Report of the Committee on Infectious Diseases.* 32nd ed. 2021:678–692
7. AAP. Group A streptococcal infections. In: Kimberlin DW, et al, eds. *Red Book: 2021–2024 Report of the Committee on Infectious Diseases.* 32nd ed. 2021:694–707
8. Bass JW, et al. *Pediatr Infect Dis J.* 1998;17(6):447–452 PMID: 9655532
9. Hatzenbuehler LA, et al. *Pediatr Infect Dis J.* 2014;33(1):89–91 PMID: 24346597
10. Muñoz-Egea MC, et al. *Expert Opin Pharmacother.* 2020;21(8):969–981 PMID: 32200657
11. Zimmermann P, et al. *J Infect.* 2017;74(suppl 1):S136–S142 PMID: 28646953
12. Tebruegge M, et al. *PLoS One.* 2016;26;11(1):e0147513 PMID: 26812154
13. Aliano D, et al. *Pediatr Infect Dis J.* 2020;39(8):671–677 PMID: 32235244
14. Neven Q, et al. *Eur Arch Otorhinolaryngol.* 2020;277(6):1785–1792 PMID: 32144570
15. Nolt D, et al. *Pediatrics.* 2021;148(6):e2021054663 PMID: 34851422
16. AAP. Tuberculosis. In: Kimberlin DW, et al, eds. *Red Book: 2021–2024 Report of the Committee on Infectious Diseases.* 32nd ed. 2021:786–814
17. Bradley JS, et al. *Pediatrics.* 2014;133(5):e1411–e1436 PMID: 24777226
18. Oehler RL, et al. *Lancet Infect Dis.* 2009;9(7):439–447 PMID: 19555903
19. Thomas N, et al. *Expert Rev Anti Infect Ther.* 2011;9(2):215–226 PMID: 21342069
20. Bula-Rudas FJ, et al. *Pediatr Rev.* 2018;39(10):490–500 PMID: 30275032
21. AAP. Bite wounds. In: Kimberlin DW, et al, eds. *Red Book: 2021–2024 Report of the Committee on Infectious Diseases.* 32nd ed. 2021:169–175
22. Talan DA, et al. *N Engl J Med.* 1999;340(2):85–92 PMID: 9887159
23. Goldstein EJ, et al. *Antimicrob Agents Chemother.* 2012;56(12):6319–6323 PMID: 23027193
24. AAP. Rabies. In: Kimberlin DW, et al, eds. *Red Book: 2021–2024 Report of the Committee on Infectious Diseases.* 32nd ed. 2021:619–627
25. Talan DA, et al. *Clin Infect Dis.* 2003;37(11):1481–1489 PMID: 14614671
26. Miller LG, et al. *N Engl J Med.* 2015;372(12):1093–1103 PMID: 25785967
27. Talan DA, et al. *N Engl J Med.* 2016;374(9):823–832 PMID: 26962903
28. Moran GJ, et al. *JAMA.* 2017;317(20):2088–2096 PMID: 28535235
29. Bradley J, et al. *Pediatrics.* 2017;139(3):e20162477 PMID: 28202770
30. AAP. *Haemophilus influenzae* infections. In: Kimberlin DW, et al, eds. *Red Book: 2021–2024 Report of the Committee on Infectious Diseases.* 32nd ed. 2021:345–354
31. Brindle R, et al. *JAMA Dermatol.* 2019;155(9):1033–1040 PMID: 31188407
32. Koning S, et al. *Cochrane Database Syst Rev.* 2012;(1):CD003261 PMID: 22258953
33. Lin HW, et al. *Clin Pediatr (Phila).* 2009;48(6):583–587 PMID: 19286617
34. Pannaraj PS, et al. *Clin Infect Dis.* 2006;43(8):953–960 PMID: 16983604
35. Young BC, et al. *Elife.* 2019;8:e42486 PMID: 30794157
36. Schröder A, et al. *BMC Infect Dis.* 2019;19(1):317 PMID: 30975101
37. Zundel S, et al. *Eur J Pediatr Surg.* 2017;27(2):127–137 PMID: 27380058
38. Totapally BR. *Pediatr Infect Dis J.* 2017;36(7):641–644 PMID: 28005689
39. Levett D, et al. *Cochrane Database Syst Rev.* 2015;(1):CD007937 PMID: 25879088
40. Stevens DL, et al. *Infect Dis Clin North Am.* 2021;35(1):135–155 PMID: 33303335
41. Daum RS. *N Engl J Med.* 2007;357(4):380–390 PMID: 17652653
42. Sharara SL, et al. *Infect Dis Clin North Am.* 2021;35(1):107–133 PMID: 33303331
43. Elliott SP. *Clin Microbiol Rev.* 2007;20(1):13–22 PMID: 17223620

44. AAP. Rat-bite fever. In: Kimberlin DW, et al, eds. *Red Book: 2021–2024 Report of the Committee on Infectious Diseases*. 32nd ed. 2021:627–628
45. Braunstein I, et al. *Pediatr Dermatol.* 2014;31(3):305–308 PMID: 24033633
46. Liy-Wong C, et al. *Pediatr Dermatol.* 2021;38(1):149–153 PMID: 33283348
47. Woods CR, et al. *J Pediatric Infect Dis Soc.* 2021:10(8):801–844 PMID: 34350458
48. Saavedra-Lozano J, et al. *Pediatr Infect Dis J.* 2017;36(8):788–799 PMID: 28708801
49. Keren R, et al. *JAMA Pediatr.* 2015;169(2):120–128 PMID: 25506733
50. McNeil JC, et al. *Pediatr Infect Dis J.* 2017;36(6):572–577 PMID: 28027279
51. Pääkkönen M. *Pediatric Health Med Ther.* 2017;8:65–68 PMID: 29388627
52. Montgomery NI, et al. *Orthop Clin North Am.* 2017;48(2):209–216 PMID: 28336043
53. Arnold JC, et al. *Pediatrics.* 2012;130(4):e821–e828 PMID: 22966033
54. Chou AC, et al. *J Pediatr Orthop.* 2016;36(2):173–177 PMID: 25929777
55. Delgado-Noguera MF, et al. *Cochrane Database Syst Rev.* 2018;(11):CD012125 PMID: 30480764
56. St Cyr S, et al. *MMWR Morb Mortal Wkly Rep.* 2020;69(50):1911–1916 PMID: 33332296
57. Workowski KA, et al. *MMWR Recomm Rep.* 2021;70(4):1–187 PMID: 34292926
58. AAP. Gonococcal infections. In: Kimberlin DW, et al, eds. *Red Book: 2021–2024 Report of the Committee on Infectious Diseases.* 32nd ed. 2021:338–344
59. Peltola H, et al. *N Engl J Med.* 2014;370(4):352–360 PMID: 24450893
60. Funk SS, et al. *Orthop Clin North Am.* 2017;48(2):199–208 PMID: 28336042
61. Messina AF, et al. *Pediatr Infect Dis J.* 2011;30(12):1019–1021 PMID: 21817950
62. Howard-Jones AR, et al. *J Paediatr Child Health.* 2013;49(9):760–768 PMID: 23745943
63. Le Vavasseur B, et al. *Antibiotics (Basel).* 2022;11(4):486 PMID: 35453237
64. Kok EY, et al. *Antimicrob Agents Chemother.* 2018;62(5):e00084–18 PMID: 29530845
65. Chen CJ, et al. *Pediatr Infect Dis J.* 2007;26(11):985–988 PMID: 17984803
66. Volk A, et al. *Pediatr Emerg Care.* 2017;33(11):724–729 PMID: 26785095
67. Kornelsen E, et al. *Cochrane Database Syst Rev.* 2021;(4):CD013535 PMID: 33908631
68. McKenna D, et al. *Clin Case Rep.* 2019;7(3):593–594 PMID: 30899507
69. Seltz LB, et al. *Pediatrics.* 2011;127(3):e566–e572 PMID: 21321025
70. Anosike BI, et al. *J Pediatric Infect Dis Soc.* 2022;11(5):214–220 PMID: 3543876671
71. Saltagi MZ, et al. *Allergy Rhinol (Providence).* 2022;13:21526575221097311 PMID: 35496892
72. McDermott SM, et al. *Otolaryngol Head Neck Surg.* 2020;194599820918832 PMID: 32396416
73. Murphy DC, et al. *J Paediatr Child Health.* 2021;57(2):227–233 PMID: 32987452
74. Williams KJ, et al. *Curr Opin Ophthalmol.* 2019;30(5):349–355 PMID: 31261188
75. Sheikh A, et al. *Cochrane Database Syst Rev.* 2012;(9):CD001211 PMID: 22972049
76. Johnson D, et al. *JAMA.* 2022;327(22):2231–2237 PMID: 35699701
77. Wilhelmus KR. *Cochrane Database Syst Rev.* 2015;(1):CD002898 PMID: 25879115
78. Sibley D, et al. *Eye (Lond).* 2020;34(12):2219–2226 PMID: 32843744
79. Azher TN, et al. *Clin Ophthalmol.* 2017;11:185–191 PMID: 28176902
80. Faden HS. *Clin Pediatr (Phila).* 2006;45(6):567–569 PMID: 16893863
81. Khan S, et al. *J Pediatr Ophthalmol Strabismus.* 2014;51(3):140–153 PMID: 24877526
82. Schwartz SG, et al. *Expert Rev Ophthalmol.* 2014;9(5):425–430 PMID: 26609317
83. Pappas PG, et al. *Clin Infect Dis.* 2016;62(4):e1–e50 PMID: 26679628
84. Munro M, et al. *Microorganisms.* 2019;8(1):55 PMID: 31905656
85. Larochelle MB, et al. *Am J Ophthalmol.* 2017;175:8–15 PMID: 27746296
86. Groth A, et al. *Int J Pediatr Otorhinolaryngol.* 2012;76(10):1494–1500 PMID: 22832239
87. Loh R, et al. *J Laryngol Otol.* 2018;132(2):96–104 PMID: 28879826
88. Laulajainen-Hongisto A, et al. *Int J Pediatr Otorhinolaryngol.* 2014;78(12):2072–2078 PMID: 25281339
89. Head K, et al. *Cochrane Database Syst Rev.* 2020;(1):CD013056 PMID: 31902139
90. Haynes DS, et al. *Otolaryngol Clin North Am.* 2007;40(3):669–683 PMID: 17544701
91. Kaushik V, et al. *Cochrane Database Syst Rev.* 2010;(1):CD004740 PMID: 20091565
92. Rosenfeld RM, et al. *Otolaryngol Head Neck Surg.* 2014;150(1)(suppl):S1–S24 PMID: 24491310
93. Izurieta P, et al. *Hum Vaccin Immunother.* 2022;18(1):2013693 PMID: 35020530
94. Vadlamudi NK, et al. *J Antimicrob Chemother.* 2021;76(9):2419–2427 PMID: 34021757
95. Wald ER, et al. *Pediatr Infect Dis J.* 2018;37(12):1255–1257 PMID: 29570583

96. Lieberthal AS, et al. *Pediatrics*. 2013;131(3):e964–e999 PMID: 23439909
97. Venekamp RP, et al. *Cochrane Database Syst Rev*. 2015;(6):CD000219 PMID: 26099233
98. Shaikh N, et al. *J Pediatr*. 2017;189:54–60.e3 PMID: 28666536
99. Suzuki HG, et al. *BMJ Open*. 2020;10(5):e035343 PMID: 32371515
100. Van Dyke MK, et al. *Pediatr Infect Dis J*. 2017;36(3):274–281 PMID: 27918383
101. Olarte L, et al. *J Clin Microbiol*. 2017;55(3):724–734 PMID: 27847379
102. Sader HS, et al. *Open Forum Infect Dis*. 2019;6(suppl 1):S14–S23 PMID: 30895211
103. Gregory J, et al. *JAMA Netw Open*. 2021;4(3):e212713 PMID: 33755168
104. Wald ER, et al. *Pediatrics*. 2013;132(1):e262–e280 PMID: 23796742
105. Shaikh N, et al. *Cochrane Database Syst Rev*. 2014;(10):CD007909 PMID: 25347280
106. Chow AW, et al. *Clin Infect Dis*. 2012;54(8):e72–e112 PMID: 22438350
107. Ogle OE. *Dent Clin North Am*. 2017;61(2):235–252 PMID: 28317564
108. Cope AL, et al. *Cochrane Database Syst Rev*. 2018;(9):CD010136 PMID: 30259968
109. AAP. Diphtheria. In: Kimberlin DW, et al, eds. *Red Book: 2021–2024 Report of the Committee on Infectious Diseases*. 32nd ed. 2021:304–307
110. Tibballs J, et al. *J Paediatr Child Health*. 2011;47(3):77–82 PMID: 21091577
111. Sobol SE, et al. *Otolaryngol Clin North Am*. 2008;41(3):551–566 PMID: 18435998
112. Nasser M, et al. *Cochrane Database Syst Rev*. 2008;(4):CD006700 PMID: 18843726
113. Amir J, et al. *BMJ*. 1997;314(7097):1800–1803 PMID: 9224082
114. Kimberlin DW, et al. *Clin Infect Dis*. 2010;50(2):221–228 PMID: 20014952
115. Riordan T. *Clin Microbiol Rev*. 2007;20(4):622–659 PMID: 17934077
116. Correia MS, et al. *J Emerg Med*. 2019;56(6):709–712 PMID: 31229258
117. Ridgway JM, et al. *Am J Otolaryngol*. 2010;31(1):38–45 PMID: 19944898
118. Lee WS, et al. *J Microbiol Immunol Infect*. 2020;53(4):513–517 PMID: 32303484
119. Valerio L, et al. *J Intern Med*. 2021;289(3):325–339 PMID: 32445216
120. Carbone PN, et al. *Int J Pediatr Otorhinolaryngol*. 2012;76(11):1647–1653 PMID: 22921604
121. Hur K, et al. *Laryngoscope*. 2018;128(1):72–77 PMID: 28561258
122. Shulman ST, et al. *Clin Infect Dis*. 2012;55(10):e86–e102 PMID: 22965026
123. van Driel ML, et al. *Cochrane Database Syst Rev*. 2021;(3):CD004406 PMID: 33728634
124. Skoog Ståhlgren G, et al. *BMJ*. 2019;367:l5337 PMID: 31585944
125. Altamimi S, et al. *Cochrane Database Syst Rev*. 2012;(8):CD004872 PMID: 22895944
126. Abdel-Haq N, et al. *Pediatr Infect Dis J*. 2012;31(7):696–699 PMID: 22481424
127. Cheng J, et al. *Otolaryngol Head Neck Surg*. 2013;148(6):1037–1042 PMID: 23520072
128. Casazza G, et al. *Otolaryngol Head Neck Surg*. 2019;160(3):546–549 PMID: 30348058
129. Lemaître C, et al. *Pediatr Infect Dis J*. 2013;32(10):1146–1149 PMID: 23722529
130. Ramgopal S, et al. *Pediatr Emerg Care*. 2017;33(2):112–115 PMID: 26785088
131. Brook I. *J Chemother*. 2016;28(3):143–150 PMID: 26365224
132. Wardlaw AJ, et al. *J Asthma Allergy*. 2021;14:557–573 PMID: 34079294
133. Agarwal R, et al. *Eur Respir J*. 2018;52(3):1801159 PMID: 30049743
134. Agarwal R, et al. *Chest*. 2018;153(3):656–664 PMID: 29331473
135. Meissner HC. *N Engl J Med*. 2016;374(1):62–72 PMID: 26735994
136. Hahn A, et al. *J Investig Med*. 2021;69(7):1350–1359 PMID: 34021052
137. Hahn A, et al. *J Pediatr Pharmacol Ther*. 2018;23(5):379–389 PMID: 30429692
138. Chmiel JF, et al. *Ann Am Thorac Soc*. 2014;11(7):1120–1129 PMID: 25102221
139. Flume PA, et al. *Am J Respir Crit Care Med*. 2009;180(9):802–808 PMID: 19729669
140. Saint GL, et al. *Arch Dis Child*. 2022;107(5):479–485 PMID: 34740877
141. Ng C, et al. *Curr Opin Pulm Med*. 2020;26(6):679–684 PMID: 32890021
142. Chmiel JF, et al. *Ann Am Thorac Soc*. 2014;11(8):1298–1306 PMID: 25167882
143. Waters V, et al. *Cochrane Database Syst Rev*. 2020;(6):CD010004 PMID: 32521055
144. Cogen JD, et al. *Ann Am Thorac Soc*. 2020;17(12):1590–1598 PMID: 32726564
145. Smith S, et al. *Cochrane Database Syst Rev*. 2020;(5):CD006961 PMID: 32412092
146. Langton Hewer SC, et al. *Cochrane Database Syst Rev*. 2017;(4):CD004197 PMID: 28440853
147. Smith S, et al. *Cochrane Database Syst Rev*. 2018;(3):CD001021 PMID: 29607494
148. Flume PA, et al. *J Cyst Fibros*. 2016;15(6):809–815 PMID: 27233377

149. Mogayzel PJ Jr, et al. *Am J Respir Crit Care Med.* 2013;187(7):680–689 PMID: 23540878
150. Southern KW, et al. *Cochrane Database Syst Rev.* 2012;(11):CD002203 PMID: 23152214
151. Conole D, et al. *Drugs.* 2014;74(3):377–387 PMID: 24510624
152. Nichols DP, et al. *Thorax.* 2022;77(6):581–588 PMID: 34706982
153. AAP. Pertussis (whooping cough). In: Kimberlin DW, et al, eds. *Red Book: 2021–2024 Report of the Committee on Infectious Diseases.* 32nd ed. 2021:578–589
154. Kilgore PE, et al. *Clin Microbiol Rev.* 2016;29(3):449–486 PMID: 27029594
155. Wang K, et al. *Cochrane Database Syst Rev.* 2014;(9):CD003257 PMID: 25243777
156. Jain S, et al. *N Engl J Med.* 2015;372(9):835–845 PMID: 25714161
157. Bradley JS, et al. *Clin Infect Dis.* 2011;53(7):e25–e76 PMID: 21880587
158. Blumer JL, et al. *Pediatr Infect Dis J.* 2016;35(7):760–766 PMID: 27078119
159. Ambroggio L, et al. *Pediatr Pulmonol.* 2016;51(5):541–548 PMID: 26367389
160. Williams DJ, et al. *JAMA Pediatr.* 2017;171(12):1184–1191 PMID: 29084336
161. Leyenaar JK, et al. *Pediatr Infect Dis J.* 2014;33(4):387–392 PMID: 24168982
162. Same RG, et al. *J Pediatric Infect Dis Soc.* 2021;10(3):267–273 PMID: 32525203
163. Dorman RM, et al. *J Pediatr Surg.* 2016;51(6):885–890 PMID: 27032611
164. Islam S, et al. *J Pediatr Surg.* 2012;47(11):2101–2110 PMID: 23164006
165. Redden MD, et al. *Cochrane Database Syst Rev.* 2017;(3):CD010651 PMID: 28304084
166. Oyetunji TA, et al. *J Pediatr Surg.* 2020;55(11):2352–2355 PMID: 31983399
167. Randolph AG, et al. *Clin Infect Dis.* 2019;68(3):365–372 PMID: 29893805
168. Bradley JS, et al. *Pediatr Infect Dis J.* 2007;26(10):868–878 PMID: 17901791
169. Hidron AI, et al. *Lancet Infect Dis.* 2009;9(6):384–392 PMID: 19467478
170. Frush JM, et al. *J Hosp Med.* 2018;13(12):848–852 PMID: 30379141
171. Wunderink RG, et al. *Clin Infect Dis.* 2012;54(5):621–629 PMID: 22247123
172. Freifeld AG, et al. *Clin Infect Dis.* 2011;52(4):e56–e93 PMID: 21258094
173. Kalil AC, et al. *Clin Infect Dis.* 2016;63(5):e61–e111 PMID: 27418577
174. Chang I, et al. *Paediatr Respir Rev.* 2016;20:10–16 PMID: 26527358
175. Sweeney DA, et al. *Clin Microbiol Infect.* 2019;25(10):1195–1199 PMID: 31035015
176. AAP. Chlamydial infections. In: Kimberlin DW, et al, eds. *Red Book: 2021–2024 Report of the Committee on Infectious Diseases.* 32nd ed. 2021:256–266
177. AAP. Cytomegalovirus infection. In: Kimberlin DW, et al, eds. *Red Book: 2021–2024 Report of the Committee on Infectious Diseases.* 32nd ed. 2021:294–300
178. Kotton CN, et al. *Transplantation.* 2018;102(6):900–931 PMID: 29596116
179. Limaye AP, et al. *Clin Microbiol Rev.* 2020;34(1):e00043-19 PMID: 33115722
180. Danziger-Isakov L, et al. *J Pediatric Infect Dis Soc.* 2018;7(suppl 2):S72–S74 PMID: 30590625
181. AAP. Tularemia. In: Kimberlin DW, et al, eds. *Red Book: 2021–2024 Report of the Committee on Infectious Diseases.* 32nd ed. 2021:822–825
182. Galgiani JN, et al. *Clin Infect Dis.* 2016;63(6):e112–e146 PMID: 27470238
183. AAP. Coccidioidomycosis. In: Kimberlin DW, et al, eds. *Red Book: 2021–2024 Report of the Committee on Infectious Diseases.* 32nd ed. 2021:277–280
184. AAP. Histoplasmosis. In: Kimberlin DW, et al, eds. *Red Book: 2021–2024 Report of the Committee on Infectious Diseases.* 32nd ed. 2021:417–421
185. Wheat LJ, et al. *Clin Infect Dis.* 2007;45(7):807–825 PMID: 17806045
186. Salmanton-García J, et al. *J Antimicrob Chemother.* 2019;74(11):3315–3327 PMID: 31393591
187. Marty FM, et al. *Lancet Infect Dis.* 2016;16(7):828–837 PMID: 26969258
188. Uyeki TM, et al. *Clin Infect Dis.* 2019;68(6):895–902 PMID: 30834445
189. AAP Committee on Infectious Diseases. *Pediatrics.* 2020;146(4):e2020024588 PMID: 32900875
190. Kimberlin DW, et al. *J Infect Dis.* 2013;207(5):709–720 PMID: 23230059
191. Stewart AG, et al. *Open Forum Infect Dis.* 2021;8(8):ofab387 PMID: 34395716
192. Harris PNA, et al. *JAMA.* 2018;320(10):984–994 PMID: 30208454
193. Daley CL, et al. *Clin Infect Dis.* 2020;71(4):905–913 PMID: 32797222
194. Gardiner SJ. *Cochrane Database Syst Rev.* 2015;(1):CD004875 PMID: 25566754
195. Lee H, et al. *Expert Rev Anti Infect Ther.* 2018;16(1):23–34 PMID: 29212389

196. Panel on the Prevention and Treatment of Opportunistic Infections in HIV-Exposed and HIV-Infected Children. Guidelines for the prevention and treatment of opportunistic infections in HIV-exposed and HIV-infected children. Updated September 2, 2022. Accessed October 3, 2022. https://clinicalinfo.hiv.gov/en/guidelines/hiv-clinical-guidelines-pediatric-opportunistic-infections/updates-guidelines-prevention
197. Caselli D, et al. *J Pediatr.* 2014;164(2):389–392.e1 PMID: 24252793
198. Micek ST, et al. *Medicine (Baltimore).* 2011;90(6):390–395 PMID: 22033455
199. Reynolds D, et al. *Drugs.* 2021;81(18):2117–2131 PMID: 34743315
200. AAP. Respiratory syncytial virus. In: Kimberlin DW, et al, eds. *Red Book: 2021–2024 Report of the Committee on Infectious Diseases.* 32nd ed. 2021:628–636
201. Berger CA, et al. *Ann Am Thorac Soc.* 2020;17(8):911–917 PMID: 32464069
202. Jaganath D, et al. *Infect Dis Clin North Am.* 2022;36(1):49–71 PMID: 35168714
203. Sterling TR, et al. *MMWR Recomm Rep.* 2020;69(1):1–11 PMID: 32053584
204. Scarfone R, et al. *J Pediatr.* 2017;187:200–205.e1 PMID: 28526220
205. Aronson PL, et al. *Pediatrics.* 2018;142(6):e20181879 PMID: 30425130
206. Aronson PL, et al. *Pediatrics.* 2019;144(1):e20183604 PMID: 31167938
207. Greenhow TL, et al. *Pediatrics.* 2017;139(4):e20162098 PMID: 28283611
208. Pantell RH, et al. *Adv Pediatr.* 2018;65(1):173–208 PMID: 30053923
209. Kuppermann N, et al. *JAMA Pediatr.* 2019;173(4):342–351 PMID: 30776077
210. McMullan BJ, et al. *JAMA Pediatr.* 2016;170(10):979–986 PMID: 27533601
211. Ruiz J, et al. *Minerva Pediatr.* 2018 PMID: 29651827
212. Russell CD, et al. *J Med Microbiol.* 2014;63(pt 6):841–848 PMID: 24623637
213. Ligon J, et al. *Pediatr Infect Dis J.* 2014;33(5):e132–e134 PMID: 24732394
214. Arrieta AC, et al. *Pediatr Infect Dis J.* 2018;37(9):893–900 PMID: 29406465
215. Baddour LM, et al. *Circulation.* 2015;132(15):1435–1486 [Erratum. *Circulation.* 2015;132(17):e215. Erratum. *Circulation.* 2016;134(8):e113] PMID: 26373316
216. Baltimore RS, et al. *Circulation.* 2015;132(15):1487–1515 PMID: 26373317
217. Eleyan L, et al. *Eur J Pediatr.* 2021;180(10):3089–3100 PMID: 33852085
218. Abdelghani M, et al. *J Am Heart Assoc.* 2018;7(13):e008163 PMID: 29934419
219. Dixon G, et al. *Curr Opin Infect Dis.* 2017;30(3):257–267 PMID: 28319472
220. Wilson WR, et al. *Circulation.* 2021;143(20):e963–e978 PMID: 33853363
221. Williams ML, et al. *Ther Adv Cardiovasc Dis.* 2021;15:17539447211002687 PMID: 33784909
222. Radovanovic M, et al. *J Cardiovasc Dev Dis.* 2022;9(4):103 PMID: 35448079
223. Abdel-Haq N, et al. *Int J Pediatr.* 2018;2018:5450697 PMID: 30532791
224. Shane AL, et al. *Clin Infect Dis.* 2017;65(12):1963–1973 PMID: 29194529
225. Denno DM, et al. *Clin Infect Dis.* 2012;55(7):897–904 PMID: 22700832
226. Freedman SB, et al. *Clin Infect Dis.* 2016;62(10):1251–1258 PMID: 26917812
227. Bennish ML, et al. *Clin Infect Dis.* 2006;42(3):356–362 PMID: 16392080
228. Smith KE, et al. *Pediatr Infect Dis J.* 2012;31(1):37–41 PMID: 21892124
229. Imdad A, et al. *Cochrane Database Syst Rev.* 2021;(7):CD012997 PMID: 34219224
230. Florez ID, et al. *Curr Infect Dis Rep.* 2020;22(2):4 PMID: 31993758
231. Ashkenazi S, et al. *Pediatr Infect Dis J.* 2016;35(6):698–700 PMID: 26986771
232. Taylor DN, et al. *J Travel Med.* 2017;24(suppl 1):S17–S22 PMID: 28520998
233. Riddle MS, et al. *J Travel Med.* 2017;24(suppl 1):S57–S74 PMID: 28521004
234. Williams PCM, et al. *Paediatr Int Child Health.* 2018;38(suppl 1):S50–S65 PMID: 29790845
235. *Med Lett Drugs Ther.* 2019;61(1582):153–160 PMID: 31599872
236. Adler AV, et al. *J Travel Med.* 2022;29(1):taab099 PMID: 34230966
237. Kantele A, et al. *Clin Infect Dis.* 2015;60(6):837–846 PMID: 25613287
238. Riddle MS, et al. *Clin Infect Dis.* 2008;47(8):1007–1014 PMID: 18781873
239. Janda JM, et al. *Clin Microbiol Rev.* 2010;23(1):35–73 PMID: 20065325
240. AAP. *Campylobacter* infections. In: Kimberlin DW, et al, eds. *Red Book: 2021–2024 Report of the Committee on Infectious Diseases.* 32nd ed. 2021:243–246
241. Same RG, et al. *Pediatr Rev.* 2018;39(11):533–541 PMID: 30385582

242. Kanungo S, et al. *Lancet*. 2022;399(10333):1429–1440 PMID: 35397865
243. Connor BA, et al. *J Travel Med*. 2019;26(8):taz085 PMID: 31804684
244. AAP. *Clostridioides difficile* (formerly *Clostridium difficile*). In: Kimberlin DW, et al, eds. *Red Book: 2021–2024 Report of the Committee on Infectious Diseases*. 32nd ed. 2021:271–276
245. McDonald LC, et al. *Clin Infect Dis*. 2018;66(7):987–994 PMID: 29562266
246. Adams DJ, et al. *J Pediatric Infect Dis Soc*. 2021;10(suppl 3):S22–S26 PMID: 34791398
247. O'Gorman MA, et al. *J Pediatric Infect Dis Soc*. 2018;7(3):210–218 PMID: 28575523
248. Weng MK, et al. *Epidemiol Infect*. 2019;147:e172 PMID: 31063097
249. Mühlen S, et al. *Antimicrob Agents Chemother*. 2020;64(4):e02159–19 PMID: 32015030
250. Jones NL, et al. *J Pediatr Gastroenterol Nutr*. 2017;64(6):991–1003 PMID: 28541262
251. Crowe SE. *N Engl J Med*. 2019;380(12):1158–1165 PMID: 30893536
252. AAP. *Helicobacter pylori* infections. In: Kimberlin DW, et al, eds. *Red Book: 2021–2024 Report of the Committee on Infectious Diseases*. 32nd ed. 2021:357–362
253. Kalach N, et al. *Helicobacter*. 2017;22(suppl 1) PMID: 28891139
254. AAP. *Giardia duodenalis* (formerly *Giardia lamblia* and *Giardia intestinalis*) infections. In: Kimberlin DW, et al, eds. *Red Book: 2021–2024 Report of the Committee on Infectious Diseases*. 32nd ed. 2021:335–338
255. Ordóñez-Mena JM, et al. *J Antimicrob Chemother*. 2018;73(3):596–606 PMID: 29186570
256. Leinert JL, et al. *Antibiotics (Basel)*. 2021;10(10):1187 PMID: 34680768
257. AAP. *Salmonella* infections. In: Kimberlin DW, et al, eds. *Red Book: 2021–2024 Report of the Committee on Infectious Diseases*. 32nd ed. 2021:655–663
258. Frenck RW Jr, et al. *Clin Infect Dis*. 2004;38(7):951–957 PMID: 15034826
259. Trivedi NA, et al. *J Postgrad Med*. 2012;58(2):112–118 PMID: 22718054
260. Effa EE, et al. *Cochrane Database Syst Rev*. 2011;(10):CD004530 PMID: 21975746
261. Begum B, et al. *Mymensingh Med J*. 2014;23(3):441–448 PMID: 25178594
262. Andrews JR, et al. *N Engl J Med*. 2018;379(16):1493–1495 PMID: 30332569
263. Centers for Disease Control and Prevention. National Antimicrobial Resistance Monitoring System for Enteric Bacteria (NARMS). Reviewed June 22, 2022. Accessed October 3, 2022. www.cdc.gov/narms/reports/index.html
264. Kotloff KL, et al. *Lancet*. 2018;391(10122):801–812 PMID: 29254859
265. AAP. *Shigella* infections. In: Kimberlin DW, et al, eds. *Red Book: 2021–2024 Report of the Committee on Infectious Diseases*. 32nd ed. 2021:668–672
266. Abdel-Haq NM, et al. *Pediatr Infect Dis J*. 2000;19(10):954–958 PMID: 11055595
267. Abdel-Haq NM, et al. *Int J Antimicrob Agents*. 2006;27(5):449–452 PMID: 16621458
268. El Qouqa IA, et al. *Int J Infect Dis*. 2011;15(1):e48–e53 PMID: 21131221
269. Yousef Y, et al. *J Pediatr Surg*. 2018;53(2):250–255 PMID: 29223673
270. Marino NE, et al. *Surg Infect (Larchmt)*. 2017;18(8):894–903 PMID: 29064344
271. Anandalwar SP, et al. *JAMA Surg*. 2018;153(11):1021–1027 PMID: 30046808
272. Solomkin JS, et al. *Clin Infect Dis*. 2010;50(2):133–164 PMID: 20034345
273. Sawyer RG, et al. *N Engl J Med*. 2015;372(21):1996–2005 PMID: 25992746
274. Fraser JD, et al. *J Pediatr Surg*. 2010;45(6):1198–1202 PMID: 20620320
275. Kronman MP, et al. *Pediatrics*. 2016;138(1):e20154547 PMID: 27354453
276. Bradley JS, et al. *Pediatr Infect Dis J*. 2019;38(8):816–824 PMID: 31306396
277. Hurst AL, et al. *J Pediatric Infect Dis Soc*. 2017;6(1):57–64 PMID: 26703242
278. Theodorou CM. *J Pediatr Surg*. 2021;56(10):1826–1830 PMID: 33223225
279. Wang C, et al. *BMC Pediatr*. 2019;19(1):407 PMID: 31684906
280. Scott C, et al. *Clin Infect Dis*. 2016;63(5):594–601 PMID: 27298329
281. Hlavsa MC, et al. *Clin Infect Dis*. 2008;47(2):168–175 PMID: 18532886
282. Sartoris G, et al. *J Pediatric Infect Dis Soc*. 2020;9(2):218–227 PMID: 31909804
283. Soni H, et al. *Infection*. 2019;47(3):387–394 PMID: 30324229
284. Arditi M, et al. *Pediatr Infect Dis J*. 1990;9(6):411–415 PMID: 2367163
285. Sethna CB, et al. *Clin J Am Soc Nephrol*. 2016;11(9):1590–1596 PMID: 27340282
286. Warady BA, et al. *Perit Dial Int*. 2012;32(suppl 2):S32–S86 PMID: 22851742
287. Preece ER, et al. *ANZ J Surg*. 2012;82(4):283–284 PMID: 22510192

288. Gkentzis A, et al. *Ann R Coll Surg Engl.* 2014;96(3):181–183 PMID: 24780779
289. George CRR, et al. *PLoS One.* 2019;14(4):e0213312 PMID: 30943199
290. Wi T, et al. *PLoS Med.* 2017;14(7):e1002344 PMID: 28686231
291. Hammad WAB, et al. *Eur J Obstet Gynecol Reprod Biol.* 2021;259:38–45 PMID: 33581405
292. *Obstet Gynecol.* 2020;135(5):e193–e202 PMID: 32332414
293. Savaris RF, et al. *Sex Transm Infect.* 2019;95(1):21–27 PMID: 30341232
294. Peeling RW, et al. *Nat Rev Dis Primers.* 2017;3:17073 PMID: 29022569
295. Jordan SJ, et al. *Sex Transm Infect.* 2020;96(4):306–311 PMID: 31515293
296. Bradshaw CS, et al. *J Infect Dis.* 2016;214(suppl 1):S14–S20 PMID: 27449869
297. Matheson A, et al. *Aust N Z J Obstet Gynaecol.* 2017;57(2):139–145 PMID: 28299777
298. Brander EPA, et al. *CMAJ.* 2018;190(26):E800 PMID: 29970369
299. Beyitler İ, et al. *World J Pediatr.* 2017;13(2):101–105 PMID: 28083751
300. Hansen MT, et al. *J Pediatr Adolesc Gynecol.* 2007;20(5):315–317 PMID: 17868900
301. Brouwer MC, et al. *N Engl J Med.* 2014;371(5):447–456 PMID: 25075836
302. Mameli C, et al. *Childs Nerv Syst.* 2019;35(7):1117–1128 PMID: 31062139
303. Boucher A, et al. *Med Mal Infect.* 2017;47(3):221–235 PMID: 28341533
304. Dalmau J, et al. *N Engl J Med.* 2018;378(9):840–851 PMID: 29490181
305. Abzug MJ, et al. *J Pediatric Infect Dis Soc.* 2016;5(1):53–62 PMID: 26407253
306. Cheng H, et al. *BMC Infect Dis.* 2020;20(1):886 PMID: 33238935
307. Stahl JP, et al. *Curr Opin Infect Dis.* 2019;32(3):239–243 PMID: 30921087
308. Ajibowo AO, et al. *Cureus.* 2021;13(4):e14579 PMID: 34036000
309. Brouwer MC, et al. *Cochrane Database Syst Rev.* 2015;(9):CD004405 PMID: 26362566
310. van de Beek D, et al. *Lancet.* 2021;398(10306):1171–1183 PMID: 34303412
311. Tunkel AR, et al. *Clin Infect Dis.* 2017;64(6):e34–e65 PMID: 28203777
312. Jhaveri R. *J Pediatric Infect Dis Soc.* 2019;8(1):92–93 PMID: 30380088
313. Bradley JS, et al. *Pediatr Infect Dis J.* 1991;10(11):871–873 PMID: 1749702
314. Prasad K, et al. *Cochrane Database Syst Rev.* 2016;(4):CD002244 PMID: 27121755
315. James G, et al. *J Neurosurg Pediatr.* 2014;13(1):101–106 PMID: 24206346
316. Cies JJ, et al. *J Pediatr Pharmacol Ther.* 2020;25(4):336–339 PMID: 32461749
317. National Institute for Health and Care Excellence. Urinary tract infection in under 16s: diagnosis and management. Updated October 31, 2018. Accessed October 3, 2022. www.nice.org.uk/guidance/CG54
318. National Institute for Health and Care Excellence. Urinary tract infection (recurrent): antimicrobial prescribing; treatment for children and young people under 16 years with recurrent UTI. Updated October 31, 2018. Accessed October 3, 2022. www.nice.org.uk/guidance/ng112/chapter/Recommendations#treatment-for-children-and-young-people-under-16-years-with-recurrent-uti
319. Tullus K, et al. *Lancet.* 2020;395(10237):1659–1668 PMID: 32446408
320. Meesters K, et al. *Antimicrob Agents Chemother.* 2018;62(9):e00517–18 PMID: 29987142
321. Chen WL, et al. *Pediatr Neonatal.* 2015;56(3):176–182 PMID: 25459491
322. Fujita Y, et al. *Pediatr Infect Dis J.* 2021;40(7):e278–e280 PMID: 34097665
323. Strohmeier Y, et al. *Cochrane Database Syst Rev.* 2014;(7):CD003772 PMID: 25066627
324. Fox MT, et al. *JAMA Netw Open.* 2020;3(5):e203951 PMID: 32364593
325. Tamma PD, et al. *Clin Infect Dis.* 2015;60(9):1319–1325 PMID: 25586681
326. Bocquet N, et al. *Pediatrics.* 2012;129(2):e269–e275 PMID: 22291112
327. AAP Subcommittee on Urinary Tract Infection and Steering Committee on Quality Improvement and Management. *Pediatrics.* 2011;128(3):595–610 PMID: 21873693
328. Craig JC, et al. *N Engl J Med.* 2009;361(18):1748–1759 PMID: 19864673
329. Williams G, et al. *Cochrane Database Syst Rev.* 2019;(4):CD001534 PMID: 30932167
330. Hoberman A, et al. *N Engl J Med.* 2014;370(25):2367–2376 PMID: 24795142
331. Craig JC. *J Pediatr.* 2015;166(3):778 PMID: 25722276
332. Hewitt IK, et al. *Pediatrics.* 2017;139(5):e20163145 PMID: 28557737
333. AAP. Actinomycosis. In: Kimberlin DW, et al, eds. *Red Book: 2021–2024 Report of the Committee on Infectious Diseases.* 32nd ed. 2021:187–188
334. Steininger C, et al. *J Antimicrob Chemother.* 2016;71(2):422–427 PMID: 26538502
335. Wacharachaisurapol N, et al. *Pediatr Infect Dis J.* 2017;36(3):e76–e79 PMID: 27870811

336. Biggs HM, et al. *MMWR Recomm Rep.* 2016;65(2):1–44 PMID: 27172113
337. Dixon DM, et al. *Ticks Tick Borne Dis.* 2021;12(6):101823 PMID: 34517150
338. AAP. Brucellosis. In: Kimberlin DW, et al, eds. *Red Book: 2021–2024 Report of the Committee on Infectious Diseases.* 32nd ed. 2021:238–240
339. Bukhari EE. *Saudi Med J.* 2018;39(4):336–341 PMID: 29619483
340. Shorbatli LA, et al. *Int J Clin Pharm.* 2018;40(6):1458–1461 PMID: 30446895
341. Zangwill KM. *Adv Exp Med Biol.* 2013;764:159–166 PMID: 23654065
342. Chang CC, et al. *Paediatr Int Child Health.* 2016;36(3):232–234 PMID: 25940800
343. Mogg M, et al. *Vector Borne Zoonotic Dis.* 2020;20(7):547–550 PMID: 32077809
344. Mukkada S, et al. *Infect Dis Clin North Am.* 2015;29(3):539–555 PMID: 26188606
345. Lehrnbecher T, et al. *J Clin Oncol.* 2017;35(18):2082–2094 PMID: 28459614
346. Taplitz RA, et al. *J Clin Oncol.* 2018;36(14):1443–1453 PMID: 29461916
347. Alali M, et al. *J Pediatr Hematol Oncol.* 2020;42(6):e445–e451 PMID: 32404688
348. Haeusler GM, et al. *EClinicalMedicine.* 2020;23:100394 PMID: 32637894
349. Miedema KG, et al. *Eur J Cancer.* 2016;53:16–24 PMID: 26700076
350. Payne JR, et al. *J Pediatr.* 2018;193:172–177 PMID: 29229452
351. Son MBF, et al. *Pediatr Rev.* 2018;39(2):78–90 PMID: 29437127
352. Green J, et al. *Cochrane Database Syst Rev.* 2022;(5):CD011188 PMID: 35622534
353. Friedman KG, et al. *Arch Dis Child.* 2021;106(3):247–252 PMID: 32943389
354. McCrindle BW, et al. *Circulation.* 2017;135(17):e927–e999 PMID: 28356445
355. Yamaji N, et al. *Cochrane Database Syst Rev.* 2019;(8):CD012448 PMID: 31425625
356. Portman MA, et al. *Pediatrics.* 2019;143(6):e20183675 PMID: 31048415
357. AAP. Leprosy. In: Kimberlin DW, et al, eds. *Red Book: 2021–2024 Report of the Committee on Infectious Diseases.* 32nd ed. 2021:472–475
358. Haake DA, et al. *Curr Top Microbiol Immunol.* 2015;387:65–97 PMID: 25388133
359. AAP. Leptospirosis. In: Kimberlin DW, et al, eds. *Red Book: 2021–2024 Report of the Committee on Infectious Diseases.* 32nd ed. 2021:475–477
360. AAP. Lyme disease. In: Kimberlin DW, et al, eds. *Red Book: 2021–2024 Report of the Committee on Infectious Diseases.* 32nd ed. 2021:482–489
361. Nguyen CT, et al. *JAMA.* 2022;327(8):772–773 PMID: 35191942
362. Wiersinga WJ, et al. *Nat Rev Dis Primers.* 2018;4:17107 PMID: 29388572
363. Chetchotisakd P, et al. *Lancet.* 2014;383(9919):807–814 PMID: 24284287
364. Philley JV, et al. *Thorac Surg Clin.* 2019;29(1):65–76 PMID: 30454923
365. Griffith DE, et al. *Chest.* 2022;161(1):64–75 PMID: 34314673
366. Pasipanodya JG, et al. *Antimicrob Agents Chemother.* 2017;61(11):e01206–17 PMID: 28807911
367. Wilson JW. *Mayo Clin Proc.* 2012;87(4):403–407 PMID: 22469352
368. AAP. Nocardiosis. In: Kimberlin DW, et al, eds. *Red Book: 2021–2024 Report of the Committee on Infectious Diseases.* 32nd ed. 2021:546–548
369. Kugeler KJ, et al. *Clin Infect Dis.* 2020;70(suppl 1):S20–S26 PMID: 32435801
370. Yang R. *J Clin Microbiol.* 2017;56(1):e01519–17 PMID: 29070654
371. Apangu T, et al. *Emerg Infect Dis.* 2017;23(3):553–555 PMID: 28125398
372. Cherry CC, et al. *Curr Infect Dis Rep.* 2020;22(4) PMID: 34135692
373. Anderson A, et al. *MMWR Recomm Rep.* 2013;62(RR-03):1–30 PMID: 23535757
374. AAP. Rocky Mountain spotted fever. In: Kimberlin DW, et al, eds. *Red Book: 2021–2024 Report of the Committee on Infectious Diseases.* 32nd ed. 2021:641–644
375. Blanton LS. *Infect Dis Clin North Am.* 2019;33(1):213–229 PMID: 30712763
376. AAP. Tetanus. In: Kimberlin DW, et al, eds. *Red Book: 2021–2024 Report of the Committee on Infectious Diseases.* 32nd ed. 2021:750–755
377. Centers for Disease Control and Prevention. Tetanus. Reviewed August 29, 2022. Accessed October 3, 2022. www.cdc.gov/tetanus/clinicians.html
378. Adalat S, et al. *Arch Dis Child.* 2014;99(12):1078–1082 PMID: 24790135
379. Cook A, et al. *Emerg Infect Dis.* 2020;26(6):1077–1083 PMID: 32442091
380. Harik NS. *Pediatr Ann.* 2013;42(7):288–292 PMID: 23805970

Chapter 2

1. Allegaert K, et al. *Acta Clin Belg.* 2019;74(3):157–163 PMID: 29745792
2. Keij FM, et al. *BMJ Open.* 2019;9(7):e026688 PMID: 31289068
3. Wagner CL, et al. *J Perinatol.* 2000;20(6):346–350 PMID: 11002871
4. Arnold CJ, et al. *Pediatr Infect Dis J.* 2015;34(9):964–968 PMID: 26376308
5. Martin E, et al. *Eur J Pediatr.* 1993;152(6):530–534 PMID: 8335024
6. Hile GB, et al. *J Pediatr Pharmacol Ther.* 2021;26(1):99–103 PMID: 33424507
7. Bradley JS, et al. *Pediatrics.* 2009;123(4):e609–e613 PMID: 19289450
8. Zikic A, et al. *J Pediatric Infect Dis Soc.* 2018;7(3):e107–e115 PMID: 30007329
9. AAP. Chlamydial infections. In: Kimberlin DW, et al, eds. *Red Book: 2021–2024 Report of the Committee on Infectious Diseases.* 32nd ed. 2021:256–266
10. Honein MA, et al. *Lancet.* 1999;354(9196):2101–2105 PMID: 10609814
11. Hammerschlag MR, et al. *Pediatr Infect Dis J.* 1998;17(11):1049–1050 PMID: 9849993
12. Abdellatif M, et al. *Eur J Pediatr.* 2019;178(3):301–314 PMID: 30470884
13. Laga M, et al. *N Engl J Med.* 1986;315(22):1382–1385 PMID: 3095641
14. Workowski KA, et al. *MMWR Recomm Rep.* 2015;64(RR-3):1–137 PMID: 26042815
15. Newman LM, et al. *Clin Infect Dis.* 2007;44(suppl 3):S84–S101 PMID: 17342672
16. MacDonald N, et al. *Adv Exp Med Biol.* 2008;609:108–130 PMID: 18193661
17. AAP. Gonococcal infections. In: Kimberlin DW, et al, eds. *Red Book: 2021–2024 Report of the Committee on Infectious Diseases.* 32nd ed. 2021:338–344
18. Cimolai N. *Am J Ophthalmol.* 2006;142(1):183–184 PMID: 16815280
19. Marangon FB, et al. *Am J Ophthalmol.* 2004;137(3):453–458 PMID: 15013867
20. AAP. Coagulase-negative staphylococcal infections. In: Kimberlin DW, et al, eds. *Red Book: 2021–2024 Report of the Committee on Infectious Diseases.* 32nd ed. 2021:692–694
21. Brito DV, et al. *Braz J Infect Dis.* 2003;7(4):234–235 PMID: 14533982
22. Chen CJ, et al. *Am J Ophthalmol.* 2008;145(6):966–970 PMID: 18378213
23. Shah SS, et al. *J Perinatol.* 1999;19(6, pt 1):462–465 PMID: 10685281
24. Kimberlin DW, et al. *J Pediatr.* 2003;143(1):16–25 PMID: 12915819
25. Kimberlin DW, et al. *J Infect Dis.* 2008;197(6):836–845 PMID: 18279073
26. AAP. Cytomegalovirus infection. In: Kimberlin DW, et al, eds. *Red Book: 2021–2024 Report of the Committee on Infectious Diseases.* 32nd ed. 2021:294–300
27. Kimberlin DW, et al. *N Engl J Med.* 2015;372(10):933–943 PMID: 25738669
28. Rawlinson WD, et al. *Lancet Infect Dis.* 2017;17(6):e177–e188 PMID: 28291720
29. Marsico C, et al. *J Infect Dis.* 2019;219(9):1398–1406 PMID: 30535363
30. AAP. Candidiasis. In: Kimberlin DW, et al, eds. *Red Book: 2021–2024 Report of the Committee on Infectious Diseases.* 32nd ed. 2021:246–252
31. Hundalani S, et al. *Expert Rev Anti Infect Ther.* 2013;11(7):709–721 PMID: 23829639
32. Saez-Llorens X, et al. *Antimicrob Agents Chemother.* 2009;53(3):869–875 PMID: 19075070
33. Ericson JE, et al. *Clin Infect Dis.* 2016;63(5):604–610 PMID: 27298330
34. Smith PB, et al. *Pediatr Infect Dis J.* 2009;28(5):412–415 PMID: 19319022
35. Wurthwein G, et al. *Antimicrob Agents Chemother.* 2005;49(12):5092–5098 PMID: 16304177
36. Heresi GP, et al. *Pediatr Infect Dis J.* 2006;25(12):1110–1115 PMID: 17133155
37. Kawaguchi C, et al. *Pediatr Int.* 2009;51(2):220–224 PMID: 19405920
38. Hsieh E, et al. *Early Hum Dev.* 2012;88(suppl 2):S6–S10 PMID: 22633516
39. Pappas PG, et al. *Clin Infect Dis.* 2016;62(4):e1–e50 PMID: 26679628
40. Hwang MF, et al. *Antimicrob Agents Chemother.* 2017;61(12):e01352–17 PMID: 28893774
41. Watt KM, et al. *Antimicrob Agents Chemother.* 2015;59(7):3935–3943 PMID: 25896706
42. Ascher SB, et al. *Pediatr Infect Dis J.* 2012;31(5):439–443 PMID: 22189522
43. Swanson JR, et al. *Pediatr Infect Dis J.* 2016;35(5):519–523 PMID: 26835970
44. Santos RP, et al. *Pediatr Infect Dis J.* 2007;26(4):364–366 PMID: 17414408
45. Frankenbusch K, et al. *J Perinatol.* 2006;26(8):511–514 PMID: 16871222
46. Thomas L, et al. *Expert Rev Anti Infect Ther.* 2009;7(4):461–472 PMID: 19400765
47. Mehler K, et al. *Pediatr Infect Dis J.* 2022;41(4):352–357 PMID: 34817413

48. Fatemizadeh R, et al. *Pediatr Infect Dis J.* 2020;39(4):310–312 PMID: 32084112
49. Verweij PE, et al. *Drug Resist Updat.* 2015;21–22:30–40 PMID: 26282594
50. Shah D, et al. *Cochrane Database Syst Rev.* 2012;(8):CD007448 PMID: 22895960
51. Cohen-Wolkowiez M, et al. *Clin Infect Dis.* 2012;55(11):1495–1502 PMID: 22955430
52. Knell J, et al. *Curr Probl Surg.* 2019;56(1):11–38 PMID: 30691547
53. Smith MJ, et al. *Pediatr Infect Dis J.* 2021;40(6):550–555 PMID: 33902072
54. Commander SJ, et al. *Pediatr Infect Dis J.* 2020;39(9):e245–e248 PMID: 32453198
55. Morgan RL, et al. *Gastroenterology.* 2020;159(2):467–480 PMID: 32592699
56. Gray KD, et al. *J Pediatr.* 2020;222:59–64.e1 PMID: 32418818
57. AAP. *Salmonella* infections. In: Kimberlin DW, et al, eds. *Red Book: 2021–2024 Report of the Committee on Infectious Diseases.* 32nd ed. 2021:655–663
58. Pinninti SG, et al. *Pediatr Clin North Am.* 2013;60(2):351–365 PMID: 23481105
59. AAP. Herpes simplex. In: Kimberlin DW, et al, eds. *Red Book: 2021–2024 Report of the Committee on Infectious Diseases.* 32nd ed. 2021:407–417
60. Jones CA, et al. *Cochrane Database Syst Rev.* 2009;(3):CD004206 PMID: 19588350
61. Downes KJ, et al. *J Pediatr.* 2020;219:126–132 PMID: 32037154
62. Kimberlin DW, et al. *N Engl J Med.* 2011;365(14):1284–1292 PMID: 21991950
63. Grondin A, et al. *Neuropediatrics.* 2020;51(3):221–224 PMID: 31887772
64. Sampson MR, et al. *Pediatr Infect Dis J.* 2014;33(1):42–49 PMID: 24346595
65. Panel on Antiretroviral Therapy and Medical Management of Children Living with HIV. Guidelines for the use of antiretroviral agents in pediatric HIV infection. Updated April 11, 2022. Accessed October 3, 2022. https://clinicalinfo.hiv.gov/en/guidelines/pediatric-arv/whats-new-guidelines
66. Panel on Treatment of Pregnant Women with HIV Infection and Prevention of Perinatal Transmission. Recommendations for the use of antiretroviral drugs in pregnant women with HIV infection and interventions to reduce perinatal HIV transmission in the United States. Updated March 17, 2022. Accessed October 3, 2022. https://clinicalinfo.hiv.gov/en/guidelines/perinatal/whats-new-guidelines
67. Luzuriaga K, et al. *N Engl J Med.* 2015;372(8):786–788 PMID: 25693029
68. AAP Committee on Infectious Diseases. *Pediatrics.* 2019;144(4):e20192478 PMID: 31477606
69. Acosta EP, et al. *J Infect Dis.* 2010;202(4):563–566 PMID: 20594104
70. McPherson C, et al. *J Infect Dis.* 2012;206(6):847–850 PMID: 22807525
71. Kamal MA, et al. *Clin Pharmacol Ther.* 2014;96(3):380–389 PMID: 24865390
72. Kimberlin DW, et al. *J Infect Dis.* 2013;207(5):709–720 PMID: 23230059
73. Bradley JS, et al. *Pediatrics.* 2017;140(5):e20162727 PMID: 29051331
74. Hayden FG, et al. *N Engl J Med.* 2018;379(10):913–923 PMID: 30184455
75. Fraser N, et al. *Acta Paediatr.* 2006;95(5):519–522 PMID: 16825129
76. Ulloa-Gutierrez R, et al. *Pediatr Emerg Care.* 2005;21(9):600–602 PMID: 16160666
77. Sawardekar KP. *Pediatr Infect Dis J.* 2004;23(1):22–26 PMID: 14743041
78. Bingol-Kologlu M, et al. *J Pediatr Surg.* 2007;42(11):1892–1897 PMID: 18022442
79. Brook I. *J Perinat Med.* 2002;30(3):197–208 PMID: 12122901
80. Kaplan SL. *Adv Exp Med Biol.* 2009;634:111–120 PMID: 19280853
81. Korakaki E, et al. *Jpn J Infect Dis.* 2007;60(2-3):129–131 PMID: 17515648
82. Dessi A, et al. *J Chemother.* 2008;20(5):542–550 PMID: 19028615
83. Berkun Y, et al. *Arch Dis Child.* 2008;93(8):690–694 PMID: 18337275
84. Greenberg D, et al. *Paediatr Drugs.* 2008;10(2):75–83 PMID: 18345717
85. Ismail EA, et al. *Pediatr Int.* 2013;55(1):60–64 PMID: 23039834
86. Megged O, et al. *J Pediatr.* 2018;196:319 PMID: 29428272
87. Engle WD, et al. *J Perinatol.* 2000;20(7):421–426 PMID: 11076325
88. Brook I. *Microbes Infect.* 2002;4(12):1271–1280 PMID: 12467770
89. Darville T. *Semin Pediatr Infect Dis.* 2005;16(4):235–244 PMID: 16210104
90. Eberly MD, et al. *Pediatrics.* 2015;135(3):483–488 PMID: 25687145
91. Waites KB, et al. *Semin Fetal Neonatal Med.* 2009;14(4):190–199 PMID: 19109084
92. Morrison W. *Pediatr Infect Dis J.* 2007;26(2):186–188 PMID: 17259889
93. AAP. Pertussis (whooping cough). In: Kimberlin DW, et al, eds. *Red Book: 2021–2024 Report of the Committee on Infectious Diseases.* 32nd ed. 2021:578–589

94. Foca MD. *Semin Perinatol.* 2002;26(5):332–339 PMID: 12452505
95. AAP Committee on Infectious Diseases and Bronchiolitis Guidelines Committee. *Pediatrics.* 2014;134(2):e620–e638 PMID: 25070304
96. Banerji A, et al. *CMAJ Open.* 2016;4(4):E623–E633 PMID: 28443266
97. Borse RH, et al. *J Pediatric Infect Dis Soc.* 2014;3(3):201–212 PMID: 26625383
98. Vergnano S, et al. *Pediatr Infect Dis J.* 2011;30(10):850–854 PMID: 21654546
99. Nelson MU, et al. *Semin Perinatol.* 2012;36(6):424–430 PMID: 23177801
100. Lyseng-Williamson KA, et al. *Paediatr Drugs.* 2003;5(6):419–431 PMID: 12765493
101. AAP. Group B streptococcal infections. In: Kimberlin DW, et al, eds. *Red Book: 2021–2024 Report of the Committee on Infectious Diseases.* 32nd ed. 2021:707–713
102. Schrag S, et al. *MMWR Recomm Rep.* 2002;51(RR-11):1–22 PMID: 12211284
103. AAP. *Ureaplasma urealyticum* and *Ureaplasma parvum* infections. In: Kimberlin DW, et al, eds. *Red Book: 2021–2024 Report of the Committee on Infectious Diseases.* 32nd ed. 2021:829–830
104. Merchan LM, et al. *Antimicrob Agents Chemother.* 2015;59(1):570–578 PMID: 25385115
105. Viscardi RM, et al. *Arch Dis Child Fetal Neonatal Ed.* 2020;105(6):615–622 PMID: 32170033
106. Lowe J, et al. *BMJ Open.* 2020;10(10):e041528 PMID: 33028566
107. AAP. *Escherichia coli* diarrhea. In: Kimberlin DW, et al, eds. *Red Book: 2021–2024 Report of the Committee on Infectious Diseases.* 32nd ed. 2021:322–328
108. Venkatesh MP, et al. *Expert Rev Anti Infect Ther.* 2008;6(6):929–938 PMID: 19053905
109. Aguilera-Alonso D, et al. *Antimicrob Agents Chemother.* 2020;64(3):e02183–19 PMID: 31844014
110. Nakwan N, et al. *Pediatr Infect Dis J.* 2019;38(11):1107–1112 PMID: 31469781
111. Abzug MJ, et al. *J Pediatric Infect Dis Soc.* 2016;5(1):53–62 PMID: 26407253
112. AAP. *Listeria monocytogenes* infections. In: Kimberlin DW, et al, eds. *Red Book: 2021–2024 Report of the Committee on Infectious Diseases.* 32nd ed. 2021:478–482
113. Workowski KA, et al. *MMWR Recomm Rep.* 2021;70(4):1–187 PMID: 34292926
114. van der Lugt NM, et al. *BMC Pediatr.* 2010;10:84 PMID: 21092087
115. Fortunov RM, et al. *Pediatrics.* 2006;118(3):874–881 PMID: 16950976
116. Fortunov RM, et al. *Pediatrics.* 2007;120(5):937–945 PMID: 17974729
117. Riccobene TA, et al. *J Clin Pharmacol.* 2017;57(3):345–355 PMID: 27510635
118. Stauffer WM, et al. *Pediatr Emerg Care.* 2003;19(3):165–166 PMID: 12813301
119. Kaufman DA, et al. *Clin Infect Dis.* 2017;64(10):1387–1395 PMID: 28158439
120. Dehority W, et al. *Pediatr Infect Dis J.* 2006;25(11):1080–1081 PMID: 17072137
121. AAP. Syphilis. In: Kimberlin DW, et al, eds. *Red Book: 2021–2024 Report of the Committee on Infectious Diseases.* 32nd ed. 2021:729–744
122. AAP. Tetanus. In: Kimberlin DW, et al, eds. *Red Book: 2021–2024 Report of the Committee on Infectious Diseases.* 32nd ed. 2021:750–755
123. AAP. *Toxoplasma gondii* infections. In: Kimberlin DW, et al, eds. *Red Book: 2021–2024 Report of the Committee on Infectious Diseases.* 32nd ed. 2021:767–775
124. Petersen E. *Semin Fetal Neonatal Med.* 2007;12(3):214–223 PMID: 17321812
125. Beetz R. *Curr Opin Pediatr.* 2012;24(2):205–211 PMID: 22227782
126. RIVUR Trial Investigators, et al. *N Engl J Med.* 2014;370(25):2367–2376 PMID: 24795142
127. Williams G, et al. *Cochrane Database Syst Rev.* 2019;(4):CD001534 PMID: 30932167
128. van Donge T, et al. *Antimicrob Agents Chemother.* 2018;62(4):e02004–17 PMID: 29358294
129. Sahin L, et al. *Clin Pharmacol Ther.* 2016;100(1):23–25 PMID: 27082701
130. Roberts SW, et al. Placental transmission of antibiotics. In: *Glob Libr Women's Med.* Updated June 2008. Accessed October 3, 2022. www.glowm.com/section_view/heading/Placental%20Transmission%20of%20Antibiotics/item/174
131. Zhang Z, et al. *Drug Metab Dispos.* 2017;45(8):939–946 PMID: 28049636
132. Pacifici GM. *Int J Clin Pharmacol Ther.* 2006;44(2):57–63 PMID: 16502764
133. Sachs HC, et al. *Pediatrics.* 2013;132(3):e796–e809 PMID: 23979084
134. Hale TW. *Medication and Mothers' Milk 2021: A Manual of Lactational Pharmacology.* 19th ed. 2021
135. Briggs GG, et al. *Briggs Drugs in Pregnancy and Lactation.* 12th ed. 2021
136. Ito S, et al. *Am J Obstet Gynecol.* 1993;168(5):1393–1399 PMID: 8498418

Chapter 3

1. Sáez-Llorens X, et al. *Pediatr Infect Dis J*. 2001;20(3):356–361 PMID: 11303850
2. Rodriguez WJ, et al. *Pediatr Infect Dis*. 1986;5(4):408–415 PMID: 3523457
3. Qureshi ZA, et al. *Clin Infect Dis*. 2015;60(9):1295–1303 PMID: 25632010
4. Chiotos K, et al. *J Pediatric Infect Dis Soc*. 2020;9(1):56–66 PMID: 31872226
5. Aguilera-Alonso D, et al. *Antimicrob Agents Chemother*. 2020;64(3):e02183–19 PMID: 31844014
6. Karakonstantis S, et al. *Infection*. 2020;48(6):835–851 PMID: 32875545
7. Mohd Sazlly Lim S, et al. *Int J Antimicrob Agents*. 2019;53(6):726–745 PMID: 30831234
8. Wacharachaisurapol N, et al. *Pediatr Infect Dis J*. 2017;36(3):e76–e79 PMID: 27870811
9. Gandhi K, et al. *Ann Otol Rhinol Laryngol*. 2021:34894211021273 PMID: 34060325
10. Janda JM, et al. *Clin Microbiol Rev*. 2010;23(1):35–73 PMID: 20065325
11. Sharma K, et al. *Ann Clin Microbiol Antimicrob*. 2017;16(1):12 PMID: 28288638
12. Maraki S, et al. *J Microbiol Immunol Infect*. 2016;49(1):119–122 PMID: 24529567
13. Sigurjonsdottir VK, et al. *Diagn Microbiol Infect Dis*. 2017;89(3):230–234 PMID: 29050793
14. Dixon DM, et al. *Ticks Tick Borne Dis*. 2021;12(6):101823 PMID: 34517150
15. Therriault BL, et al. *Ann Pharmacother*. 2008;42(11):1697–1702 PMID: 18812563
16. Bradley JS, et al. *Pediatrics*. 2014;133(5):e1411–e1436 PMID: 24777226
17. AAP. *Bacillus cereus* infections and intoxications. In: Kimberlin DW, et al, eds. *Red Book: 2021–2024 Report of the Committee on Infectious Diseases*. 32nd ed. 2021:219–221
18. Bottone EJ. *Clin Microbiol Rev*. 2010;23(2):382–398 PMID: 20375358
19. Wexler HM. *Clin Microbiol Rev*. 2007;20(4):593–621 PMID: 17934076
20. Snydman DR, et al. *Anaerobe*. 2017;43:21–26 PMID: 27867083
21. Shorbatli LA, et al. *Int J Clin Pharm*. 2018;40(6):1458–1461 PMID: 30446895
22. Zangwill KM. *Adv Exp Med Biol*. 2013;764:159–166 PMID: 23654065
23. Angelakis E, et al. *Int J Antimicrob Agents*. 2014;44(1):16–25 PMID: 24933445
24. Kilgore PE, et al. *Clin Microbiol Rev*. 2016;29(3):449–486 PMID: 27029594
25. AAP. Pertussis (whooping cough). In: Kimberlin DW, et al, eds. *Red Book: 2021–2024 Report of the Committee on Infectious Diseases*. 32nd ed. 2021:578–589
26. Nguyen CT, et al. *JAMA*. 2022;327(8):772–773 PMID: 35191942
27. AAP. Lyme disease. In: Kimberlin DW, et al, eds. *Red Book: 2021–2024 Report of the Committee on Infectious Diseases*. 32nd ed. 2021:482–489
28. AAP. *Borrelia* infections other than Lyme disease. In: Kimberlin DW, et al, eds. *Red Book: 2021–2024 Report of the Committee on Infectious Diseases*. 32nd ed. 2021:235–237
29. Dworkin MS, et al. *Infect Dis Clin North Am*. 2008;22(3):449–468 PMID: 18755384
30. AAP. Brucellosis. In: Kimberlin DW, et al, eds. *Red Book: 2021–2024 Report of the Committee on Infectious Diseases*. 32nd ed. 2021:238–240
31. Bukhari EE. *Saudi Med J*. 2018;39(4):336–341 PMID: 29619483
32. Yagupsky P. *Adv Exp Med Biol*. 2011;719:123–132 PMID: 22125040
33. AAP. *Burkholderia* infections. In: Kimberlin DW, et al, eds. *Red Book: 2021–2024 Report of the Committee on Infectious Diseases*. 32nd ed. 2021:240–243
34. Massip C, et al. *J Antimicrob Chemother*. 2019;74(2):525–528 PMID: 30312409
35. Mazer DM, et al. *Antimicrob Agents Chemother*. 2017;61(9):e00766–17 PMID: 28674053
36. Lord R, et al. *Cochrane Database Syst Rev*. 2020;(4):CD009529 PMID: 32239690
37. Wiersinga WJ, et al. *N Engl J Med*. 2012;367(11):1035–1044 PMID: 22970946
38. Wiersinga WJ, et al. *Nat Rev Dis Primers*. 2018;4:17107 PMID: 29388572
39. Chetchotisakd P, et al. *Lancet*. 2014;383(9919):807–814 PMID: 24284287
40. Same RG, et al. *Pediatr Rev*. 2018;39(11):533–541 PMID: 30385582
41. Wagenaar JA, et al. *Clin Infect Dis*. 2014;58(11):1579–1586 PMID: 24550377
42. AAP. *Campylobacter* infections. In: Kimberlin DW, et al, eds. *Red Book: 2021–2024 Report of the Committee on Infectious Diseases*. 32nd ed. 2021:243–246
43. Schiaffino F, et al. *Antimicrob Agents Chemother*. 2019;63(2):e01911–18 PMID: 30420482
44. Bula-Rudas FJ, et al. *Pediatr Rev*. 2018;39(10):490–500 PMID: 30275032
45. Jolivet-Gougeon A, et al. *Int J Antimicrob Agents*. 2007;29(4):367–373 PMID: 17250994
46. Wang HK, et al. *J Clin Microbiol*. 2007;45(2):645–647 PMID: 17135428

47. Alhifany AA, et al. *Am J Case Rep.* 2017;18:674–667 PMID: 28620153
48. Rivero M, et al. *BMC Infect Dis.* 2019;19(1):816 PMID: 31533642
49. Kohlhoff SA, et al. *Expert Opin Pharmacother.* 2015;16(2):205–212 PMID: 25579069
50. AAP. Chlamydial infections. In: Kimberlin DW, et al, eds. *Red Book: 2021–2024 Report of the Committee on Infectious Diseases.* 32nd ed. 2021:256–266
51. Workowski KA, et al. *MMWR Recomm Rep.* 2015;64(RR-03):1–137 PMID: 26042815
52. Blasi F, et al. *Clin Microbiol Infect.* 2009;15(1):29–35 PMID: 19220337
53. Knittler MR, et al. *Pathog Dis.* 2015;73(1):1–15 PMID: 25853998
54. Campbell JI, et al. *BMC Infect Dis.* 2013;13:4 PMID: 23286235
55. Alisjahbana B, et al. *Int J Gen Med.* 2021;14:3259–3270 PMID: 3426754456
56. Richard KR, et al. *Am J Case Rep.* 2015;16:740–744 PMID: 26477750
57. Paterson DL, et al. *Curr Opin Infect Dis.* 2020;33(2):214–223 PMID: 32068644
58. Harris PN, et al. *J Antimicrob Chemother.* 2016;71(2):296–306 PMID: 26542304
59. Clostridioides difficile *Infection: Antimicrobial Prescribing.* National Institute for Health and Care Excellence; 2021 PMID: 3446404060
60. AAP. *Clostridioides difficile* (formerly *Clostridium difficile*). In: Kimberlin DW, et al, eds. *Red Book: 2021–2024 Report of the Committee on Infectious Diseases.* 32nd ed. 2021:271–276
61. McDonald LC, et al. *Clin Infect Dis.* 2018;66(7):987–994 PMID: 29562266
62. O'Gorman MA, et al. *J Pediatric Infect Dis Soc.* 2018;7(3):210–218 PMID: 28575523
63. Carrillo-Marquez MA. *Pediatr Rev.* 2016;37(5):183–192 PMID: 27139326
64. AAP. Botulism and infant botulism. In: Kimberlin DW, et al, eds. *Red Book: 2021–2024 Report of the Committee on Infectious Diseases.* 32nd ed. 2021:266–269
65. Hill SE, et al. *Ann Pharmacother.* 2013;47(2):e12 PMID: 23362041
66. AAP. Clostridial myonecrosis. In: Kimberlin DW, et al, eds. *Red Book: 2021–2024 Report of the Committee on Infectious Diseases.* 32nd ed. 2021:269–271
67. AAP. *Clostridium perfringens* foodborne illness. In: Kimberlin DW, et al, eds. *Red Book: 2021–2024 Report of the Committee on Infectious Diseases.* 32nd ed. 2021:276–277
68. AAP. Tetanus. In: Kimberlin DW, et al, eds. *Red Book: 2021–2024 Report of the Committee on Infectious Diseases.* 32nd ed. 2021:750–755
69. Yen LM, et al. *Lancet.* 2019;393(10181):1657–1668 PMID: 30935736
70. Rhinesmith E, et al. *Pediatr Rev.* 2018;39(8):430–432 PMID: 30068747
71. AAP. Diphtheria. In: Kimberlin DW, et al, eds. *Red Book: 2021–2024 Report of the Committee on Infectious Diseases.* 32nd ed. 2021:304–307
72. Fernandez-Roblas R, et al. *Int J Antimicrob Agents.* 2009;33(5):453–455 PMID: 19153032
73. Gupta R, et al. *Cardiol Rev.* 2021;29(5):259–262 PMID: 32976125
74. Forouzan P, et al. *Cureus.* 2020;12(9):e10733 PMID: 33145138
75. Dalal A, et al. *J Infect.* 2008;56(1):77–79 PMID: 18036665
76. Eldin C, et al. *Clin Microbiol Rev.* 2017;30(1):115–190 PMID: 27856520
77. Cherry CC, et al. *Curr Infect Dis Rep.* 2020;22(4):10.1007/s11908-020-0719-0 PMID: 34135692
78. Mayslich C, et al. *Microorganisms.* 2021;9(2):303 PMID: 33540667
79. Lin ZX, et al. *Orthopedics.* 2020;43(1):52–61 PMID: 31958341
80. Madison-Antenucci S, et al. *Clin Microbiol Rev.* 2020;33(2):e00083–18 PMID: 31896541
81. Xu G, et al. *Emerg Infect Dis.* 2018;24(6):1143–1144 PMID: 29774863
82. Paul K, et al. *Clin Infect Dis.* 2001;33(1):54–61 PMID: 11389495
83. Tricard T, et al. *Arch Pediatr.* 2016;23(11):1146–1149 PMID: 27663465
84. Huang YC, et al. *Int J Antimicrob Agents.* 2018;51(1):47–51 PMID: 28668676
85. Dziuban EJ, et al. *Clin Infect Dis.* 2018;67(1):144–149 PMID: 29211821
86. Siedner MJ, et al. *Clin Infect Dis.* 2014;58(11):1554–1563 PMID: 24647022
87. Tamma PD, et al. *Clin Infect Dis.* 2013;57(6):781–788 PMID: 23759352
88. Tamma PD, et al. *Clin Infect Dis.* 2021;72(7):1109–1116 PMID: 33830222
89. Iovleva A, et al. *Clin Lab Med.* 2017;37(2):303–315 PMID: 2845735290
90. Arias CA, et al. *Nat Rev Microbiol.* 2012;10(4):266–278 PMID: 22421879
91. Yim J, et al. *Pharmacotherapy.* 2017;37(5):579–592 PMID: 28273381
92. Beganovic M, et al. *Clin Infect Dis.* 2018;67(2):303–309 PMID: 29390132

93. Shah NH, et al. *Open Forum Infect Dis.* 2021;8(4):ofab102 PMID: 34805443
94. Principe L, et al. *Infect Dis Rep.* 2016;8(1):6368 PMID: 27103974
95. AAP. Tularemia. In: Kimberlin DW, et al, eds. *Red Book: 2021–2024 Report of the Committee on Infectious Diseases.* 32nd ed. 2021:822–825
96. Mittal S, et al. *Pediatr Rev.* 2019;40(4):197–201 PMID: 30936402
97. Van TT, et al. *J Clin Microbiol.* 2018;56(12):e00487–18 PMID: 30482869
98. Riordan T. *Clin Microbiol Rev.* 2007;20(4):622–659 PMID: 17934077
99. Valerio L, et al. *J Intern Med.* 2020 PMID: 32445216
100. Abou Chacra L, et al. *Front Cell Infect Microbiol.* 2022;11:672429 PMID: 35118003
101. Butler DF, et al. *Infect Dis Clin North Am.* 2018;32(1):119–128 PMID: 29233576
102. AAP. *Helicobacter pylori* infections. In: Kimberlin DW, et al, eds. *Red Book: 2021–2024 Report of the Committee on Infectious Diseases.* 32nd ed. 2021:357–362
103. Jones NL, et al. *J Pediatr Gastroenterol Nutr.* 2017;64(6):991–1003 PMID: 28541262
104. Crowe SE. *N Engl J Med.* 2019;380(12):1158–1165 PMID: 30893536
105. Yagupsky P. *Clin Microbiol Rev.* 2015;28(1):54–79 PMID: 25567222
106. Gouveia C, et al. *Pediatr Infect Dis J.* 2021;40(7):623–627 PMID: 33657599
107. Livermore DM, et al. *Clin Infect Dis.* 2020;71(7):1776–1782 PMID: 32025698
108. Mesini A, et al. *Clin Infect Dis.* 2018;66(5):808–809 PMID: 29020309
109. Bradley JS, et al. *Pediatr Infect Dis J.* 2019;38(9):920–928 PMID: 31335570
110. van Duin D, et al. *Clin Infect Dis.* 2018;66(2):163–171 PMID: 29020404
111. Cunha CB, et al. *Infect Dis Clin North Am.* 2017;31(1):179–191 PMID: 28159174
112. Jiménez JIS, et al. *J Crit Care.* 2018;43:361–365 PMID: 29129539
113. Florescu D, et al. *Pediatr Infect Dis J.* 2008;27(11):1013–1019 PMID: 18833028
114. Schlech WF. *Microbiol Spectr.* 2019;7(3) PMID: 31837132
115. Dickstein Y, et al. *Eur J Clin Microbiol Infect Dis.* 2019;38(12):2243–2251 PMID: 31399915
116. Murphy TF, et al. *Clin Infect Dis.* 2009;49(1):124–131 PMID: 19480579
117. Shi H, et al. *J Clin Lab Anal.* 2022;36(5):e24399 PMID: 35349730
118. Milligan KL, et al. *Clin Pediatr (Phila).* 2013;52(5):462–464 PMID: 22267858
119. AAP. Nontuberculous mycobacteria. In: Kimberlin DW, et al, eds. *Red Book: 2021–2024 Report of the Committee on Infectious Diseases.* 32nd ed. 2021:814–822
120. Daley CL, et al. *Clin Infect Dis.* 2020;71(4):905–913 PMID: 32797222
121. Koh WJ, et al. *Clin Infect Dis.* 2017;64(3):309–316 PMID: 28011608
122. Waters V, et al. *Cochrane Database Syst Rev.* 2020;(6):CD010004 PMID: 32521055
123. Haworth CS, et al. *BMJ Open Respir Res.* 2017;4(1):e000242 PMID: 29449949
124. Adelman MH, et al. *Curr Opin Pulm Med.* 2018;24(3):212–219 PMID: 29470253
125. Muñoz-Egea MC. *Expert Opin Pharmacother.* 2020;21(8):969–981 PMID: 32200657
126. AAP. Tuberculosis. In: Kimberlin DW, et al, eds. *Red Book: 2021–2024 Report of the Committee on Infectious Diseases.* 32nd ed. 2021:786–814
127. Scott C, et al. *Clin Infect Dis.* 2016;63(5):594–601 PMID: 27298329
128. Sartoris G, et al. *J Pediatric Infect Dis Soc.* 2020;9(2):218–227 PMID: 31909804129
129. Brown-Elliott BA, et al. *J Clin Microbiol.* 2016;54(6):1586–1592 PMID: 27053677
130. Centers for Disease Control and Prevention. Hansen's disease (leprosy). Reviewed February 10, 2017. Accessed October 3, 2022. www.cdc.gov/leprosy/health-care-workers/treatment.html
131. Johnson MG, et al. *Infection.* 2015;43(6):655–662 PMID: 25869820
132. Jaganath D, et al. *Infect Dis Clin North Am.* 2022;36(1):49–71 PMID: 35168714
133. Scaggs Huang FA, et al. *Pediatr Infect Dis J.* 2019;38(7):749–751 PMID: 30985508
134. Watt KM, et al. *Pediatr Infect Dis J.* 2012;31(2):197–199 PMID: 22016080
135. Waites KB, et al. *Clin Microbiol Rev.* 2017;30(3):747–809 PMID: 28539503
136. Gardiner SJ, et al. *Cochrane Database Syst Rev.* 2015;(1):CD004875 PMID: 25566754
137. Lee H, et al. *Expert Rev Anti Infect Ther.* 2018;16(1):23–34 PMID: 29212389
138. St Cyr S, et al. *MMWR Morb Mortal Wkly Rep.* 2020;69(50):1911–1916 PMID: 33332296
139. Brady RC. *Adv Pediatr.* 2020;67:29–46 PMID: 32591062
140. Nadel S, et al. *Front Pediatr.* 2018;6:321 PMID: 30474022
141. Wilson JW. *Mayo Clin Proc.* 2012;87(4):403–407 PMID: 22469352

142. AAP. Nocardiosis. In: Kimberlin DW, et al, eds. *Red Book: 2021–2024 Report of the Committee on Infectious Diseases*. 32nd ed. 2021:546–548
143. Wilson BA, et al. *Clin Microbiol Rev*. 2013;26(3):631–655 PMID: 23824375
144. Mogilner L, et al. *Pediatr Rev*. 2019;40(2):90–92 PMID: 30709978
145. Murphy EC, et al. *FEMS Microbiol Rev*. 2013;37(4):520–553 PMID: 23030831
146. Ozdemir O, et al. *J Microbiol Immunol Infect*. 2010;43(4):344–346 PMID: 20688296
147. Janda JM, et al. *Clin Microbiol Rev*. 2016;29(2):349–374 PMID: 26960939
148. Brook I, et al. *Clin Microbiol Rev*. 2013;26(3):526–546 PMID: 23824372
149. Schaffer JN, et al. *Microbiol Spectr*. 2015;3(5) PMID: 26542036
150. Abdallah M, et al. *New Microbes New Infect*. 2018;25:16–23 PMID: 29983987
151. Kunz Coyne AJ, et al. *Infect Dis Ther*. 2022;11(2):661–682 PMID: 35150435
152. Kalil AC, et al. *Clin Infect Dis*. 2016;63(5):e61–e111 PMID: 27418577
153. Alali M, et al. *J Pediatr Hematol Oncol*. 2020;42(6):e445–e451 PMID: 32404688
154. Paterson DL, et al. *Curr Opin Infect Dis*. 2020;33(2):214–223 PMID: 32068644
155. McCarthy KL, et al. *Infect Dis (Lond)*. 2018;50(5):403–406 PMID: 29205079
156. Kim HS, et al. *BMC Infect Dis*. 2017;17(1):500 PMID: 28716109
157. Ng C, et al. *Curr Opin Pulm Med*. 2020;26(6):679–684 PMID: 32890021
158. Epps QJ, et al. *Pediatr Pulmonol*. 2021;56(6):1784–1788 PMID: 33524241
159. Langton Hewer SC, et al. *Cochrane Database Syst Rev*. 2017;(4):CD004197 PMID: 28440853
160. Mogayzel PJ Jr, et al. *Ann Am Thorac Soc*. 2014;11(10):1640–1650 PMID: 25549030
161. Lin WV, et al. *Clin Microbiol Infect*. 2019;25(3):310–315 PMID: 29777923
162. AAP. Rickettsial diseases. In: Kimberlin DW, et al, eds. *Red Book: 2021–2024 Report of the Committee on Infectious Diseases*. 32nd ed. 2021:638–640
163. Blanton LS. *Infect Dis Clin North Am*. 2019;33(1):213–229 PMID: 30712763
164. AAP. *Salmonella* infections. In: Kimberlin DW, et al, eds. *Red Book: 2021–2024 Report of the Committee on Infectious Diseases*. 32nd ed. 2021:655–663
165. Leinert JL, et al. *Antibiotics (Basel)*. 2021;10(10):1187 PMID: 34680768
166. Onwuezobe IA, et al. *Cochrane Database Syst Rev*. 2012;(11):CD001167 PMID: 23152205
167. Karkey A, et al. *Curr Opin Gastroenterol*. 2018;34(1):25–30 PMID: 29059070
168. Wain J, et al. *Lancet*. 2015;385(9973):1136–1145 PMID: 25458731
169. Yousfi K, et al. *Eur J Clin Microbiol Infect Dis*. 2017;36(8):1353–1362 PMID: 28299457
170. Janda JM, et al. *Crit Rev Microbiol*. 2014;40(4):293–312 PMID: 23043419
171. Klontz KC, et al. *Expert Rev Anti Infect Ther*. 2015;13(1):69–80 PMID: 25399653
172. AAP. *Shigella* infections. In: Kimberlin DW, et al, eds. *Red Book: 2021–2024 Report of the Committee on Infectious Diseases*. 32nd ed. 2021:668–672
173. Kotloff KL, et al. *Lancet*. 2018;391(10122):801–812 PMID: 29254859174
174. Centers for Disease Control and Prevention. NARMS Now: Human Data. Updated September 30, 2022. Accessed October 3, 2022. wwwn.cdc.gov/narmsnow
175. Rognrud K, et al. *Case Rep Infect Dis*. 2020;2020:7185834 PMID: 33101743
176. El Beaino M, et al. *Int J Infect Dis*. 2018;77:68–73 PMID: 30267938
177. AAP. Rat-bite fever. In: Kimberlin DW, et al, eds. *Red Book: 2021–2024 Report of the Committee on Infectious Diseases*. 32nd ed. 2021:627–628
178. Stevens DL, et al. *Clin Infect Dis*. 2014;59(2):e10–e52 [Erratum. *Clin Infect Dis*. 20151;60(9):1448] PMID: 24973422
179. Sharma R, et al. *Curr Infect Dis Rep*. 2019;21(10):37 PMID: 31486979
180. Korczowski B, et al. *Pediatr Infect Dis J*. 2016;35(8):e239–e247 PMID: 27164462
181. Bradley J, et al. *Pediatrics*. 2017;139(3):e20162477 PMID: 28202770
182. Rybak MJ, et al. *Am J Health Syst Pharm*. 2020;77(11):835–864 PMID: 32191793
183. Arrieta AC, et al. *Pediatr Infect Dis J*. 2018;37(9):893–900 PMID: 29406465
184. Becker K, et al. *Clin Microbiol Rev*. 2014;27(4):870–926 PMID: 25278577
185. Sader HS, et al. *Diagn Microbiol Infect Dis*. 2016;85(1):80–84 PMID: 26971182
186. Mojica MF, et al. *JAC Antimicrob Resist*. 2022;4(3):dlac040 PMID: 35529051
187. Anđelković MV, et al. *J Chemother*. 2019:1–10 PMID: 31130079
188. Delgado-Valverde M, et al. *J Antimicrob Chemother*. 2020;75(7):1840–1849 PMID: 32277821

189. Crews JD, et al. *JAMA Pediatr*. 2014;168(12):1165–1166 PMID: 25436846
190. Gerber MA, et al. *Circulation*. 2009;119(11):1541–1551 PMID: 19246689
191. AAP. Group B streptococcal infections. In: Kimberlin DW, et al, eds. *Red Book: 2021–2024 Report of the Committee on Infectious Diseases*. 32nd ed. 2021:707–713
192. Faden H, et al. *Pediatr Infect Dis J*. 2017;36(11):1099–1100 PMID: 28640003
193. Furuichi M, et al. *J Infect Chemother*. 2018;24(2):99–102 PMID: 29050796
194. Otto WR, et al. *J Pediatric Infect Dis Soc*. 2021;10(3):309–316 PMID: 32955086
195. Dodson DS, et al. *Open Forum Infect Dis*. 2022;9(1):ofab628 PMID: 35028336
196. Baltimore RS, et al. *Circulation*. 2015;132(15):1487–1515 PMID: 26373317
197. Bradley JS, et al. *Clin Infect Dis*. 2011;53(7):e25–e76 PMID: 21880587
198. Mendes RE, et al. *Diagn Microbiol Infect Dis*. 2014;80(1):19–25 PMID: 24974272
199. Kaplan SL, et al. *Pediatrics*. 2019;144(3):e20190567 PMID: 31420369
200. AAP. Syphilis. In: Kimberlin DW, et al, eds. *Red Book: 2021–2024 Report of the Committee on Infectious Diseases*. 32nd ed. 2021:729–744
201. Viscardi RM, et al. *Arch Dis Child Fetal Neonatal Ed*. 2020;105(6):615–622 PMID: 32170033
202. Centers for Disease Control and Prevention. Cholera - *Vibrio cholerae* infection. Reviewed June 1, 2022. Accessed October 3, 2022. www.cdc.gov/cholera/treatment/antibiotic-treatment.html
203. Kanungo S, et al. *Lancet*. 2022;399(10333):1429–1440 PMID: 35397865
204. Trinh SA, et al. *Antimicrob Agents Chemother*. 2017;61(12):e01106-17 PMID: 28971862
205. Coerdt KM, et al. *Cutis*. 2021;107(2):E12–E17 PMID: 33891847
206. Leng F, et al. *Eur J Clin Microbiol Infect Dis*. 2019;38(11):1999–2004 PMID: 31325061
207. AAP. *Yersinia enterocolitica* and *Yersinia pseudotuberculosis* infections. In: Kimberlin DW, et al, eds. *Red Book: 2021–2024 Report of the Committee on Infectious Diseases*. 32nd ed. 2021:851–854
208. Kato H, et al. *Medicine (Baltimore)*. 2016;95(26):e3988 PMID: 27368001
209. Yang R. *J Clin Microbiol*. 2017;56(1):e01519-17 PMID: 29070654
210. Barbieri R, et al. *Clin Microbiol Rev*. 2020;34(1):e00044-19 PMID: 33298527
211. Centers for Disease Control and Prevention. Plague. Clinicians. Reviewed February 25, 2022. Accessed October 3, 2022. www.cdc.gov/plague/healthcare/clinicians.html
212. Somova LM, et al. *Pathogens*. 2020;9(6):436 PMID: 32498317

Chapter 4

1. Cannavino CR, et al. *Pediatr Infect Dis J*. 2016;35(7):752–759 PMID: 27093162
2. Smyth AR, et al. *Cochrane Database Syst Rev*. 2017;(3):CD002009 PMID: 28349527
3. Zhanel GG, et al. *Drugs*. 2019;79(3):271–289 PMID: 30712199
4. Yu PH, et al. *BMC Pediatr*. 2020;20(1):64 PMID: 32046672
5. Wirth S, et al. *Pediatr Infect Dis J*. 2018;37(8):e207–e213 PMID: 29356761
6. Jackson MA, et al. *Pediatrics*. 2016;138(5):e20162706 PMID: 27940800
7. Bradley JS, et al. *Pediatrics*. 2014;134(1):e146–e153 PMID: 24918220

Chapter 5

1. Groll AH, et al. *Lancet Oncol*. 2014;15(8):e327–e340 PMID: 24988936
2. Wingard JR, et al. *Blood*. 2010;116(24):5111–5118 PMID: 20826719
3. Van Burik JA, et al. *Clin Infect Dis*. 2004;39(10):1407–1416 PMID: 15546073
4. Cornely OA, et al. *N Engl J Med*. 2007;356(4):348–359 PMID: 17251531
5. Kung HC, et al. *Cancer Med*. 2014;3(3):667–673 PMID: 24644249
6. Science M, et al. *Pediatr Blood Cancer*. 2014;61(3):393–400 PMID: 24424789
7. Bow EJ, et al. *BMC Infect Dis*. 2015;15:128 PMID: 25887385
8. Tacke D, et al. *Ann Hematol*. 2014;93(9):1449–1456 PMID: 24951122
9. Almyroudis NG, et al. *Curr Opin Infect Dis*. 2009;22(4):385–393 PMID: 19506476
10. Maschmeyer G. *J Antimicrob Chemother*. 2009;63(suppl 1):i27–i30 PMID: 19372178
11. Freifeld AG, et al. *Clin Infect Dis*. 2011;52(4):e56–e93 PMID: 21258094
12. Fisher BT. *JAMA*. 2019;322(17):1673–1681 PMID: 31688884
13. Dvorak CC, et al. *J Pediatric Infect Dis Soc*. 2021;10(4):417–425 PMID: 33136159
14. Kim BK, et al. *Children (Basel)*. 2022;9(3):372 PMID: 35327744

15. De Pauw BE, et al. *N Engl J Med.* 2007;356(4):409–411 PMID: 17251538
16. Salavert M. *Int J Antimicrob Agents.* 2008;32(suppl 2):S149–S153 PMID: 19013340
17. Eschenauer GA, et al. *Liver Transpl.* 2009;15(8):842–858 PMID: 19642130
18. Winston DJ, et al. *Am J Transplant.* 2014;14(12):2758–2764 PMID: 25376267
19. Sun HY, et al. *Transplantation.* 2013;96(6):573–578 PMID: 23842191
20. Radack KP, et al. *Curr Infect Dis Rep.* 2009;11(6):427–434 PMID: 19857381
21. Patterson TF, et al. *Clin Infect Dis.* 2016;63(4):e1–e60 PMID: 27365388
22. Thomas L, et al. *Expert Rev Anti Infect Ther.* 2009;7(4):461–472 PMID: 19400765
23. Friberg LE, et al. *Antimicrob Agents Chemother.* 2012;56(6):3032–3042 PMID: 22430956
24. Burgos A, et al. *Pediatrics.* 2008;121(5):e1286–e1294 PMID: 18450871
25. Herbrecht R, et al. *N Engl J Med.* 2002;347(6):408–415 PMID: 12167683
26. Mousset S, et al. *Ann Hematol.* 2014;93(1):13–32 PMID: 24026426
27. Blyth CC, et al. *Intern Med J.* 2014;44(12b):1333–1349 PMID: 25482744
28. Denning DW, et al. *Eur Respir J.* 2016;47(1):45–68 PMID: 26699723
29. Cornely OA, et al. *Clin Infect Dis.* 2007;44(10):1289–1297 PMID: 17443465
30. Maertens JA, et al. *Lancet.* 2016;387(10020):760–769 PMID: 26684607
31. Tissot F, et al. *Haematologica.* 2017;102(3):433–444 PMID: 28011902
32. Ullmann AJ, et al. *Clin Microbiol Infect.* 2018;24(suppl 1):e1–e38 PMID: 29544767
33. Walsh TJ, et al. *Antimicrob Agents Chemother.* 2010;54(10):4116–4123 PMID: 20660687
34. Arrieta AC, et al. *Antimicrob Agents Chemother.* 2021;65(8):e0029021 PMID: 34031051
35. Maertens JA, et al. *Lancet.* 2021;397(10273):499–509 PMID: 33549194
36. Bartelink IH, et al. *Antimicrob Agents Chemother.* 2013;57(1):235–240 PMID: 23114771
37. Slavin MA, et al. *J Antimicrob Chemother.* 2022;77(1):16–23 PMID: 34508633
38. Marr KA, et al. *Ann Intern Med.* 2015;162(2):81–89 PMID: 25599346
39. Verweij PE, et al. *Drug Resist Updat.* 2015;21–22:30–40 PMID: 26282594
40. Kohno S, et al. *Eur J Clin Microbiol Infect Dis.* 2013;32(3):387–397 PMID: 23052987
41. Naggie S, et al. *Clin Chest Med.* 2009;30(2):337–353 PMID: 19375639
42. Revankar SG, et al. *Clin Microbiol Rev.* 2010;23(4):884–928 PMID: 20930077
43. Wong EH, et al. *Infect Dis Clin North Am.* 2016;30(1):165–178 PMID: 26897066
44. Revankar SG, et al. *Clin Infect Dis.* 2004;38(2):206–216 PMID: 14699452
45. Li DM, et al. *Lancet Infect Dis.* 2009;9(6):376–383 PMID: 19467477
46. Chowdhary A, et al. *Clin Microbiol Infect.* 2014;20(suppl 3):47–75 PMID: 24483780
47. McCarty TP, et al. *Med Mycol.* 2015;53(5):440–446 PMID: 25908651
48. Schieffelin JS, et al. *Transplant Infect Dis.* 2014;16(2):270–278 PMID: 24628809
49. Chapman SW, et al. *Clin Infect Dis.* 2008;46(12):1801–1812 PMID: 18462107
50. McKinnell JA, et al. *Clin Chest Med.* 2009;30(2):227–239 PMID: 19375630
51. Walsh CM, et al. *Pediatr Infect Dis J.* 2006;25(7):656–658 PMID: 16804444
52. Fanella S, et al. *Med Mycol.* 2011;49(6):627–632 PMID: 21208027
53. Smith JA, et al. *Proc Am Thorac Soc.* 2010;7(3):173–180 PMID: 20463245
54. Bariola JR, et al. *Clin Infect Dis.* 2010;50(6):797–804 PMID: 20166817
55. Limper AH, et al. *Am J Respir Crit Care Med.* 2011;183(1):96–128 PMID: 21193785
56. Thompson GR, et al. *Lancet Infect Dis.* 2021;21(12):e364–e374 PMID: 34364529
57. Pappas PG, et al. *Clin Infect Dis.* 2016;62(4):e1–e50 PMID: 26679628
58. Lortholary O, et al. *Clin Microbiol Infect.* 2012;18(suppl 7):68–77 PMID: 23137138
59. Ullman AJ, et al. *Clin Microbiol Infect.* 2012;18(suppl 7):53–67 PMID: 23137137
60. Hope WW, et al. *Clin Microbiol Infect.* 2012;18(suppl 7):38–52 PMID: 23137136
61. Cornely OA, et al. *Clin Microbiol Infect.* 2012;18(suppl 7):19–37 PMID: 23137135
62. Hope WW, et al. *Antimicrob Agents Chemother.* 2015;59(2):905–913 PMID: 25421470
63. Piper L, et al. *Pediatr Infect Dis J.* 2011;30(5):375–378 PMID: 21085048
64. Watt KM, et al. *Antimicrob Agents Chemother.* 2015;59(7):3935–3943 PMID: 25896706
65. Ascher SB, et al. *Pediatr Infect Dis J.* 2012;31(5):439–443 PMID: 22189522
66. Sobel JD. *Lancet.* 2007;369(9577):1961–1971 PMID: 17560449
67. Kim J, et al. *J Antimicrob Chemother.* 2020;75(1):215–220 PMID: 31586424
68. Almangour TA, et al. *Saudi Pharm J.* 2021;29(4):315–323 PMID: 33994826

69. Barnes KN, et al. *Ann Pharmacother.* 2022;10600280221091301 PMID: 35502451
70. Lopez Martinez R, et al. *Clin Dermatol.* 2007;25(2):188–194 PMID: 17350498
71. Ameen M. *Clin Exp Dermatol.* 2009;34(8):849–854 PMID: 19575735
72. Chowdhary A, et al. *Clin Microbiol Infect.* 2014;20(suppl 3):47–75 PMID: 24483780
73. Queiroz-Telles F. *Rev Inst Med Trop Sao Paulo.* 2015;57(suppl 19):46–50 PMID: 26465369
74. Queiroz-Telles F, et al. *Clin Microbiol Rev.* 2017;30(1):233–276 PMID: 27856522
75. Galgiani JN, et al. *Clin Infect Dis.* 2016;63(6):717–722 PMID: 27559032
76. Anstead GM, et al. *Infect Dis Clin North Am.* 2006;20(3):621–643 PMID: 16984872
77. Williams PL. *Ann N Y Acad Sci.* 2007;1111:377–384 PMID: 17363442
78. Homans JD, et al. *Pediatr Infect Dis J.* 2010;29(1):65–67 PMID: 19884875
79. Kauffman CA, et al. *Transplant Infectious Diseases.* 2014;16(2):213–224 PMID: 24589027
80. McCarty JM, et al. *Clin Infect Dis.* 2013;56(11):1579–1585 PMID: 23463637
81. Bravo R, et al. *J Pediatr Hematol Oncol.* 2012;34(5):389–394 PMID: 22510771
82. Catanzaro A, et al. *Clin Infect Dis.* 2007;45(5):562–568 PMID: 17682989
83. Thompson GR, et al. *Clin Infect Dis.* 2016;63(3):356–362 PMID: 27169478
84. Thompson GR III, et al. *Clin Infect Dis.* 2017;65(2):338–341 PMID: 28419259
85. Chayakulkeeree M, et al. *Infect Dis Clin North Am.* 2006;20(3):507–544 PMID: 16984867
86. Jarvis JN, et al. *Semin Respir Crit Care Med.* 2008;29(2):141–150 PMID: 18365996
87. Perfect JR, et al. *Clin Infect Dis.* 2010;50(3):291–322 PMID: 20047480
88. Joshi NS, et al. *Pediatr Infect Dis J.* 2010;29(12):e91–e95 PMID: 20935590
89. Day JN, et al. *N Engl J Med.* 2013;368(14):1291–1302 PMID: 23550668
90. Jarvis JN, et al. *N Engl J Med.* 2022;386(12):1109–1120 PMID: 3532064
91. Cortez KJ, et al. *Clin Microbiol Rev.* 2008;21(1):157–197 PMID: 18202441
92. Tortorano AM, et al. *Clin Microbiol Infect.* 2014;20(suppl 3):27–46 PMID: 24548001
93. Horn DL, et al. *Mycoses.* 2014;57(11):652–658 PMID: 24943384
94. Muhammed M, et al. *Medicine (Baltimore).* 2013;92(6):305–316 PMID: 24145697
95. Rodriguez-Tudela JL, et al. *Med Mycol.* 2009;47(4):359–370 PMID: 19031336
96. Wheat LJ, et al. *Clin Infect Dis.* 2007;45(7):807–825 PMID: 17806045
97. Myint T, et al. *Medicine (Baltimore).* 2014;93(1):11–18 PMID: 24378739
98. Assi M, et al. *Clin Infect Dis.* 2013;57(11):1542–1549 PMID: 24046304
99. Chayakulkeeree M, et al. *Eur J Clin Microbiol Infect Dis.* 2006;25(4):215–229 PMID: 16568297
100. Spellberg B, et al. *Clin Infect Dis.* 2009;48(12):1743–1751 PMID: 19435437
101. Reed C, et al. *Clin Infect Dis.* 2008;47(3):364–371 PMID: 18558882
102. Cornely OA, et al. *Clin Microbiol Infect.* 2014;20(suppl 3):5–26 PMID: 24479848
103. Spellberg B, et al. *Clin Infect Dis.* 2012;54(suppl 1):S73–S78 PMID: 22247449
104. Chitasombat MN, et al. *Curr Opin Infect Dis.* 2016;29(4):340–345 PMID: 27191199
105. Pana ZD, et al. *BMC Infect Dis.* 2016;16(1):667 PMID: 27832748
106. Pagano L, et al. *Haematologica.* 2013;98(10):e127–e130 PMID: 23716556
107. Kyvernitakis A, et al. *Clin Microbiol Infect.* 2016;22(9):811.e1–811.e8 PMID: 27085727
108. Marty FM, et al. *Lancet Infect Dis.* 2016;16(7):828–837 PMID: 26969258
109. Cornely OA. *Lancet Infect Dis.* 2019;19(12):e405–e421 PMID: 31699664
110. Queiroz-Telles F, et al. *Clin Infect Dis.* 2007;45(11):1462–1469 PMID: 17990229
111. Menezes VM, et al. *Cochrane Database Syst Rev.* 2006;(2):CD004967 PMID: 16625617
112. Marques SA. *An Bras Dermatol.* 2013;88(5):700–711 PMID: 24173174
113. Borges SR, et al. *Med Mycol.* 2014;52(3):303–310 PMID: 24577007
114. Panel on the Prevention and Treatment of Opportunistic Infections in HIV-Exposed and HIV-Infected Children. Guidelines for the prevention and treatment of opportunistic infections in HIV-exposed and HIV-infected children. Updated September 2, 2022. Accessed October 3, 2022. https://clinicalinfo.hiv.gov/en/guidelines/hiv-clinical-guidelines-pediatric-opportunistic-infections/updates-guidelines-prevention
115. Siberry GK, et al. *Pediatr Infect Dis J.* 2013;32(suppl 2):i–KK4 PMID: 24569199
116. Maschmeyer G, et al. *J Antimicrob Chemother.* 2016;71(9):2405–2413 PMID: 27550993
117. Kauffman CA, et al. *Clin Infect Dis.* 2007;45(10):1255–1265 PMID: 17968818
118. Aung AK, et al. *Med Mycol.* 2013;51(5):534–544 PMID: 23286352

119. Ali S, et al. *Pediatr Emerg Care.* 2007;23(9):662–668 PMID: 17876261
120. Shy R. *Pediatr Rev.* 2007;28(5):164–174 PMID: 17473121
121. Andrews MD, et al. *Am Fam Physician.* 2008;77(10):1415–1420 PMID: 18533375
122. Kakourou T, et al. *Pediatr Dermatol.* 2010;27(3):226–228 PMID: 20609140
123. Gupta AK, et al. *Pediatr Dermatol.* 2013;30(1):1–6 PMID: 22994156
124. Chen X, et al. *J Am Acad Dermatol.* 2017;76(2):368–374 PMID: 27816294
125. Gupta AK, et al. *Pediatr Dermatol.* 2020;37(6):1014–1022 PMID: 32897584
126. de Berker D. *N Engl J Med.* 2009;360(20):2108–2116 PMID: 19439745
127. Ameen M, et al. *Br J Dermatol.* 2014;171(5):937–958 PMID: 25409999
128. Gupta AK. *J Eur Acad Dermatol Venereol.* 2020;34(3):580–588 PMID: 31746067
129. Sprenger AB. *J Fungi (Basel).* 2019;5(3):82 PMID: 31487828
130. Pantazidou A, et al. *Arch Dis Child.* 2007;92(11):1040–1042 PMID: 17954488
131. Gupta AK, et al. *J Cutan Med Surg.* 2014;18(2):79–90 PMID: 24636433

Chapter 6

1. Cornely OA, et al. *Clin Infect Dis.* 2007;44(10):1289–1297 PMID: 17443465
2. Lestner JM, et al. *Antimicrob Agents Chemother*. 2016;60(12):7340–7346 PMID: 27697762
3. Seibel NL, et al. *Antimicrob Agents Chemother*. 2017;61(2):e01477–16 PMID: 27855062
4. Azoulay E, et al. *PLoS One.* 2017;12(5):e0177093 PMID: 28531175
5. Ascher SB, et al. *Pediatr Infect Dis J.* 2012;31(5):439–443 PMID: 22189522
6. Piper L, et al. *Pediatr Infect Dis J.* 2011;30(5):375–378 PMID: 21085048
7. Gerhart JG, et al. *CPT Pharmacometrics Syst Pharmacol.* 2019;8(7):500–510 PMID: 31087536
8. Watt KM, et al. *Antimicrob Agents Chemother*. 2015;59(7):3935–3943 PMID: 25896706
9. Watt KM, et al. *CPT Pharmacometrics Syst Pharmacol.* 2018;7(10):629–637 PMID: 30033691
10. Friberg LE, et al. *Antimicrob Agents Chemother.* 2012;56(6):3032–3042 PMID: 22430956
11. Zembles TN, et al. *Pharmacotherapy.* 2016;36(10):1102–1108 PMID: 27548272
12. Moriyama B, et al. *Clin Pharmacol Ther.* 2017;102(1):45–51 PMID: 27981572
13. Arrieta AC, et al. *PLoS One.* 2019;14(3):e0212837 PMID: 30913226
14. Groll AH, et al. *Int J Antimicrob Agents.* 2020;56(3):106084 PMID: 32682946
15. Bernardo V, et al. *Pediatr Transplant.* 2020;24(6):e13777 PMID: 32639095
16. Maertens JA, et al. *Lancet.* 2016;387(10020):760–769 PMID: 26684607
17. Marty FM, et al. *Lancet Infect Dis.* 2016;16(7):828–837 PMID: 26969258
18. Cornely OA, et al. *Lancet Infect Dis.* 2019;19(12):e405–e421 PMID: 31699664
19. Arrieta AC, et al. *Antimicrob Agents Chemother.* 2021;65(8):e0029021 PMID: 34031051
20. Furfaro E, et al. *J Antimicrob Chemother.* 2019;74(8):2341–2346 PMID: 31119272
21. Fisher BT, et al. *JAMA*. 2019;322(17):1673–1681 PMID: 31688884
22. Dvorak CC, et al. *J Pediatric Infect Dis Soc.* 2021;10(4):417–425 PMID: 33136159
23. Niu CH, et al. *Front Pharmacol.* 2020;11:184 PMID: 32194415
24. Smith PB, et al. *Pediatr Infect Dis J.* 2009;28(5):412–415 PMID: 19319022
25. Hope WW, et al. *Antimicrob Agents Chemother.* 2010;54(6):2633–2637 PMID: 20308367
26. Benjamin DK Jr, et al. *Clin Pharmacol Ther.* 2010;87(1):93–99 PMID: 19890251
27. Auriti C, et al. *Antimicrob Agents Chemother.* 2021;65(4):e02494-20 PMID: 33558294
28. Kim BK, et al. *Children (Basel).* 2022;9(3):372 PMID: 35327744
29. Cohen-Wolkowiez M, et al. *Clin Pharmacol Ther.* 2011;89(5):702–707 PMID: 21412233
30. Roilides E, et al. *Pediatr Infect Dis J.* 2019;38(3):275–279 PMID: 30418357
31. Roilides E, et al. *Pediatr Infect Dis J.* 2020;39(4):305–309 PMID: 32032174
32. Spec A, et al. *J Antimicrob Chemother.* 2019;74(10):3056–3062 PMID: 31304536

Chapter 7

1. Lenaerts L, et al. *Rev Med Virol.* 2008;18(6):357–374 PMID: 18655013
2. Michaels MG. *Expert Rev Anti Infect Ther.* 2007;5(3):441–448 PMID: 17547508
3. Biron KK. *Antiviral Res.* 2006;71(2–3):154–163 PMID: 16765457
4. Boeckh M, et al. *Blood.* 2009;113(23):5711–5719 PMID: 19299333
5. Vaudry W, et al. *Am J Transplant.* 2009;9(3):636–643 PMID: 19260840

6. Emanuel D, et al. *Ann Intern Med.* 1988;109(10):777–782 PMID: 2847609
7. Reed EC, et al. *Ann Intern Med.* 1988;109(10):783–788 PMID: 2847610
8. *Ophthalmology.* 1994;101(7):1250–1261 PMID: 8035989
9. Singh N, et al. *JAMA*. 2020;323(14):1378–1387 PMID: 32286644
10. Martin DF, et al. *N Engl J Med.* 2002;346(15):1119–1126 PMID: 11948271
11. Kempen JH, et al. *Arch Ophthalmol.* 2003;121(4):466–476 PMID: 12695243
12. Studies of Ocular Complications of AIDS Research Group. The AIDS Clinical Trials Group. *Am J Ophthalmol.* 2001;131(4):457–467 PMID: 11292409
13. Dieterich DT, et al. *J Infect Dis.* 1993;167(2):278–282 PMID: 8380610
14. Gerna G, et al. *Antiviral Res.* 1997;34(1):39–50 PMID: 9107384
15. Markham A, et al. *Drugs.* 1994;48(3):455–484 PMID: 7527763
16. Kimberlin DW, et al. *J Infect Dis.* 2008;197(6):836–845 PMID: 18279073
17. Kimberlin DW, et al. *N Engl J Med.* 2015;372(10):933–943 PMID: 25738669
18. Griffiths P, et al. *Herpes.* 2008;15(1):4–12 PMID: 18983762
19. Panel on the Prevention and Treatment of Opportunistic Infections in HIV-Exposed and HIV-Infected Children. Guidelines for the prevention and treatment of opportunistic infections in HIV-exposed and HIV-infected children. Updated September 2, 2022. Accessed October 3, 2022. https://clinicalinfo.hiv.gov/en/guidelines/hiv-clinical-guidelines-pediatric-opportunistic-infections/updates-guidelines-prevention
20. Marty FM, et al. *N Engl J Med.* 2017;377(25):2433–2444 PMID: 29211658
21. Abzug MJ, et al. *J Pediatric Infect Dis Soc.* 2016;5(1):53–62 PMID: 26407253
22. Biebl A, et al. *Nat Clin Pract Neurol.* 2009;5(3):171–174 PMID: 19262593
23. Chadaide Z, et al. *J Med Virol.* 2008;80(11):1930–1932 PMID: 18814244
24. AAP. Epstein-Barr virus infections. In: Kimberlin DW, et al, eds. *Red Book: 2021–2024 Report of the Committee on Infectious Diseases*. 32nd ed. 2021:318–322
25. Gross TG. *Herpes.* 2009;15(3):64–67 PMID: 19306606
26. Styczynski J, et al. *Bone Marrow Transplant.* 2009;43(10):757–770 PMID: 19043458
27. Jonas MM, et al. *Hepatology.* 2016;63(2):377–387 PMID: 26223345
28. Marcellin P, et al. *Gastroenterology.* 2016;150(1):134–144.e10 PMID: 26453773
29. Chen HL, et al. *Hepatology.* 2015;62(2):375–386 PMID: 25851052
30. Wu Q, et al. *Clin Gastroenterol Hepatol.* 2015;13(6):1170–1176 PMID: 25251571
31. Hou JL, et al. *J Viral Hepat.* 2015;22(2):85–93 PMID: 25243325
32. Kurbegov AC, et al. *Expert Rev Gastroenterol Hepatol.* 2009;3(1):39–49 PMID: 19210112
33. Jonas MM, et al. *Hepatology.* 2008;47(6):1863–1871 PMID: 18433023
34. Lai CL, et al. *Gastroenterology.* 2002;123(6):1831–1838 PMID: 12454840
35. Honkoop P, et al. *Expert Opin Investig Drugs.* 2003;12(4):683–688 PMID: 12665423
36. Shaw T, et al. *Expert Rev Anti Infect Ther.* 2004;2(6):853–871 PMID: 15566330
37. Elisofon SA, et al. *Clin Liver Dis.* 2006;10(1):133–148 PMID: 16376798
38. Jonas MM, et al. *Hepatology.* 2010;52(6):2192–2205 PMID: 20890947
39. Haber BA, et al. *Pediatrics.* 2009;124(5):e1007–e1013 PMID: 19805457
40. Shneider BL, et al. *Hepatology.* 2006;44(5):1344–1354 PMID: 17058223
41. Jain MK, et al. *J Viral Hepat.* 2007;14(3):176–182 PMID: 17305883
42. Sokal EM, et al. *Gastroenterology.* 1998;114(5):988–995 PMID: 9558288
43. Jonas MM, et al. *N Engl J Med.* 2002;346(22):1706–1713 PMID: 12037150
44. Chang TT, et al. *N Engl J Med.* 2006;354(10):1001–1010 PMID: 16525137
45. Liaw YF, et al. *Gastroenterology.* 2009;136(2):486–495 PMID: 19027013
46. Terrault NA, et al. *Hepatology*. 2018;67(4):1560–1599 PMID: 29405329
47. Keam SJ, et al. *Drugs.* 2008;68(9):1273–1317 PMID: 18547135
48. Marcellin P, et al. *Gastroenterology.* 2011;140(2):459–468 PMID: 21034744
49. Poordad F, et al. *N Engl J Med.* 2011;364(13):1195–1206 PMID: 21449783
50. Schwarz KB, et al. *Gastroenterology.* 2011;140(2):450–458 PMID: 21036173
51. Nelson DR. *Liver Int.* 2011;31(suppl 1):53–57 PMID: 21205138
52. Strader DB, et al. *Hepatology.* 2004;39(4):1147–1171 PMID: 15057920
53. Soriano V, et al. *AIDS.* 2007;21(9):1073–1089 PMID: 17502718

54. Murray KF, et al. *Hepatology*. 2018;68(6):2158–2166 PMID: 30070726
55. Feld JJ, et al. *N Engl J Med.* 2014;370(17):1594–1603 PMID: 24720703
56. Zeuzem S, et al. *N Engl J Med.* 2014;370(17):1604–1614 PMID: 24720679
57. Andreone P, et al. *Gastroenterology.* 2014;147(2):359–365.e1 PMID: 24818763
58. Ferenci P, et al. *N Engl J Med.* 2014;370(21):1983–1992 PMID: 24795200
59. Poordad F, et al. *N Engl J Med.* 2014;370(21):1973–1982 PMID: 24725237
60. Jacobson IM, et al. *Lancet.* 2014;384(9941):403–413 PMID: 24907225
61. Manns M, et al. *Lancet.* 2014;384(9941):414–426 PMID: 24907224
62. Forns X, et al. *Gastroenterology.* 2014;146(7):1669–1679.e3 PMID: 24602923
63. Zeuzem S, et al. *Gastroenterology.* 2014;146(2):430–441.e6 PMID: 24184810
64. Lawitz E, et al. *Lancet.* 2014;384(9956):1756–1765 PMID: 25078309
65. Afdhal N, et al. *N Engl J Med.* 2014;370(20):1889–1898 PMID: 24725239
66. Afdhal N, et al. *N Engl J Med.* 2014;370(16):1483–1493 PMID: 24725238
67. Kowdley KV, et al. *N Engl J Med.* 2014;370(20):1879–1888 PMID: 24720702
68. Lawitz E, et al. *N Engl J Med.* 2013;368(20):1878–1887 PMID: 23607594
69. Jacobson IM, et al. *N Engl J Med.* 2013;368(20):1867–1877 PMID: 23607593
70. Zeuzem S, et al. *N Engl J Med.* 2014;370(21):1993–2001 PMID: 24795201
71. American Association for the Study of Liver Diseases, Infectious Diseases Society of America. HCV in children. Updated September 29, 2021. Accessed October 3, 2022. www.hcvguidelines.org/unique-populations/children
72. Hollier LM, et al. *Cochrane Database Syst Rev.* 2008;(1):CD004946 PMID: 18254066
73. Pinninti SG, et al. *J Pediatr.* 2012;161(1):134–138 PMID: 22336576
74. ACOG. *Obstet Gynecol.* 2020;135(5):e193–e202 PMID: 32332414
75. Kimberlin DW, et al. *Clin Infect Dis.* 2010;50(2):221–228 PMID: 20014952
76. Abdel Massih RC, et al. *World J Gastroenterol.* 2009;15(21):2561–2569 PMID: 19496184
77. Mofenson LM, et al. *MMWR Recomm Rep.* 2009;58(RR-11):1–166 PMID: 19730409
78. Kuhar DT, et al. *Infect Control Hosp Epidemiol.* 2013;34(9):875–892 PMID: 23917901
79. Acosta EP, et al. *J Infect Dis.* 2010;202(4):563–566 PMID: 20594104
80. Kimberlin DW, et al. *J Infect Dis.* 2013;207(5):709–720 PMID: 23230059
81. McPherson C, et al. *J Infect Dis.* 2012;206(6):847–850 PMID: 22807525
82. Bradley JS, et al. *Pediatrics.* 2017;140(5):e20162727 PMID: 29051331
83. AAP. Measles. In: Kimberlin DW, et al, eds. *Red Book: 2021–2024 Report of the Committee on Infectious Diseases.* 32nd ed. 2021:503–519
84. AAP Committee on Infectious Diseases and Bronchiolitis Guidelines Committee. *Pediatrics.* 2014;134(2):415–420 PMID: 25070315
85. AAP Committee on Infectious Diseases and Bronchiolitis Guidelines Committee. *Pediatrics.* 2014;134(2):e620–e638 PMID: 25070304
86. Whitley RJ. *Adv Exp Med Biol.* 2008;609:216–232 PMID: 18193668

Chapter 9

1. Gonzales MLM, et al. *Cochrane Database Syst Rev.* 2019;(1):CD006085 PMID: 30624763
2. Haque R, et al. *N Engl J Med.* 2003;348(16):1565–1573 PMID: 1270037
3. Rossignol JF, et al. *Trans R Soc Trop Med Hyg.* 2007;101(10):1025–1031 PMID: 17658567
4. Mackey-Lawrence NM, et al. *BMJ Clin Evid.* 2011;2011:0918 PMID: 21477391
5. Fox LM, et al. *Clin Infect Dis.* 2005;40(8):1173–1180 PMID: 15791519
6. Cope JR, et al. *Clin Infect Dis.* 2016;62(6):774–776 PMID: 26679626
7. Vargas-Zepeda J, et al. *Arch Med Res.* 2005;36(1):83–86 PMID: 15900627
8. Linam WM, et al. *Pediatrics.* 2015;135(3):e744–e748 PMID: 25667249
9. Visvesvara GS, et al. *FEMS Immunol Med Microbiol.* 2007;50(1):1–26 PMID: 17428307
10. Martínez DY, et al. *Clin Infect Dis.* 2010;51(2):e7–e11 PMID: 20550438
11. Chotmongkol V, et al. *Am J Trop Med Hyg.* 2009;81(3):443–445 PMID: 19706911
12. Lo Re V III, et al. *Am J Med.* 2003;114(3):217–223 PMID: 12637136
13. Jitpimolmard S, et al. *Parasitol Res.* 2007;100(6):1293–1296 PMID: 17177056
14. Checkley AM, et al. *J Infect.* 2010;60(1):1–20 PMID: 19931558

15. Bethony J, et al. *Lancet.* 2006;367(9521):1521–1532 PMID: 16679166
16. Krause PJ, et al. *N Engl J Med.* 2000;343(20):1454–1458 PMID: 11078770
17. Vannier E, et al. *Infect Dis Clin North Am.* 2008;22(3):469–488 PMID: 18755385
18. Krause PJ, et al. *Clin Infect Dis.* 2021;72(2):185–189 PMID: 33501959
19. Sanchez E, et al. *JAMA.* 2016;315(16):1767–1777 PMID: 27115378
20. Kletsova EA, et al. *Ann Clin Microbiol Antimicrob.* 2017;16(1):26 PMID: 28399851
21. Schuster FL, et al. *Clin Microbiol Rev.* 2008;21(4):626–638 PMID: 18854484
22. Murray WJ, et al. *Clin Infect Dis.* 2004;39(10):1484–1492 PMID: 15546085
23. Sircar AD, et al. *MMWR Morb Mortal Wkly Rep.* 2016;65(35):930–933 PMID: 27608169
24. Rossignol JF, et al. *Clin Gastroenterol Hepatol.* 2005;3(10):987–991 PMID: 16234044
25. Nigro L, et al. *J Travel Med.* 2003;10(2):128–130 PMID: 12650658
26. Bern C, et al. *JAMA.* 2007;298(18):2171–2181 PMID: 18000201
27. Salvador F, et al. *Clin Infect Dis.* 2015;61(11):1688–1694 PMID: 26265500
28. Miller DA, et al. *Clin Infect Dis.* 2015;60(8):1237–1240 PMID: 25601454
29. Smith HV, et al. *Curr Opin Infect Dis.* 2004;17(6):557–564 PMID: 15640710
30. Davies AP, et al. *BMJ.* 2009;339:b4168 PMID: 19841008
31. Krause I, et al. *Pediatr Infect Dis J.* 2012;31(11):1135–1138 PMID: 22810017
32. Abubakar I, et al. *Cochrane Database Syst Rev.* 2007;(1):CD004932 PMID: 17253532
33. Jelinek T, et al. *Clin Infect Dis.* 1994;19(6):1062–1066 PMID: 7534125
34. Schuster A, et al. *Clin Infect Dis.* 2013;57(8):1155–1157 PMID: 23811416
35. Hoge CW, et al. *Lancet.* 1995;345(8951):691–693 PMID: 7885125
36. Ortega YR, et al. *Clin Microbiol Rev.* 2010;23(1):218–234 PMID: 20065331
37. Steffen R, et al. *J Travel Med.* 2018;25(1):tay116 PMID: 30462260
38. Nash TE, et al. *Neurology.* 2006;67(7):1120–1127 PMID: 17030744
39. Garcia HH, et al. *Lancet Neurol.* 2014;13(12):1202–1215 PMID: 25453460
40. Lillie P, et al. *J Infect.* 2010;60(5):403–404 PMID: 20153773
41. White AC Jr, et al. *Clin Infect Dis.* 2018;66(8):1159–1163 PMID: 29617787
42. Verdier RI, et al. *Ann Intern Med.* 2000;132(11):885–888 PMID: 10836915
43. Stark DJ, et al. *Trends Parasitol.* 2006;22(2):92–96 PMID: 16380293
44. Röser D, et al. *Clin Infect Dis.* 2014;58(12):1692–1699 PMID: 24647023
45. Smego RA Jr, et al. *Clin Infect Dis.* 2003;37(8):1073–1083 PMID: 14523772
46. Brunetti E, et al. *Acta Trop.* 2010;114(1):1–16 PMID: 19931502
47. Fernando SD, et al. *J Trop Med.* 2011;2011:175941 PMID: 21234244
48. Walker M, et al. *Clin Infect Dis.* 2015;60(8):1199–2017 PMID: 25537873
49. Debrah AY, et al. *Clin Infect Dis.* 2015;61(4):517–526 PMID: 25948064
50. Mand S, et al. *Clin Infect Dis.* 2012;55(5):621–630 PMID: 22610930
51. Ottesen EA, et al. *Annu Rev Med.* 1992;43:417–424 PMID: 1580599
52. Jong EC, et al. *J Infect Dis.* 1985;152(3):637–640 PMID: 3897401
53. Sayasone S, et al. *Clin Infect Dis.* 2017;64(4):451–458 PMID: 28174906
54. Calvopina M, et al. *Trans R Soc Trop Med Hyg.* 1998;92(5):566–569 PMID: 9861383
55. Johnson RJ, et al. *Rev Infect Dis.* 1985;7(2):200–206 PMID: 4001715
56. Graham CS, et al. *Clin Infect Dis.* 2001;33(1):1–5 PMID: 11389487
57. Granados CE, et al. *Cochrane Database Syst Rev.* 2012;(12):CD007787 PMID: 23235648
58. Ross AG, et al. *N Engl J Med.* 2013;368(19):1817–1825 PMID: 23656647
59. Requena-Mendez A, et al. *J Infect Dis.* 2017;215(6):946–953 PMID: 28453841
60. Hotez PJ, et al. *N Engl J Med.* 2004;351(8):799–807 PMID: 15317893
61. Keiser J, et al. *JAMA.* 2008;299(16):1937–1948 PMID: 18430913
62. Steinmann P, et al. *PLoS One.* 2011;6(9):e25003 PMID: 21980373
63. Aronson N, et al. *Clin Infect Dis.* 2016;63(12):e202–e264 PMID: 27941151
64. Control of the leishmaniases: a report of a meeting of the WHO Expert Committee on the Control of Leishmaniases, Geneva, 22–26 March 2010. World Health Organization. 2010. Accessed October 3, 2022. https://apps.who.int/iris/handle/10665/44412
65. Alrajhi AA, et al. *N Engl J Med.* 2002;346(12):891–895 PMID: 11907288
66. Bern C, et al. *Clin Infect Dis.* 2006;43(7):917–924 PMID: 16941377

67. Ritmeijer K, et al. *Clin Infect Dis.* 2006;43(3):357–364 PMID: 16804852
68. Monge-Maillo B, et al. *Clin Infect Dis.* 2015;60(9):1398–1404 PMID: 25601455
69. Sundar S, et al. *N Engl J Med.* 2002;347(22):1739–1746 PMID: 12456849
70. Sundar S, et al. *N Engl J Med.* 2007;356(25):2571–2581 PMID: 17582067
71. Drugs for head lice. *JAMA.* 2017;317(19):2010–2011 PMID: 28510677
72. AAP. Drugs for parasitic infections. In: Kimberlin DW, et al, eds. *Red Book: 2021–2024 Report of the Committee on Infectious Diseases.* 32nd ed. 2021:949–989
73. Ashley EA, et al. *Lancet Child Adolesc Health.* 2020;4(10):775–789 PMID: 32946831
74. Tan KR, et al. Malaria. In: Brunette GW, Nemhauser JB, eds. *Yellow Book 2020: CDC Health Information for International Travel.* 2019:267–287
75. Usha V, et al. *J Am Acad Dermatol.* 2000;42(2, pt 1):236–240 PMID: 10642678
76. Brodine SK, et al. *Am J Trop Med Hyg.* 2009;80(3):425–430 PMID: 19270293
77. Doenhoff MJ, et al. *Expert Rev Anti Infect Ther.* 2006;4(2):199–210 PMID: 16597202
78. Fenwick A, et al. *Curr Opin Infect Dis.* 2006;19(6):577–582 PMID: 17075334
79. Marti H, et al. *Am J Trop Med Hyg.* 1996;55(5):477–481 PMID: 8940976
80. Segarra-Newnham M. *Ann Pharmacother.* 2007;41(12):1992–2001 PMID: 17940124
81. Barisani-Asenbauer T, et al. *J Ocul Pharmacol Ther.* 2001;17(3):287–294 PMID: 11436948
82. McAuley JB. *Pediatr Infect Dis J.* 2008;27(2):161–162 PMID: 18227714
83. Maldonado YA, et al. *Pediatrics.* 2017;139(2):e20163860 PMID: 28138010
84. de-la-Torre A, et al. *Ocul Immunol Inflamm.* 2011;19(5):314–320 PMID: 21970662
85. Shane AL, et al. *Clin Infect Dis.* 2017;65(12):e45–e80 PMID: 29053792
86. DuPont HL. *Clin Infect Dis.* 2007;45(suppl 1):S78–S84 PMID: 17582576
87. Riddle MS, et al. *J Travel Med.* 2017;24(suppl 1):S57–S74 PMID: 28521004
88. Gottstein B, et al. *Clin Microbiol Rev.* 2009;22(1):127–145 PMID: 19136437
89. Workowski KA, et al. *MMWR Recomm Rep.* 2015;64(RR-03):1–137 PMID: 26042815
90. Fairlamb AH. *Trends Parasitol.* 2003;19(11):488–494 PMID: 14580959
91. Schmid C, et al. *Lancet.* 2004;364(9436):789–790 PMID: 15337407
92. Bisser S, et al. *J Infect Dis.* 2007;195(3):322–329 PMID: 17205469
93. Priotto G, et al. *Lancet.* 2009;374(9683):56–64 PMID: 19559476
94. Buscher P, et al. *Lancet.* 2017;390(10110):2397–2409 PMID: 28673422
95. World Health Organization and WHO Expert Committee on the Control and Surveillance of Human African Trypanosomiasis. Control and surveillance of human African trypanosomiasis: report of a WHO expert committee. World Health Organization. 2013. Accessed October 3, 2022. https://apps.who.int/iris/handle/10665/95732

Chapter 12

1. Wu W, et al. *Clin Microbiol Rev.* 2019;32(2):e00115-18 PMID: 30700432
2. Hultén KG, et al. *Pediatr Infect Dis J.* 2018;37(3):235–241 PMID: 28859018
3. Acree ME, et al. *Infect Control Hosp Epidemiol.* 2017;38(10):1226–1234 PMID: 28903801
4. Liu C, et al. *Clin Infect Dis.* 2011;52(3):e18–e55 PMID: 21208910
5. Rybak MJ. *Am J Health Syst Pharm.* 2020;77(11):835–864 PMID: 32191793
6. Le J, et al. *Pediatr Infect Dis J.* 2013;32(4):e155–e163 PMID: 23340565
7. McNeil JC, et al. *Pediatr Infect Dis J.* 2016;35(3):263–268 PMID: 26646549
8. Sader HS, et al. *Antimicrob Agents Chemother.* 2017;61(9):e01043-17 PMID: 28630196
9. Depardieu F, et al. *Clin Microbiol Rev.* 2007;20(1):79–114 PMID: 17223624
10. Miller LG, et al. *N Engl J Med.* 2015;372(12):1093–1103 PMID: 25785967
11. Bradley J, et al. *Pediatrics.* 2017;139(3):e20162477 PMID: 28202770
12. Arrieta AC, et al. *Pediatr Infect Dis J.* 2018;37(9):890–900 PMID: 29406465
13. Bradley JS, et al. *Pediatr Infect Dis J.* 2020;39(9):814–823 PMID: 32639465
14. Korczowski B, et al. *Pediatr Infect Dis J.* 2016;35(8):e239–e247 PMID: 27164462
15. Cannavino CR, et al. *Pediatr Infect Dis J.* 2016;35(7):752–759 PMID: 27093162
16. Blumer JL, et al. *Pediatr Infect Dis J.* 2016;35(7):760–766 PMID: 27078119
17. Bradley JS. *Pediatr Infect Dis J.* 2020;39(5):411–418 PMID: 32091493

18. Huang JT, et al. *Pediatrics.* 2009;123(5):e808–e814 PMID: 19403473
19. Finnell SM, et al. *Clin Pediatr (Phila).* 2015;54(5):445–450 PMID: 25385929
20. Kaplan SL, et al. *Clin Infect Dis.* 2014;58(5):679–682 PMID: 24265356
21. McNeil JC, et al. *Curr Infect Dis Rep.* 2019;21(4):12 PMID: 30859379

Chapter 14

1. Nelson JD. *J Pediatr.* 1978;92(1):175–176 PMID: 619073
2. Nelson JD, et al. *J Pediatr.* 1978;92(1):131–134 PMID: 619055
3. Tetzlaff TR, et al. *J Pediatr.* 1978;92(3):485–490 PMID: 632997
4. Ballock RT, et al. *J Pediatr Orthop.* 2009;29(6):636–642 PMID: 19700997
5. Peltola H, et al. *N Engl J Med.* 2014;370(4):352–360 PMID: 24450893
6. Bradley JS, et al. *Pediatrics.* 2011;128(4):e1034–e1045 PMID: 21949152
7. Rice HE, et al. *Arch Surg.* 2001;136(12):1391–1395 PMID: 11735866
8. Fraser JD, et al. *J Pediatr Surg.* 2010;45(6):1198–1202 PMID: 20620320
9. Strohmeier Y, et al. *Cochrane Database Syst Rev.* 2014;(7):CD003772 PMID: 25066627
10. Drusano GL, et al. *J Infect Dis.* 2014;210(8):1319–1324 PMID: 24760199
11. Arnold JC, et al. *Pediatrics.* 2012;130(4):e821–e828 PMID: 22966033
12. Zaoutis T, et al. *Pediatrics.* 2009;123(2):636–642 PMID: 19171632
13. Keren R, et al. *JAMA Pediatr.* 2015;169(2):120–128 PMID: 25506733
14. Desai AA, et al. *J Pediatr Surg.* 2015;50(6):912–914 PMID: 25812441
15. Marino NE, et al. *Surg Infect (Larchmt).* 2017;8(8):894–903 PMID: 29064344
16. Liu C, et al. *Clin Infect Dis.* 2011;52(3):e18–e55 [Erratum. *Clin Infect Dis.* 2011;53(3):319] PMID: 21208910
17. Thaden JT, et al. *Int J Antimicrob Agents.* 2021;58(6):106451 PMID: 34653617
18. Syrogiannopoulos GA, et al. *Lancet.* 1988;1(8575–8576):37–40 PMID: 2891899

Chapter 15

1. Oehler RL, et al. *Lancet Infect Dis.* 2009;9(7):439–447 PMID: 19555903
2. Bula-Rudas FJ, et al. *Pediatr Rev.* 2018;39(10):490–500 PMID: 30275032
3. Elcock KL, et al. *Injury.* 2022;53(2):227–236 PMID: 34838260
4. Talan DA, et al. *Clin Infect Dis.* 2003;37(11):1481–1489 PMID: 14614671
5. Aziz H, et al. *J Trauma Acute Care Surg.* 2015;78(3):641–648 PMID: 25710440
6. Centers for Disease Control and Prevention. Rabies. State and local rabies consultation contacts. Reviewed July 29, 2022. Accessed October 3, 2022. www.cdc.gov/rabies/resources/contacts.html
7. AAP. Tetanus. In: Kimberlin DW, et al, eds. *Red Book: 2021–2024 Report of the Committee on Infectious Diseases.* 32nd ed. 2021:750–755
8. Wilson W, et al. *Circulation.* 2007;116(15):1736–1754 PMID: 17446442
9. Baltimore RS, et al. *Circulation.* 2015;132(15):1487–1515 PMID: 26373317
10. Sakai Bizmark R, et al. *Am Heart J.* 2017;189:110–119 PMID: 28625367
11. Gupta S, et al. *Congenit Heart Dis.* 2017;12(2):196–201 PMID: 27885814
12. Cahill TJ, et al. *Heart.* 2017;103(12):937–944 PMID: 28213367
13. Dayer M, et al. *J Infect Chemother.* 2018;24(1):18–24 PMID: 29107651
14. AAP. Lyme disease. In: Kimberlin DW, et al, eds. *Red Book: 2021–2024 Report of the Committee on Infectious Diseases.* 32nd ed. 2021:482–489
15. Cohn AC, et al. *MMWR Recomm Rep.* 2013;62(RR-2):1–28 PMID: 23515099
16. McNamara LA, et al. *Lancet Infect Dis.* 2018;18(9):e272–e281 PMID: 29858150
17. AAP. Pertussis (whooping cough). In: Kimberlin DW, et al, eds. *Red Book: 2021–2024 Report of the Committee on Infectious Diseases.* 32nd ed. 2021:578–589
18. Centers for Disease Control and Prevention. Pertussis (whooping cough). Postexposure antimicrobial prophylaxis. Reviewed August 4, 2022. Accessed October 3, 2022. www.cdc.gov/pertussis/pep.html
19. Brook I. *Expert Rev Anti Infect Ther.* 2008;6(3):327–336 PMID: 18588497
20. Centers for Disease Control and Prevention. Tuberculosis (TB). Treatment regimens for latent TB infection (LBTI). Reviewed February 13, 2020. Accessed October 3, 2022. www.cdc.gov/tb/topic/treatment/ltbi.htm

21. AAP. Tuberculosis. In: Kimberlin DW, et al, eds. *Red Book: 2021–2024 Report of the Committee on Infectious Diseases*. 32nd ed. 2021:786–814
22. Borisov AS, et al. *MMWR Morb Mortal Wkly Rep*. 2018;67(25):723–726 PMID: 29953429
23. ACOG. *Obstet Gynecol*. 2020;135(5):e193–e202 PMID: 32332414
24. Pinninti SG, et al. *Semin Perinatol*. 2018;42(3):168–175 PMID: 29544668
25. AAP. Herpes simplex. In: Kimberlin DW, et al, eds. *Red Book: 2021–2024 Report of the Committee on Infectious Diseases*. 32nd ed. 2021:407–417
26. AAP Committee on Infectious Diseases. *Pediatrics*. 2020;146(4):e2020024588 PMID: 32900875
27. Kimberlin DW, et al. *J Infect Dis*. 2013;207(5):709–720 PMID: 23230059
28. AAP. Rabies. In: Kimberlin DW, et al, eds. *Red Book: 2021–2024 Report of the Committee on Infectious Diseases*. 32nd ed. 2021:619–627
29. AAP. Varicella-zoster virus infections. In: Kimberlin DW, et al, eds. *Red Book: 2021–2024 Report of the Committee on Infectious Diseases*. 32nd ed. 2021:831–838
30. Leach AJ, et al. *Cochrane Database Syst Rev*. 2006;(4):CD004401 PMID: 17054203
31. Schilder AGM, et al. *Nat Rev Dis Primers*. 2016;2(1):16063 PMID: 27604644
32. Williams GJ, et al. *Adv Exp Med Biol*. 2013;764:211–218 PMID: 23654070
33. Craig JC, et al. *N Engl J Med*. 2009;361(18):1748–1759 PMID: 19864673
34. RIVUR Trial Investigators, et al. *N Engl J Med*. 2014;370(25):2367–2376 PMID: 24795142
35. AAP Subcommittee on Urinary Tract Infection and Steering Committee on Quality Improvement and Management. *Pediatrics*. 2011;128(3):595–610 PMID: 21873693
36. Craig JC. *J Pediatr*. 2015;166(3):778 PMID: 25722276
37. National Institute for Health and Care Excellence. Urinary tract infection in under 16s: diagnosis and management. Updated October 31, 2018. Accessed October 3, 2022. www.nice.org.uk/guidance/CG54
38. Williams G, et al. *Cochrane Database Syst Rev*. 2019;(4):CD001534 PMID: 30932167
39. AAP. *Pneumocystis jirovecii* infections. In: Kimberlin DW, et al, eds. *Red Book: 2021–2024 Report of the Committee on Infectious Diseases*. 32nd ed. 2021:595–601
40. Caselli D, et al. *J Pediatr*. 2014;164(2):389–392.e1 PMID: 24252793
41. Proudfoot R, et al. *J Pediatr Hematol Oncol*. 2017;39(3):194–202 PMID: 28267082
42. Stern A, et al. *Cochrane Database Syst Rev*. 2014;(10):CD005590 PMID: 25269391
43. Delaplain PT, et al. *Surg Infect (Larchmt)*. 2022;23(3):232–247 PMID: 35196154
44. *Med Lett Drugs Ther*. 2016;58(1495):63–68 PMID: 27192618
45. Mangram AJ, et al. *Infect Control Hosp Epidemiol*. 1999;20(4):250–280 PMID: 10219875
46. Engelman R, et al. *Ann Thorac Surg*. 2007;83(4):1569–1576 PMID: 17383396
47. Paruk F, et al. *Int J Antimicrob Agents*. 2017;49(4):395–402 PMID: 28254373
48. Hansen E, et al. *J Orthop Res*. 2014;32(suppl 1):S31–S59 PMID: 24464896
49. Branch-Elliman W, et al. *JAMA Surg*. 2019;154(7):590–598 PMID: 31017647
50. Franco LM, et al. *Am J Infect Control*. 2017;45(4):343–349 PMID: 28109628
51. Berríos-Torres SI, et al. *JAMA Surg*. 2017;152(8):784–791 PMID: 28467526
52. Hawn MT, et al. *JAMA Surg*. 2013;148(7):649–657 PMID: 23552769
53. Shaffer WO, et al. *Spine J*. 2013;13(10):1387–1392 PMID: 23988461
54. Bratzler DW, et al. *Am J Health Syst Pharm*. 2013;70(3):195–283 PMID: 23327981
55. Lador A, et al. *J Antimicrob Chemother*. 2012;67(3):541–550 PMID: 22083832
56. De Cock PA, et al. *J Antimicrob Chemother*. 2017;72(3):791–800 PMID: 27999040
57. Marino NE, et al. *Surg Infect (Larchmt)*. 2017;18(8):894–903 PMID: 29064344
58. Andersen BR, et al. *Cochrane Database Syst Rev*. 2005;(3):CD001439 PMID: 16034862

Chapter 17

1. Merriam-Webster. Stewardship. Accessed October 3, 2022. www.merriam-webster.com/dictionary/stewardship
2. Centers for Disease Control and Prevention. Infection control. Guideline library. Reviewed September 2, 2020. Accessed October 3, 2022. www.cdc.gov/infectioncontrol/guidelines/index.html
3. Farnaes L, et al. *Diagn Microbiol Infect Dis*. 2019;94(2):188–191 PMID: 30819624

Index

B

D

E

F

H

O

Index

Q

R

U

V

W